Essential General Surgical Operations

To our families:

Peggy, Valentine, Jeremy and Louise (RMK)

and

Esther, Kitty, Harold and Jonah (MCW)

Commissioning Editor: Sue Hodgson
Project Development Manager: Francesca Lumkin
Project Manager: Hilary Hewitt
Designer: Jayne Jones

Essential General Surgical Operations

R. M. Kirk MS, FRCS

Honorary Consulting Surgeon, The Royal Free Hospital, London, UK

M. C. Winslet MS, FRCS

Professor of Surgery and Head of Department, The Royal Free Hospital, London, UK

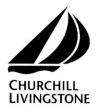

CHURCHILL
LIVINGSTONE

LONDON • EDINBURGH • NEW YORK • PHILADELPHIA • ST LOUIS • SYDNEY • TORONTO 2001

CHURCHILL LIVINGSTONE
An imprint of Harcourt Publishers Limited

© R. M. Kirk 2001

is a registered trademark of Harcourt Publishers Limited

ISBN 0 443 06398 2

BRITISH LIBRARY CATALOGUING IN PUBLICATION DATA
A catalogue record for this book is available from the British Library

LIBRARY OF CONGRESS CATALOGING IN PUBLICATION DATA
A catalog record for this book is available from the Library of Congress

NOTE
Medical knowledge is constantly changing. As new information becomes available,
changes in treatment, procedures, equipment and the use of drugs become necessary.
The editors/authors/contributors and the publishers have taken care to ensure that
the information given in this text is accurate and up to date. However, readers are
strongly advised to confirm that the information, especially with regard to drug usage,
complies with the latest legislation and standards of practice.

Existing UK nomenclature is changing to the system of Recommended International
Nonproprietary Names (rINNs). Until the UK names are no longer in use, these more
familiar names are used in this book in preference to rINNs, details of which may be
obtained from the *British National Formulary*.

Printed in Hong Kong

The
Publisher's
policy is to use
**paper manufactured
from sustainable forests**

Contents

Contents

Contributors

David Abrams MA, MD, FRCS, DO
Consulting Ophthalmic Surgeon, The Royal Free
Hospital, London, UK

Hiroshi Akiyama MD, FRCS(Eng)(Hon), FACS(Hon)
President, Toranomon Hospital, Tokyo, Japan

Shaun Appleton FRCS
Surgical Specialist Registrar, Chelsea and Westminster
Hospital, London, UK

John Bancewicz BSc(Hons), ChM, FRCS
Reader in Surgery and Consultant Surgeon, Department
of Surgery, University of Manchester, Hope Hospital,
Salford, UK

Michael Baum MB, ChM, FRCS, MD, FRCR
Professor of Surgery, Academic Department of Surgery,
The Royal Free and University College Medical School,
London, UK

Satyajit Bhattacharya MS, MPhil, FRCS
Consultant Surgeon, The Royal London Hospital,
London, UK

Michael D. Brough MA, MB, BChir, FRCS
Consultant Plastic Surgeon, University College London
Hospitals, Royal Free Hospital and Whittington
Hospital, London, UK

Kevin G. Burnand MS, FRCS
Professor of Surgery, Academic Department of Surgery,
St Thomas' Hospital, London, UK

Frank W. Cross MS(Lond), FRCS(Eng)
Consultant Vascular and Trauma Surgeon, Royal
London Hospital, London, UK

Ara Darzi MD, FRCS, FRCSI, FACS
Professor of Surgery and Head of Department, Imperial
College of Science, Technology and Medicine, St
Mary's Hospital, London, UK

John R. Farndon BSc, MD, FRCS(Eng), FRCS(Ed)
Professor of Surgery, Department of Surgery, University
of Bristol, Bristol, UK

Roy W. R. Farrell MA, MB, BAO BCL, FRCSI, FRCS
Consultant Otolaryngologist and Head and Neck
Surgeon, Northwick Park Hospital, Harrow, Middlesex,
UK

Chris Fowler BSc, MA, MS, FRCP, FRCS(Urol), FEBU
Director of Surgical Education, Academic Urological
Unit, St Bartholomew's and the Royal London School of
Medicine and Dentistry, Royal London Hospital,
London, UK

Clare A. Fowler MBBS, FRCS
Specialist Registrar General Surgery, Department of
Surgery, Bristol Royal Infirmary, Bristol, UK

Nicholas Goddard MB, BS, FRCS
Consultant Orthopaedic Surgeon, The Royal Free
Hospital, London, UK

Gareth Harper MA, BM, BChir, FRCS(Orth)
Consultant Orthopaedic Surgeon, Queen Alexandra
Hospital, Portsmouth, UK

Peter L. Harris MB, ChB, MD, FRCS(Eng)
Consultant Vascular Surgeon and Director of Vascular
and Transplant Services, Regional Vascular Unit, Royal
Liverpool University Hospital, Liverpool, UK

Peter Hawley MS, FRCS
Surgeon (retired), St Mark's Hospital, Northwick Park
Hospital, Harrow, UK

K. E. F. Hobbs ChM, FRCS
Emeritus Professor, University Department of Surgery,
The Royal Free and University College Medical School,
London, UK

Michael Hobsley MA, MB, Mchir, PhD, DSc, FRCS
Emeritus Professor, Department of Surgery, University
College London Medical School, London, UK

Jonathan D. Jagger MBBS, FRCS, Do, FRCOphth
Consultant Ophthalmic Surgeon, Eye Department, The
Royal Free Hospital, London, UK

David Johnston MD, ChM, FRCS(Edin, Eng, Glasg)
Professor Emeritus; *formerly* Professor of Surgery,
University of Leeds and Surgeon, Leeds General
Infirmary, Leeds, UK

Islam Junaid MBBS, FRCS(Urol)
Specialist Registrar and Honorary Lecturer, Academic
Urological Unit, St Bartholomew's and the Royal
London School of Medicine and Dentistry, Royal
London Hospital, London, UK

Ajay K. Kakkar MBBS(Hons), BSc, PhD, FRCS
Senior Lecturer and Consultant Surgeon, Department of
Gastrointestinal Surgery, Imperial College School of
Medicine, Hammersmith Hospital, London, UK

Robin R. Kanagasabay BSc, MRCP, FRCS
Specialist Registrar Cardiothoracic Surgery,
Cardiothoracic Unit, St George's Hospital, London, UK

R. M. Kirk MS, FRCS
Honorary Consulting Surgeon, The Royal Free Hospital,
London, UK

Iain M. Laws TD, MB, ChB, FDSRCS
Emeritus Consultant in Oral and Maxillofacial Surgery,
The Royal Free Hospital, London, UK

Roger J. Leicester OBE, MB, FRCS (Edinburgh & England)
Consultant Colorectal Surgeon, St George's Hospital,
London; Endoscopy Tutor, Raven Department of
Education, Royal College of Surgeons of England,
London, UK

Arthur R. Makey MS, FRCS
Emeritus Cardiothoracic Surgeon Charing Cross
Hospital, London; Emeritus Cardiothoracic Consultant
to the Royal Air Force

R. S. Maurice-Williams MA, MB, BChir, FRCP, FRCS
Consultant Neurosurgeon, Neurosurgical Unit, The
Royal Free Hospital, London, UK

P. A. Paraskeva BSc(Hons), MBBS(Hons), FRCS
Lecturer in Surgery, Imperial College of Science,
Technology and Medicine, St Mary's Hospital, London,
UK

Robin Phillips MS, FRCS
Consultant Surgeon, St Mark's Hospital, Northwick Park
Hospital, Harrow, UK

Keith Rolles MA, MS, FRCS
Consultant Surgeon, The Royal Free Hospital, London,
UK

James Ryan MB, MCh, FRCS, DMCC
Leonard Cheshire Professor of Conflict Recovery,
Department of Surgery, University College London
Hospitals Trust, London, UK

Christobel Saunders FRCS(Gen)
Senior Lecturer and Consultant Surgeon, Department of
Surgery, Perth Royal Infirmary, Perth, Australia

Marcus E. Setchell MA, MB, BChir, FRCS(Eng), FRCS(Edin), FRCOG
Consultant Obstetrician and Gynaecologist, St
Bartholomew's Hospital, London and Homerton
Hospital, London, UK

Robert S. Simons QHP(C), MB, ChB, FRCA, FANZCA
Consultant Anaesthetist, The Royal Free Hospital,
London, UK

Lewis Spitz MBChB, PhD, FRCS, FRCS(Ed), FAAP(Hon), FRCPCH
Nuffield Professor of Paediatric Surgery, Institute of
Child Health (University College London); Consultant
Paediatric Surgeon, Great Ormond Street Hospital for
Children, London, UK

Michael P. Stearns MB, BS, BDS, FRCS
Consultant Otolaryngologist/Head and Neck Surgeon,
The Royal Free Hospital, London, UK

Ian D. Sugarman MB, ChB, FRCS(Ed), FRCS(Paeds)
Consultant Paediatric Surgeon, Leeds General Infirmary,
Leeds, UK

Jeremy Thompson MA, MB, MChir, FRCS
Consultant Surgeon, Chelsea and Westminster Hospital,
London, UK

James P. S. Thomson DM, MS, FRCS
Surgeon (retired), St Mark's Hospital, Northwick Park
Hospital, Harrow: Honorary Consultant Surgeon, St
Mary's Hospital; Civil Consultant in Surgery, Royal
Air Force; Civilian Consultant in Colorectal Surgery,
Royal Navy; Honorary Lecturer in Surgery, The
Medical College of St Bartholomew's Hospital,
London, UK

Tom Treasure MD, MS, FRCS
Professor of Cardiothoracic Surgery, Cardiothoracic
Unit, St George's Hospital, London, UK

Harushi Udagawa MD, FACS
Chief of Gastroenterological Surgery, Toranomon
Hospital, Tokyo, Japan

Valery Usatoff MBBS(Hon), FRACS
Consultant Surgeon, Department of Surgery,
Hammersmith Hospital, Imperial College School of
Medicine, London, UK

Matthew Waltham MA, FRCS
Clinical Lecturer, Academic Department of Surgery, St
Thomas' Hospital, London, UK

David F. L. Watkin MChir, FRCS
Consultant Surgeon, Leicester Royal Infirmary,
Leicester, UK

R. C. N. Williamson MA, MD, MChir, FRCS
Professor of Surgery, Department of Gastrointestinal
Surgery, Imperial College School of Medicine,
Hammersmith Hospital, London, UK

Alastair C. J. Windsor MD, FRCS, FRCS(Ed)
Consultant Surgeon, St Mark's Hospital, Northwick Park
Hospital, Harrow, UK

Timothy R. Worthington MB, ChB, FRCS
Royal College of Surgeons Research Fellow, Department
of Gastrointestinal Surgery, Imperial College School of
Medicine, Hammersmith Hospital, London, UK

Preface

This is a selection from *General Surgical Operations*, 4th edition. We have extracted sections from the main book as far as possible without changing the words of the expert contributors. The emphasis is on principles, with detailed, step-by-step instructions on performing specific procedures. We have retained as far as possible the standardized format of the main text. In particular, we have tried to emphasize the key points and given advice on recognizing, avoiding and dealing with difficulties.

Basic surgical trainees are required to spend only six months in general surgery. It could be claimed that more emphasis should be given to orthopaedics, to urology or the other specialities within surgery. We have taken into account the need for experience in dealing with trauma and have included the whole of the outstanding new chapter on dealing with the severely-injured patient. Most trainees spend some time in the accident and emergency department, so we have included short accounts on how to deal with problems likely to be encountered that may demand urgent treatment.

Keen aspiring surgeons wish to know about the major procedures at which they will assist. For this reason we have included brief outlines of some of the major operations.

This is a 'What to do' book. Do not embark on surgical operations without being competent in performing the basic skills. 'How to do it' is described in *Basic Surgical Techniques*. In order to reduce the size of the book we have excluded perioperative management but this is described in detail in *Clinical Surgery in General*. They are both published by Churchill Livingstone.

We are well aware of the reduced practical experience to which modern young surgeons are exposed compared with former years. Textbooks offer guidance but they do not supervise your observance of the principles of good surgical practice. Make the most of the only true way to acquire surgical skills – that is by attaching yourself as an apprentice to a master. The trainer is often not aware of much of the specific practical wisdom that he or she has acquired. Much of what you learn from your teacher you learn unconsciously. If you concentrate on watching what is done and how it is done, when you come to do it, you automatically follow the same approach.

If your length of training is short, remember the statement of the novelist Thomas Hardy, 'Experience is as to intensity, not as to duration.'

APOLOGY

We apologize to women surgeons and women in general for the frequent use of the male pronoun. Constant reference to 'he or she' and inappropriate use of plural pronouns are clumsy and irritating. There is no epicene third person pronoun.

Acknowledgements

It is a pleasure to work once more with Miranda Bromage, Sue Hodgson and Francesca Lumkin in the Editorial Offices. Hilary Hewitt is the Senior Project Manager. Once again, Angela Christie has expertly drawn additional line illustrations.

Thanks also go to Sukie Hunter, copyeditor and typesetter, Austin Guest, proofreader and Annette Musker, indexer.

R. M. Kirk and M. C. Winslet
London 2001

Choose well, cut well, get well

R. M. Kirk

Contents

Choose well
Cut well
Get well

The six-word, succinct American aphorism sums up almost the whole of surgery. As in so many complex procedures, the whole is dependent upon every single step. The old adage, 'Complications are made in the operating room', is not altogether true. Although an incompetently performed, botched operation is likely to bring disaster, it is equally dangerous to perform inappropriate procedures expertly on ill-prepared patients and fail to monitor their recovery closely. The American surgeon Spencer stated that good surgery is 75% decision-making and only 25% manual dexterity.[1]

Public expectations, which were previously low, have risen, driving the medical profession towards greater intraprofessional surveillance, more evidence-based treatments, with review of outcomes. Because operation is a specific event in management, it is too easily and un-critically used to compare results between surgeons. We shall need to pay as much attention to the outcome in those patients we decide not to submit to operation, especially since there is now a choice in many traditional surgical fields between effective drugs and treatment using endoscopic and interventional radiological methods.

CHOOSE WELL

Decide

1. The existence of double-blind, controlled clinical trials is well known. Our patients reasonably expect us to choose the correct management for their surgical conditions. Of the treatment methods available, surely, they will say, it is possible, after testing them, to conclude that one is better than the others. Ideally, there should be but one variable, the treatment. Unfortunately, biological variability is so great that very often a conclusive answer cannot be given. The physical and psychological condition of patients, the extent and virulence of diseases, make it difficult or impossible to study matched groups of people with matched disease severity. As new methods become available conflicting evidence emerges about their effectiveness and safety compared with existing methods.

2. Our selection of facts from the available evidence varies as individuals and between surgeons. An apparently inconsequential fact leads one investigator along one path, while another may direct the focus to other evidence. In reaching a decision about a particular

patient, not all pieces of evidence are of equal value. Some features may be common to many conditions, but we need to be influenced more by those that are discriminant. As individual surgeons we may be influenced by recent experience, perhaps of a run of successes or disasters, to change our viewpoint. Moreover, we favour evidence that fits our existing beliefs.

3. In some cases we may not have a diagnosis but only a clinical feature that demands action on our part. This is particularly true for some emergencies, when the exact cause of a life-threatening haemorrhage, cardiorespiratory failure or peritonitis may not be clear, but urgent treatment is necessary.

4. We cannot concentrate on a single patient in circumstances where many people are ill. This is particularly true in wartime or a civilian disaster. In such cases we must make urgent, sometimes agonizing, decisions. This process of *triage* (Old French = to pick, select) involves choosing to treat first those who can be saved by quick action, deferring treatment of those with multiple injuries and those with injuries of the extremities. In many such cases we may need to pass by those with peripheral injuries, even though this will mean loss of the extremity, in favour of those whose survival depends on quick, effective action – 'life comes before limb'.

5. Even in elective circumstances we need to make decisions with incomplete information. We never have all the necessary facts available about the physical and mental state of our patient but make the best guess, based on our general knowledge and the results of appropriately selected investigations. Thereafter we must monitor the effects of our actions, to determine if they are correct.

6. Success does not necessarily indicate good judgement; the patient

may improve in spite of inappropriate treatment. Conversely, the patient may deteriorate despite the best treatment. Nevertheless, some surgeons get better results than others; they may have greater technical skills but probably they make a higher percentage of correct decisions.

7. When seeking a solution to a difficult problem, if possible take the opportunity to set it aside while you do something else. It is remarkable how solutions often appear spontaneously, or as a result of a shift in the way you view the problem. It is also valuable to re-examine, after an interval, the patient who presents with, for example, an acute abdomen – the physical signs can change rapidly.

8. If you reach a decision, regard it as only provisional. Since it is based on incomplete knowledge, you may discover further facts, or the observed effects of your management may suggest that you review and revise the course of action. Too often, initially good management fails because it is inexorably pursued when the circumstances change. Your initial plan is comparable with the *strategy* of a general before battle, but he may need to alter his *tactics* as the battle develops.

> **Key point**
>
> ● Be flexible. React to changed circumstances.

9. Attempts to rationalize decisions have resulted in the development of *algorithms*, or standard, step-by-step actions, and *protocols*, which provide a standard approach leading to an expected optimum outcome. Especially in the USA, pressure from managed care organizations and 'stakeholders' (insurers and those who pay the bills) have resulted in *guidelines* and *clinical pathways*, although some of them have not been verified. Such methods have been worked out and evaluated by experts in the particular fields where they can be applied. They do not necessarily fit every circumstance but provide a routine approach that has been shown to give the best results in most cases. Such methods need to be re-evaluated from time to time as views change, with improvements in diagnosis and therapeutics, and in the light of follow-up. *Decision analysis*, another aid in evaluating the best course of action, is discussed later.

> **Key point**
>
> ● If you are about to make a heterodox decision, ask yourself, 'If my selected course of management fails, can I justify my actions to the patient, to my peers and, most importantly, to myself?'

10. Do not be too proud to take advice. The very action of arranging and presenting the problem to another person often clarifies it.

11. When you have reached a decision, you must discuss it with the patient, who has the right to participate. However much we try to offer a balanced judgement, it is inevitable that the presentation to our patients is biased. Our decision is the one in which we believe, and inevitably we weight the evidence towards our selected management. There is nothing dishonest about this. Indeed, it would be cowardly not to give positive advice. We have access to the available facts and have to weigh them, reach a decision and place that decision before the patient. It is our professional duty to take responsibility for our

decisions and irresolute to place the whole burden on to the patient. This does not, of course, excuse us if we ignore or override the patient's wishes. Patients faced with treatment decisions look at different criteria from us, such as quality of life; our anxieties revolve more closely around survival.[2,3]

12. Decision analysis offers a means of weighing all the factors and possible outcomes.[4]

13. In most cases the probable outcome of operation can be estimated from a study of the relevant literature. However, the outcome of withholding operation in circumstances where it is routinely offered is often not known and must be estimated from reports written before surgery was possible, or from the records of patients who have refused operation.

14. Added into the equation are the value judgements placed by you and the patient on the sequelae of surgical versus conservative management, and the likelihood of benefit from different operations. These subjective values are termed *utilities*. The possibility of curing a threatening condition by major operation has to be placed against the mortality and morbidity associated with it. If the condition is likely to be fatal, life expectation has to be balanced against the quality of life. There are a number of terms used in assessing this. One such is quality adjusted life year (*QALY*). One year of life in perfect health is 1 QALY and a lower figure is allocated for a portion of a year in perfect health or a full year spent with a disability. Also added in are the economic implications – the *cost-benefit* analysis. Decision analyses have been published for a number of common conditions.

15. The main value of such analyses is in bringing into focus all the possibilities. In the distant past, surgery was often carried out as the last resort. As new methods of management become available, as the effects of various treatments become known, and as the knowledge and desire of patients to participate in the decision-making process increases, so we need to consider and evaluate all the choices.

> **Key point**
>
> ● Although investigations, protocols, guidelines, risk and decision analyses are useful, the decision of an experienced clinician must be paramount.[5]

REFERENCES

1. Spencer FC 1979 Competence and compassion; two qualities of surgical excellence. Bulletin of the American College of Surgeons 64: 15–22
2. Mazur DJ, Hickam DH 1996 Five-year survival curves: how much data are enough for patient–physician decision making in general surgery? European Journal of Surgery 162: 101–104
3. Newton-Howes PA, Bedford ND, Dobbs BR, Frizelle FA 1998 Informed consent: what do patients want to know? New Zealand Medical Journal 111: 340–342
4. Kirk RM 1999 Decision making. In: Kirk RM, Mansfield AO, Cochrane JPS, eds. Clinical surgery in general, 3rd edn. Churchill Livingstone, Edinburgh, pp 153–157
5. Jewell ER, Persson AV 1985 Preoperative evaluation of the high risk patient. Surgical Clinics of North America 65: 3–19

CUT WELL

🔑 **Key point**

- If operation is indicated, should you perform it? Except in an emergency, avoid carrying out operations that can be better performed by someone else who is available.

Routines

1. Sterile techniques in the operating theatre have been worked out over many years. Most, but not all, have been subjected to scientific evaluation. Although experienced people carry out the correct procedures instinctively, many of us acquire bad habits that go uncorrected. Accept the need to follow strict routines and so be free to concentrate on other aspects of the operation. Question the routines from time to time to decide if they are really valuable. Discuss them with the senior theatre users. Thoughtless disparagement undermines training.

🔑 **Key points**

- Do not rush! Hurried movements result in mistakes and the need to repeat actions.

- **Concentrate on getting everything right first time.**

- A major operation is merely a series of small operations, but a successful outcome depends upon each step being accomplished perfectly.

2. Standardized operative techniques result from the pooled experience of many surgeons. If you are still an assistant, adopt the accepted and orthodox procedures followed by your chief. In this way you will at least have the consolation, if anything goes wrong, that you can justify your actions. Later in your career you may question certain points of technique and have the courage to adopt your own methods, usually a synthesis of points acquired from your teachers.

3. 'Set up' standard procedures, for example when applying a series of ligatures, suturing and mobilizing structures. Take time to place yourself in the best position; arrange the structures so that you can carry out each manoeuvre in a controlled and natural manner.

4. Never relax your vigilance over instruments, swabs and other materials placed into the wound. There is no single, once-for-all action that will prevent articles from being left inside, bringing distress and often tragedy both for the patient and yourself. Worry about the possibility without a moment's let up, and accept full responsibility. Check everything, every time. Do not let your acceptance of responsibility prevent you from involving as many others as possible in the check. They may save you from a momentary lapse.

5. Use as few swabs as possible and always use the largest ones compatible with the task. Avoid burying all the swab or pack in the wound; leave a portion, or attached tape, protruding to be clipped to the wound towels.

6. Whatever decision you made before operation, react to unexpected findings and to difficulties you may encounter. Do not doggedly persist with your original procedure but be flexible in your

🔑 **Key points**

- Unless you are intimately familiar with the anatomy you tend to wander out of the correct tissue plane.

- If you handle the tissues roughly they will swell, ooze tissue fluid and heal imperfectly.

- If your haemostasis is imperfect, you leave a potential culture medium for microorganisms.

- If your apposition of anastomoses is poor, they will leak or cause obstruction.

- If your sutures are too tight they will cut out. If they are too slack they will not retain tissue contact.

- If you tie knots slickly but casually they will fail.

approach. If appropriate, stop the operation or perform a routine part while turning over the possibilities. Do not hesitate to discuss it with the other people in the operating theatre or seek another opinion directly or over the telephone. Stating the problem to others often clarifies it in your own mind.

Haemostasis

Prepare

1. Does the patient have a bleeding tendency? If so, did you correct it or arrange for replacement blood and clotting factors to be available?

2. If the patient is already bleeding, as following trauma or local disease, are you replacing the lost blood as far as possible? Have you ordered further supplies and, if necessary, fresh frozen plasma?

3. Are you able to identify the site clinically or by suitable investigation? Can you control it before taking the patient to the operating theatre? If the bleeding is iatrogenic following inappropriate administration of anticoagulants, has the clotting mechanism been restored?

4. Ensure that the operating theatre staff are warned to have necessary equipment to hand. For calamitous thoracoabdominal bleeding you may need very large packs and at least two efficient suckers and vascular surgical instruments.

5. In some cases, operation is not the best method of controlling bleeding. Endoscopy and interventional radiology are sometimes preferable.

Action

1. Whenever possible, seal the tissues with the diathermy before cutting them. Identify, isolate and doubly ligate blood vessels before dividing them, using haemostatic forceps, aneurysm needles, mechanical stapling devices and, if necessary, suture ligation. In some cases it is possible to use cutting diathermy current, an ultrasonic dissector or a laser beam to incise the tissues and at the same time seal the vessels.

2. If the operation is carried out to control bleeding following trauma or local disease, do not expose the site until you have everything you need at hand, with suckers working and packs ready. Intra-abdominal bleeding is reduced as the abdomen distends and becomes tense but when you perform laparotomy the tension is released and

bleeding restarts. Immediately place very large packs into each quadrant of the abdomen. Aspirate residual blood, then gently remove the packs one by one, a little at a time, starting with the ones you suspect are furthest from the bleeding site. You hope to end with a dry abdomen and the last pack controlling the bleeding point, so that you can cautiously peel it away, identify the vessels and control them.

3. When you encounter unexpected bleeding, apply pressure from fingers or a swab, maintain it for a few moments while you consider how to control it, and prepare to do so. If the bleeding is calamitous, maintain the pressure for 5 minutes timed by the clock. Often, when you carefully remove the source of pressure you discover that the bleeding has stopped or is easily controlled. Whatever you do, avoid panicky stabs with haemostats plunged blindly into a lake of blood.

4. Anticipate oozing from raw surfaces and consider first infiltrating the tissues with a solution of 1:250 000 adrenaline (epinephrine) in physiological saline solution.

5. Small oozing areas can often be sealed by applying gelatin foam, a resorbable mesh graft of polyglycolic acid or by folding the tissue so that the raw surfaces come into contact. If necessary, maintain the contact using a few sutures.

6. Do not rely upon drains when bleeding occurs. It is much better to achieve perfect haemostasis, followed by meticulous removal of all spilt blood.

7. There are times when you cannot control bleeding from a raw area in, for instance, the abdomen. Do not hesitate to pack the area with sterile gauze. Preferably use a long length, folded back and forth like a 'jumping jack' cracker. Sometimes the end can be left protruding from the wound, sometimes it is convenient to close the wound over it. In 24–48 hours you may cautiously withdraw the pack, fold by fold. The bleeding will usually have stopped. If it has not, or if bleeding continues after packing it, the pack has not been properly placed. Repeat the procedure and ensure that it is effective.

Contaminated wounds

Appraise

1. Contamination of healthy tissues with moderate numbers of pathogenic bacteria does not necessarily prevent healing. Even if the organisms invade the living tissues – infection – they do not always retard healing. The effects depend on the heaviness of contamination, the virulence of the organisms and the viability of the tissues. Large numbers of virulent organisms in tissues with reduced viability, as after burns, may cause cellulitis, abscess, lymphangitis and possible progression to bacteraemia, pyaemia and septicaemia.

2. Dirty wounds are often cleaned with 1% cetrimide. This may damage the tissues. Another favoured solution is 3% hydrogen peroxide, which effervesces. Simple washing with sterile physiological saline is probably as effective.

3. Infection is increased in the presence of slough, which is adherent fibrin, dead tissue and pus. Remove it surgically when it forms a coherent sheet, which usually blackens. The traditional nonsurgical method of treating slough is with Eusol (Edinburgh University solution of lime). It is particularly used as a local application to deslough areas prior to skin grafting. Eusol has been condemned on experimental evidence that it delays healing, but no controlled clinical trials have been performed. Enzyme mixtures containing streptokinase and streptodornase are not demonstrably more effective than other substances.

4. The application of local antiseptics to contaminated wounds is controversial. Chlorhexidine as a 0.05% aqueous solution and potassium permanganate as a 0.01% solution are often used. Povidone-iodine 5% solution is valuable against *Staphylococcus aureus*. Acetic acid as a 5% solution helps eradicate *Pseudomonas* spp.

5. Locally applied antibiotics are often ineffective. They encourage the emergence of resistant bacterial strains and frequently produce allergic reactions. The only one that is effective is silver sulphadiazine cream to prevent infection of severe burns. As a rule, if antibiotics are needed, give them systemically.

6. Meleney's spreading gangrene of the skin of the abdominal wall, necrotizing fasciitis and Fournier's scrotal gangrene result from synergism between micro-aerophilic streptococci and other organisms. Excise the whole of the gangrenous area without delay, to leave no trace of the disease but only healthy clean tissue. Do not carry out a single excision but repeat it as often as is necessary to eradicate the spreading infection. Give high doses of intravenous antibiotics depending on the likely source of infection until you have been guided by the microbiologist. Penicillin, metronidazole and third-generation cephalosporins are usual choices.

Action

1. Always start by taking swabs for aerobic and anaerobic culture and tests for antibiotic sensitivity.

2. Do not close a wound that is contaminated, that has ischaemic tissues within it forming a potential source of infection, or one in which body fluids are likely to collect that will form a good culture medium for microorganisms. In case of doubt, insert sutures but delay tying them until you are sure that the wound is clean – delayed primary closure.

3. If there is considerable swelling and tension of the deep tissues, as may occur in cellulitis, burns or following trauma, do not hesitate to debride (unbridle) the wound by laying open the constricting tissues, taking care to avoid injury to important structures. In the limbs this is accomplished by making longitudinal incisions through the skin and deep fascia.

4. Excise from traumatized or infected wounds all dead or dying tissue, in particular muscle that has been crushed, is ischaemic or has been devitalized by the close passage of a high-velocity missile. Remove all foreign material, since it is potentially infected (see Ch. 3). Preserve important structures such as major blood vessels and nerves, remembering that they may be displaced following injury. Do not remove attached bone fragments unless they are grossly displaced. Do not over-aggressively excise damaged skin, especially of the hands and face.

5. In the presence of swelling, when there may be tension after closure, employ delayed primary closure. Leave the wound open, elevate the part if possible and close it when the swelling has diminished.

Viral transmission

Ensure that you are immunized against hepatitis B (HBV). You remain at risk from hepatitis C (HCV) and from human immunodeficiency virus (HIV). Adapt your technique to protect yourself, your team and patients from risk of transmitting these viruses during your management of them. This applies not just to the operating theatre but to every encounter with patients.

High-risk patients

1. If you suspect that a patient has hepatitis B or HIV, or has overt clinical features suggesting they have AIDS, you should advise them to accept antibody testing. The HIV test must be preceded by counselling.

2. Manage those you consider to have, or who are proven to have, transmissible viral infection such as HBV and HIV in a modified manner. However, they are no longer placed at the end of the operating list and are treated in the usual manner on arrival in the anaesthetic room. The anaesthetist wears eye protection and surgical gloves during induction.

3. Ensure that the operating table is covered with an impervious sheet to avoid contamination of the mattress.

4. Wear eye protection, and a completely impervious gown over a plastic apron that covers impervious boots and overshoes. Wear an impervious mask. Wear two pairs of gloves.

5. After cleaning the skin, apply impervious wound drapes.

6. At the end of the operation, ensure that the 'sharps' container and disposable gowns, drapes and swabs are placed in separate bags to be sent for disposal. Re-usable instruments are placed in containers for separate washing and sterilization.

All patients

> **Key points**
>
> - Do not delude yourself that the precautions you have taken for 'high-risk' patients protect you from contracting hepatitis virus or HIV. It is the patients you assume not to be infectious that pose the greatest threat to you.
>
> - The most dangerous substances with which you come into contact are human blood and blood products. The best way to avoid contact with the patient's blood is to avoid spilling it.

1. Adopt a standard technique that protects you and your team from contact with the blood and body secretions of all patients at all times.

2. Never allow 'sharps', such as knives, needles, trocars, spikes or hooks, to be passed from hand to hand. Have them placed in a dish. When you use them, take them from the dish and return them to it after use.

3. Avoid contact with the sharp portions of knives and needles. When suturing use a strictly 'no touch' technique – hold needles in a needle-holder, recover them after they have passed through the tissues with dissecting forceps, from which they are passed back to the needle-holder. Make sure as you draw the needle through that you do not injure yourself or anyone in the team. Grasp the thread away from the needle with your fingers (an instrument will damage the thread) and draw it through. This also prevents you from pulling the thread from the swaged needle.

4. Never use your unprotected finger as a guide for a needle or knife, as when penetrating the abdominal or chest wall. Either evert

the tissues in order to see the emerging point, or place a flat metal plate over the deeper tissues at risk, or wear a sterile metal thimble on your finger.

5. You must, from time to time, deal with active bleeding. Indeed, the operation may be performed in order to control it. As soon as you have stopped the bleeding, aspirate all the blood. Discard the blood-stained swabs, replace the bloodstained drapes.

6. If your gloves are damaged, change them immediately. If they become heavily bloodstained do not hesitate to change them; as you do so, observe your hands and fingers for blood that may have seeped through a defect, and the elastic cuff of your gown to note if it is blood-stained. If you see such evidence of contact with the patient's blood, rescrub and apply a clean gown and gloves.

7. At the end of the operation, peel off your gloves so they are turned inside out and you can then inspect them for tears. An altern-ative is first to wash your gloved hands in methylene blue solution, then remove your gloves to see if your fingers are stained blue. Inspect your fingers for pricks and cuts.

8. If you have sustained an injury during the operation you should immediately report it to the Occupational Health Officer. At present such injuries are under-reported, and in turn the risks to surgeons and other theatre staff are underestimated.

9. Disposable sharps are carefully placed in a self-locking, disposal carrier.

Surgeon with HIV

A surgeon infected with HIV must cease duties that involve the risk of contact with patients' blood or tissues. This effectively precludes a continuing career in surgery.

Closure

1. Do not close the wound until you have checked that the procedure has been accomplished perfectly, that there is no continuing bleeding and that you have not inadvertently damaged other structures.

2. Did you intend to carry out any ancillary procedure?

3. Have you aspirated any fluid collections?

4. Do you need to insert drains or other apparatus?

5. Can you reduce postoperative pain by carrying out a nerve block? This is particularly valuable for short-stay or day case patients. Following inguinal herniorrhaphy, consider carrying out inguinal field block using bupivacaine. Do not use more than 100 mg in dilute solution, such as 40 ml of 0.25%. Instillation into the wound of 10 ml 0.5% (50 mg) plain bupivacaine has been shown to be effective in reducing postoperative pain.

6. Observe the basic principles of surgical closure. Do not leave continuing cause for complications, do not close under tension and attain perfect apposition of the tissues you bring together.

7. Do not use hand-held needles. The risk of skin injuries is probably less with skin staples or clips than with sutured closure. Whenever possible close with subcuticular stitches, preferably of fine absorbable synthetic material that does not require attendance by the patient for removal. Alternatively, use adhesive strips. The newer fibrin tissue adhesives may come into common use.

8. Occasionally the wound needs to be packed because of bleeding that cannot be controlled by any other method. It can occur as a result of an uncorrected or uncorrectable bleeding diathesis,

from a localized cause such as a vascular tumour that cannot be removed or following trauma.

9. An oedematous wound, or one from which superficial tissue is lost, as following trauma or ablative surgery, may be better treated by delayed primary closure after swelling has subsided. After ensuring that the remaining tissues are viable, clean and dry, apply a single layer of non-adherent net, over which apply gauze to seal off the wound.

10. Primary closure of some defects is achieved using grafts or flaps (see Ch. 32).

Dressings

1. Make sure you know why you are applying dressings and what function they will serve. They may merely protect the wound from damage, prevent the patient from inspecting it or picking at it, protect it from becoming infected (or spreading infection elsewhere), soak up exudate, compress the wound to reduce or prevent swelling and act as a supporting corset to reduce tension.

2. Perfectly closed clean minor wounds require no dressing, since they seal within a few hours. Apply a strip of adhesive tape or a varnish if it is necessary to protect the area.

3. If oozing or exudation are expected, apply sufficient sterile gauze to absorb it, ensuring that the gauze is changed before the exudate soaks through and forms a moist pathway for organisms to track down to the wound.

4. If you wish to apply compression, ensure that this is evenly distributed. First apply gauze to absorb any exudate, then evenly laid cotton wool. Do not use the cotton wool as an extra absorbent – it will form a hard, useless cake. Alternatively, use sponge or an inflatable air cushion.

5. If you intend leaving the wound open, apply a single layer of non-adherent net or tulle gras, followed by an absorbent layer of sterile gauze. Cavities may be packed with gauze soaked in flavine emulsion.

6. Cavities can also be filled with polymerized foam formed within the cavity. These can be removed for wound cleaning, then washed and re-applied on some exposed areas, as after laying open a pilonidal sinus.

7. New wound dressings such as hydrogels and hydrocolloids absorb exudate, maintain a moist environment, protect the area from secondary infection and are non-adherent.

8. To hold dressings in place and exert compression, apply if possible an encircling bandage such as crepe bandage. If you use this method on limbs, always encase the limb with bandage from the extremity up to the site of the wound to avoid producing a garter effect, which would ensue if the bandage were applied only proximally, thus causing venous congestion and distal swelling. Always leave the tips of fingers and toes visible and inspect them regularly to ensure that they are not rendered ischaemic. For the abdomen, many-tailed bandages have been replaced by disposable elastic corsets. Adhesive elastic strips may be applied across the wound under slight tension but they tend to cause excoriation. However, when a wound needs frequent changes of dressing, adhesive strips may be placed on each side of the wound and can be laced together over the dressings to retain them.

GET WELL

1. It is not sufficient to carry out the correct procedure perfectly. However well the operation has been performed, the patient has undergone a physiological and psychological disturbance. Your aim must be to help the patient achieve maximum functional recovery and satisfaction with the procedure, as soon as possible. The more ill the patient before operation, the bigger the operation, the greater the risk of complications, both in the short and long term.

2. As a rule you will not carry out all the procedures yourself. Following a general anaesthetic the anaesthetist continues to supervise the general care of patients until they have safely recovered from the effects of the anaesthetic and are in a stable condition.

3. The recovery room nurses observe the patient and call for assistance as necessary. Nevertheless you must give clear oral and written instructions about the procedure, the likely sequelae and any special observations or actions you require.

4. Always make a full record as soon as possible of the operative findings, giving details of the procedure carried out and any special points, such as the insertion of drains. In complicated cases ensure that drains are labelled; in addition provide a sketch of the incisions and of attached drains, cannulas or other apparatus, with clear instructions about the management of each one.

5. Following a major operation, or one carried out on a poor-risk patient, inform the relatives and the general practitioner as soon as it is convenient, personally or by telephone. It is usually best to defer passing on the full impact of distressing news to relatives until you can speak under less stressful circumstances.

Recovery phase

Regard the patient who has just been submitted to an operation in the same light as one brought into the hospital following an acute illness or trauma.

Monitor

1. Airway, Breathing, Circulation (ABC) are vital functions to observe during the recovery from anaesthesia.

2. Frequently check the consciousness level of the patient by noting the response to stimuli such as calling the name. In case of doubt note pupillary and other reflexes, and peripheral tone.

3. Do not have a fixed attitude to the amount of pain the patient is likely to suffer. Be willing to administer small, repeated doses of analgesics if the patient recovering consciousness is in pain.

4. In appropriate circumstances check the wound and drains. If blood emerges from an abdominal or chest drain it may be because intra-abdominal or intrathoracic tension has increased as the patient strains. It may also signify that straining has dislodged a ligature. If you suspect that severe bleeding has restarted, do not hesitate to return the patient to the operating theatre.

5. Restlessness of the patient may have other causes than wound pain. Check that the bladder is not overfull, that the patient is lying comfortably and is not pressed upon by any sharp or hard apparatus.

6. As soon as the patient is responsive, offer information as reassuring as possible about the operation and the present situation.

7. Encourage the wakened patient to breathe deeply, cough and

exercise the legs, within the limits posed by the procedure. Moisten the patient's lips or give a mouth wash.

8. Check aspects particular to the patient or the operation. For example, monitor the electrocardiogram (ECG) in patients with cardiac disease, the central nervous system following neurosurgical procedures, the urinary output if renal function is impaired, and the blood sugar in diabetics.

9. Following a general anaesthetic the conscious, stable patient is returned to the ward on instructions from the anaesthetist. The pharyngeal airway is removed before the patient leaves the recovery room. Ill, unstable patients are transferred to the intensive care unit.

Intermediate phase

1. Transfer to the ward can be unsettling and uncomfortable.

2. Carefully check airway, breathing, circulation, temperature and other appropriate measurements and record them as a baseline. As the patient recovers, the frequency of monitoring is progressively reduced and stopped.

3. Maintain adequate analgesia. Pain will be reduced if you carried out a field block or instilled long-acting local anaesthetic such as bupivacaine into the wound before closing. The anaesthetist may have inserted an epidural catheter for the instillation of local anaesthetics or opiates. Intramuscular opiates may be titrated, or analgesics may be controlled by the patient. Ensure that the patient's discomfort and pain are reduced to a minimum. Anxiety about respiratory depression or fixed ideas on how much analgesic is needed often leads to inadequate control of pain.

4. Mobilize the patient as quickly as possible, giving breathing and coughing exercises to prevent pulmonary collapse. Encourage leg and foot movement to reduce venous stasis, and frequent changes of posture to prevent pressure sores and allow drainage of the lung bases. Depending upon the operation, aim to have the patient ambulant as soon as possible. In recent years the length of time patients stay in bed after almost all operations has been drastically reduced.

5. Maintain fluid, electrolyte and acid/base balance. This is particularly important in patients who were out of balance before operation, those who must have parenteral intake following, for example, gastrointestinal surgery, and those with renal failure.

6. Following gastrointestinal surgery, aspiration of the digestive tract is usually needed. Check the volumes and character of the aspirate.

7. Frequently check the wound and the function of the system subjected to operation.

8. Check the discharge from drains. Most wound drains are removed after 24–48 hours unless they are draining profusely. Chest drains are also removed after 1 or 2 days unless they are draining profusely, or there is a pulmonary leak as evidenced by persistent bubbling through the underwater seal.

9. Insulin-dependent diabetes is usually treated throughout the operation with an infusion of 10% dextrose containing 20 mmol potassium chloride and 300 units of insulin. Approximately 100 ml an hour is given, with frequent checks on blood glucose. It is usually possible to return progressively to the preoperative regime within 2–3 days. Some non-insulin-dependent diabetics need to be given soluble insulin over the operative period but should soon be able to return to their diet or oral islet-cell-stimulant drugs.

10. Long-term drugs often need to be given in a modified form over the perioperative period, and the drugs are restored as the patient recovers. Those on steroid drugs need to have hydrocortisone over the operative period and this is continued, usually in a dose of 100 mg hydrocortisone intravenously by slow infusion every 6 hours, with progressive diminution of the dose so that the preoperative maintenance dose can be restored after 3–5 days. Ensure that there is adequate fluid and salt replacement and urinary output, and monitor the serum electrolytes and blood glucose. Patients with renal failure taking fludrocortisone should have it restarted, preferably within 3–5 days.

11. Patients with prosthetic heart valves who take long-term warfarin will have been given heparin over the operative period, usually as a slow intravenous infusion, controlled by maintaining the activated partial thromboplastin time (APTT) 1.5–2.5 times normal. After operation, warfarin is restarted, to overlap the heparin; now also check the international normalized ratio (INR).

12. Antidepressant, anxiolytic, anticonvulsant and anti-parkinsonian drugs need to be restored. Drugs of abuse, including alcohol and opiates, must also be restored or alternative treatment given.

13. Most patients develop a mild pyrexia during the first 24 hours after operation. If it remains there may be a known reason but if not, thoroughly investigate the cause. A swinging pyrexia denotes sepsis and this is most likely to be at the site of operation. Interpret the pyrexia in association with other features, such as the general condition of the patient and any associated circulatory disorder. If you cannot discover the cause, routinely check the possibilities:

a. Remember that patients may develop upper respiratory infection, including tonsillitis and ear infections, incidentally. Consider these, especially in young children.

b. Clinical examination, chest X-ray and sputum culture may suggest pulmonary collapse, pneumonia or pulmonary embolus. Improvement following inhalations and physiotherapy may confirm a pulmonary cause.

c. Apart from the presence of unilateral leg oedema, clinical detection of deep vein thrombosis is unreliable. Clinical evidence of pulmonary embolus may be supported by chest X-ray and electrocardiography.

d. Examine the cardiovascular system for features of myocardial infarction and check the ECG and cardiac enzymes.

e. Examine the wound and, in the case of abdominal surgery, carefully examine the abdomen and perform a rectal examination. Plain X-ray of the abdomen may reveal air or fluid levels under the diaphragm, dilatation of small and large bowel suggesting adynamic ileus, and thickening of the interfaces between bowel segments – so-called 'layering', which is indicative of peritonitis. Order a white blood cell count.

f. Send a midstream urine (MSU) specimen for microscopy and culture.

g. Examine intravenous injection and infusion sites for phlebitis.

14. Look at the whole skin surface to exclude raw areas, including pressure sores.

15. Has the patient an artificial cardiac valve? You will have known this before operation and should have given the patient prophylactic antibiotics. Nevertheless, order a blood culture.

16. You may still be uncertain. If you have already sent blood for culture that was unrevealing, send another one: a single specimen may not culture organisms successfully. Re-examine the patient after an interval.

17. Consider what is the likely cause in this patient after the operation that was carried out. Do not order a battery of investigations in the hope that 'something will turn up'. First call in a senior, experienced colleague to examine the patient.

Day case

1. The monitoring of recovery from a general anaesthetic must be as thorough as that of an inpatient. Sedation with benzodiazepines and administration of analgesics may depress respiration, so this must be monitored for 2 hours.

2. The normal assessment of recovery has to be compressed into a shorter period, but ensure that the cardiovascular and respiratory functions are normal before discharge.

3. Check the wound.

4. Fully inform the patient of the procedure, the likely sequelae, danger signs and what to do about them. It is wise to give written instructions for later reference.

5. If a follow-up appointment is to be given, arrange it now.

6. Ensure that those who have had a general anaesthetic or sedation are accompanied home.

7. Record the findings and procedure immediately. Because series of day cases are often arranged, it is easy to confuse the details if they are not recorded individually, between procedures.

Audit

1. Remarkable changes have occurred during the last 10 years, and especially during the last 5 years, from changes in public expectation and from media coverage of the complications that developed following the general adoption of minimal access techniques, often by surgeons with minimal training. However the investigation in 1998 of the results of paediatric cardiac surgery in Bristol brought matters to a head.

2. We should all ensure our results are open to scrutiny – not, as formerly, just to our own consciences, but also to our patients and peers.

Follow-up

1. You follow up patients to ensure that they recover without complications, to reassure them, to give further treatment, to assess your own results for comparison with published figures, and to detect long-term sequelae.

2. Make sure that you know why each patient is returning to your clinic. If patients attend unnecessarily the clinic becomes overfilled. Those who need attention are deprived of it. Sometimes attendance at the clinic can be averted by allowing patients to write in or telephone when they have a problem or at fixed intervals.

FURTHER READING

Bell D, Shapiro C 1992 The health care worker with HIV infection or AIDS. Clinical Care 4: 9–16.

Birkmeyer JD, Welch HG 1997 A reader's guide to surgical decision making. Journal of the American College of Surgeons 184: 589–595

Bunker JP, Barnes BA, Mosteller F 1977 Costs, risks, and benefits of surgery. Oxford University Press, Oxford

Clarke JR 1989 Decision making in surgical practice. World Journal of Surgery 13: 245–251

Finlayson SRG, Birkmeyer JD 1998 Cost effectiveness analysis in surgery. Surgery 123: 151–156

Jeffries DJ 1999 The risks to surgeons of nosocomial virus transmission. In: Kirk RM, Mansfield AO, Cochrane JPS (eds) Clinical surgery in general, 4th edn. Churchill Livingstone, Edinburgh

Kirk RM 1994 Basic surgical techniques, 4th edn. Churchill Livingstone, Edinburgh

Tate JJT 1999 Postoperative care. In: Kirk RM, Mansfield AO, Cochrane JPS (eds) Clinical surgery in general, 4th edn. Churchill Livingstone, Edinburgh, pp 318–325

UK Health Departments 1998 Guidance for clinical health care workers. Protection from infection with bloodborne viruses. Department of Health, London

CHAPTER

Anaesthesia-related techniques | 2

R. S. Simons

Contents

Certain basic principles of management and several practical techniques commonly practised by the anaesthetist should be within the competence of all surgeons. These skills include the ability to:

1. Provide and secure a patent airway
2. Sustain artificial ventilation when necessary
3. Use oxygen therapy to maintain tissue oxygenation
4. Confidently undertake peripheral and central venous access
5. Maintain adequate circulation by control of circulating blood volume, vascular tone and cardiac output
6. Use local anaesthetic drugs and techniques where general anaesthesia is unnecessary or inappropriate
7. Provide effective pain relief, particularly in the postoperative period
8. Utilize intensive therapy facilities in a co-ordinated and efficient manner.

RESPIRATORY SUPPORT

To maintain the heart and the brain,
Give oxygen now and again.
Not now and again, but NOW, AND AGAIN, AND AGAIN, AND AGAIN, AND AGAIN.
Adapted from a well-known limerick

Key point

- Failure of oxygen supply can damage the brain within 3–4 minutes. It is vital that you ensure a patent airway, satisfactory exchange of gases and adequate circulation.

All doctors in clinical practice, regardless of speciality, should receive training and certification in cardiopulmonary resuscitation (CPR) to the level of basic life support (BLS). Ensure that you attend an advanced trauma life support (ATLS) course; advanced cardiac life support (ALS) requirements are just as simple to learn and perform (see Further Reading).

Assess

1. A clear airway is essential. In patients with altered consciousness (intracranial damage, drug excess or overdose, profound shock, etc.), the airway may be compromised by obstruction in the oro- or laryngo-pharynx. In the supine patient this is typically caused by the tongue falling back against the posterior pharyngeal wall.
2. Assess level of consciousness by response to speech or painful stimulus. If the patient is unconscious, determine the cause.

Action

1. Remove any dentures and clear the pharynx and mouth of any gross contamination by blood, gastric contents or foreign material. Have Magill forceps and suction equipment available at all times. The latter should have a semirigid Yankauer handpiece already attached.
2. If trauma has occurred, be suspicious of cervical spine injury. Conduct manoeuvres to ensure airway patency with the head centrally aligned. The head and neck must not be flexed or extended. Stabilize the head with a firm cervical collar, supports or straps to prevent axial rotation of the spine.
3. Assess whether simple airway adjuncts (e.g. the Guedel oropharyngeal airway or soft curved nasopharyngeal tube) will secure patency. A Guedel airway is inserted 'upside down' under the upper teeth and then rotated downwards behind the tongue. After insertion, continue to support the jaw by jaw lift or jaw thrust. A nasopharyngeal airway should be well lubricated and inserted into the nose parallel to the hard palate to lie behind the soft palate and tongue. Put a safety pin through the tube to ensure it cannot migrate into the nose.
4. If ventilation is adequate, nurse the patient in the lateral or semiprone recovery position with head dependent to avoid regurgitation and aspiration into the trachea. This posture may be impracticable while examination or treatment (including resuscitation) is in progress or if spinal trauma is present or suspected.
5. If necessary, reverse the effect of opioid or benzodiazepine drugs with their respective specific antagonists – 0.2–0.4 mg naloxone or 0.3–0.6 mg flumazenil given intravenously.
6. If spontaneous ventilation is inadequate despite the insertion of an oropharyngeal airway, apply the mask (adult sizes 4–6) of a self-inflating bag-mask resuscitator to the nose and mouth.

Hold it securely on the face with one hand while lifting the jaw upwards and forwards (with airway still in place) and ensure a tight seal. Try to achieve tidal volumes of 800–1000 ml at a rate of

10–15/min. Common problems encountered are an obstructed airway or failure to obtain an adequate seal. If the former is the case, elevate the jaw further and extend the head (providing cervical spine injury is not suspected). If mask seal is a problem, reapply the mask more evenly or ask an assistant to squeeze the bag while you use both hands to hold the mask firmly in position.

7. Add oxygen to the bag at 8–10 l/min to increase the inspired oxygen concentration to 40–60%. Where possible, add a reservoir bag to the resuscitation device. This increases the inspired oxygen to 80–90%.

8. If chest movement cannot be achieved at all, consider the possibility of a foreign body obstructing the hypopharynx, larynx or trachea. Attempt the Heimlich manoeuvre if appropriate and/or use a laryngoscope and Magill forceps to remove the offending foreign body if it can be seen at laryngoscopy. If this fails or if severe maxillofacial trauma prevents effective ventilation by conventional methods, prepare for cricothyrotomy as an emergency procedure.

9. *Cricothyrotomy*. Make an incision horizontally in the cricothyroid membrane and insert a suitable hollow device through the membrane into the trachea, below the level of the vocal cords. Although a 5 mm internal diameter tube is adequate for resuscitation purposes, replace it with a 6–7 mm tube if prolonged ventilation is needed. If still required after 1–2 days, convert the cricothyrotomy to a formal tracheostomy. Do not attempt tracheostomy as a primary emergency procedure as it is difficult to perform under emergency conditions in inadequate surroundings on hypoxic patients.

SEMICONSCIOUS PATIENTS

1. Partial or broken dentures, food and foreign debris, blood (active bleeding or clots) and vomited or regurgitated stomach contents represent additional sources from which airway obstruction may occur or by which material may be inhaled into the lungs.

2. Regurgitation with pulmonary aspiration is not uncommon in semiconscious patients and usually develops insidiously. It more commonly occurs in the presence of a full stomach, ileus, pregnancy, hiatus hernia, maxillofacial trauma or muscle relaxants, and may be compounded by air blown into the stomach during mask ventilation. Use cricoid pressure (Sellick manoeuvre) during resuscitation and intubation to avoid or minimize this risk. An assistant presses firmly with three fingers straddling the cricoid ring to compress the oesophagus between the cricoid ring and the body of the sixth cervical vertebra.

3. Vomiting, unlike regurgitation, is an active process and usually occurs at lighter levels of unconsciousness. If you observe prodromal retching or vomiting, release cricoid pressure to avoid gastric rupture. Turn the patient quickly into the recovery position with head dependent if possible.

> **Key point**
>
> ● Always have functioning suction equipment available for unconscious patients.

4. The hazard of pulmonary aspiration is accentuated if the aspirate has a pH of less than 3, when the risk of a chemical pneumonitis from acid aspiration (Mendelson's syndrome) is considerable. Should pulmonary contamination be suspected, immediately intubate the patient (see below) to secure airway isolation and if possible set aside a suction trap specimen from the lungs or pharynx to measure the acidity of the aspirate with wide-range pH paper (not litmus). Immediately lavage the lungs several times with aliquots of 20–30 ml saline, using 100% oxygen, large tidal volumes and tracheal suction. The procedure may well avert a full-blown aspiration syndrome, which can develop within 2–4 hours and resemble acute adult respiratory distress syndrome (ARDS). Give broad-spectrum antibiotic therapy. Intravenous steroids and tracheal bicarbonate instillation are of doubtful benefit. Involve anaesthetists or intensivists in the further care of such patients as soon as possible.

TRACHEAL INTUBATION

Appraise
1. Achieve competence at tracheal intubation.

2. Patients tolerate tracheal intubation only at deep levels of unconsciousness, typically associated with general anaesthesia or 'coma'. Intubation ensures the patency of the upper airway, avoiding obstruction from haemorrhage or swelling, and prevents entry of blood, gastric contents, secretions and other foreign matter into the tracheobronchial tree. It is the most effective form of airway isolation when undertaking positive pressure ventilation.

3. When deciding whether an unconscious patient requires tracheal intubation in order to safeguard the airway, be guided by the state of the laryngeal reflexes and the degree of muscle tone. If these are such that intubation is unlikely to be tolerated without great difficulty or sedation, then abandon intubation and use an oral or nasal pharyngeal airway instead.

4. Acquire skill in tracheal intubation by practice under supervision during induction of anaesthesia for routine surgery or practise on an intubation training simulator.

Prepare
1. *Laryngoscope*. The Macintosh-pattern curved laryngoscope blade is the most popular and the easiest to learn to use. The standard adult size 3 Macintosh blade is suitable for most patients over 5 years of age, although a size 4 may be required for large males. Check that the laryngoscope bulb and blade are well secured.

2. *Endotracheal tube*. These slightly curved plastic tubes have a range of internal diameters (ID) – 2.5–10.0 mm in 0.5 mm increments. They are presented as disposable, prepacked items complete with one bevelled end (cuffed above 6.0 mm) and a 15 mm plastic connector lightly inserted into the other end. The tube is stamped with the internal diameter in millimetres near the bevel and the length is often marked in centimetres at the connector end, which requires cutting to length before use. Use 7.0–8.0 mm ID for adult females and 8.0–9.5 mm for adult males. Cuffed tubes are used for patients over 7–8 years, uncuffed below that age. A convenient guide to tube *diameter* can be based on:
a. the tip of the patient's little finger – this is a good measure of overall tube size as it closely matches the size of the cricoid ring
b. for children, ID (mm) = age in years/4 + 4.5.

Length for adults ranges from 22 cm (females) to 24 cm (males). For nasal intubation add 2–4 cm. A convenient guide to length is gauged by:

a. holding the tube alongside the patient's face, allowing for the curvature in the mouth and measuring the distance from lips to cricoid ring; add an allowance for the portion outside the mouth and a safe length in the trachea
b. for children, Length (cm) = age in years/2 + 12 cm.

3. *Connections* (Fig. 2.1).

Having cut the tube to the recommended length, fit the tapered tube connector tightly into the cut end. The 15 mm end connector is a standard fit for use with a catheter mount to adapt it to a resuscitation device, anaesthetic circuit or ventilator. It will also fit directly to a self-inflating bag-valve resuscitator if the catheter mount is not available.

4. Test the cuff of the tube with a few millilitres of air from a 10 ml syringe, deflate and apply water-miscible lubricant over the cuffed portion of the tube. Have ready a small clamp to seal the cuff (if a valve is not included in the pilot tube assembly) and a curved malleable metal stylet or a long gum-elastic bougie to assist in difficult intubation.

5. Test that suction equipment is in good working order. Yankauer semirigid handpieces are required in addition to a range of plastic suction catheters.

6. Correctly position the patient. Moderately flex the cervical spine

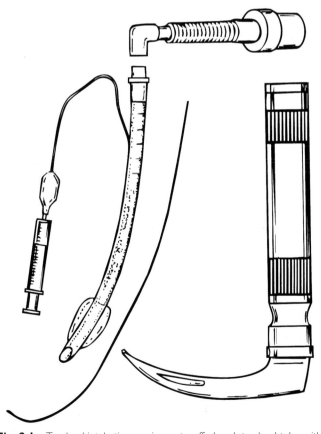

Fig. 2.1 Tracheal intubation equipment: cuffed endotracheal tube with inflation syringe, catheter mount, gum-elastic bougie and laryngoscope.

by raising the head on one pillow, and then extend the head at the atlanto-occipital joint – as when 'sniffing the morning air'.

7. Inspect the mouth. Remove any dentures and look for loose teeth, crowns or bridges, especially in the upper incisor area, so as to avoid damage or dislodgement during intubation.

Action

1. Hold the laryngoscope handle vertical in the left hand with the blade downward and the light shining towards the patient's feet. Open the mouth by gently extending the head with the right hand. Maximum opening can be obtained by placing your right index finger along the line of upper right premolars and molars and further extending the head. Avoid damage to the incisors. With the head extended, insert the blade into the right side of the mouth in an arc over the tongue, directing the blade tip towards the uvula. The laryngoscope blade holds the bulk of the tongue out of the way to the left and allows you a clear view down the right side of the mouth. Continue advancing the blade in a gentle curve along the back of the tongue until you see the epiglottis. Then pass the blade anterior to the epiglottis, between it and the base of the tongue, and lodge the tip firmly in the vallecula. The vocal cords may be visible now but it is usually necessary to lift the tongue and jaw together vertically to adequately visualize the glottis. Do not lever on the upper teeth or gums. This causes damage and does not improve the view.

2. If you cannot see the epiglottis, either the laryngoscope blade is not in the midline or it may have passed over the epiglottis into the laryngopharynx. Withdraw the blade to about two thirds along the tongue and readvance it.

3. When you see the glottis, hold the tracheal tube near its connector in the right hand, concavity forward, and pass it via the right side of the mouth, so that the tip comes into the midline immediately above the laryngeal opening. Insert the bevel between the vocal cords and slide the tube onwards through the larynx so that the cuff lies below the level of the vocal cords. Hold the tube firmly while gently withdrawing the laryngoscope.

4. To check that the tube is in the correct position, press firmly on the subject's chest. A puff of air emerging from the tube gives some reassurance that it has entered the trachea (rather than the oesophagus). Connect it to a ventilating device (self-inflating bag or anaesthetic circuit) and apply positive pressure to ventilate the patient's lungs. If you use a cuffed tube, slowly inflate the cuff with an air-filled 10 ml syringe until audible leakage ceases during inspiration. Check for reasonable tension in the pilot cuff. Clamp the distal end of the pilot tube with an artery forceps over its reinforced section near the syringe tip, avoiding the thin pilot tube itself. Recently, self-sealing Luer-lock valves have been introduced that avoid the need for clamping.

5. Uniform expansion of the chest indicates correct placement. Confirm correct placement by auscultation with a stethoscope while ventilating the lungs. Also auscultate the epigastrium to ensure that the tube was not inadvertently placed in the oesophagus. If one side of the chest expands more than the other then the tube may have passed too far into a main bronchus (usually the right). Deflate the cuff and withdraw the tube until chest expansion is uniform. Reinflate the cuff. Exclude less frequent causes of unilateral chest expansion such as pneumo- or haemothorax.

6. Secure the tube with strapping to the patient's face or by means of a loop of tape or bandage around the neck, having first knotted it securely around the tube. Avoid constricting the jugular or facial veins by tying too tightly.

Alternative

The laryngeal mask airway (Fig. 2.2) has a curved tube with a hollow, soft rubber spoon at one end bearing an inflatable rim. The device is inserted via the mouth into the laryngopharynx, concavity forward, and the cuff is inflated to 'seal' the rim against the laryngeal inlet, so maintaining patency and providing a degree of airway isolation. It is tolerated at lighter levels of consciousness than a standard tracheal tube and may allow positive pressure ventilation, though some leakage is likely. Its ability to reliably isolate the trachea against aspiration cannot be guaranteed, but with practice it is easy to use and is likely to prove a useful adjunct in situations where conventional intubation would be impracticable.

ARTIFICIAL VENTILATION

1. Institute intermittent positive pressure ventilation (IPPV) without delay whenever spontaneous breathing is inadequate to provide effective gas exchange. Room air contains 21% oxygen, and the immediate application of 35–60% oxygen via an oxygen mask is a useful emergency measure to compensate for the hypoxia associated with impaired ventilation while preparing for intubation and ventilation. If breathing is totally absent, immediately institute artificial ventilation.

2. In lay emergency situations start expired air resuscitation using mouth-to-mouth, mouth-to-nose or mouth-to-airway adjuncts, using the 16% oxygen available in expired air. Mouth-to-mouth ventilation may be hazardous in the presence of oral trauma, and resuscitation equipment for health-care professionals should include self-inflating resuscitation bags with oxygen reservoirs in addition to a range of airway adjuncts – Guedel oropharyngeal airways and soft rubber or plastic nasopharyngeal tubes.

3. Ensure airway patency and ventilate the patient with a bag-mask device. As soon as possible add oxygen from a pipeline or portable cylinder to the inlet valve of the resuscitation bag. At oxygen flows of 6–10 l/min the inspired oxygen level can be increased from 35% to 80% by the addition of an oxygen reservoir bag to the self-inflating resuscitator. When using portable oxygen cylinders ensure

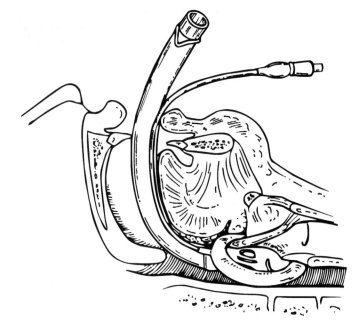

Fig. 2.2 Laryngeal mask airway.

you have adequate reserves for unexpected delays, especially during transport.

4. Isolate the trachea by passing a tracheal tube or similar device and continue bag-mask ventilation until the patient is connected to a functioning ventilator. Semiconscious patients may need sedation to tolerate airway isolation and IPPV (see below).

5. Aim for a minute volume of 8–10 litres in an adult by ventilating at a rate of 10–15 breaths per minute with tidal volumes of 600–800ml. Commence ventilation with 60% inspired oxygen. Inflate the lungs over 1–1.5 seconds and allow 2–2.5 seconds for expiration to occur passively. The expiratory pause is necessary as IPPV raises intrathoracic pressure and impairs venous return.

6. If a prolonged period of ventilation is anticipated, switch to an automatic ventilator as soon as possible. Compact oxygen-powered ventilators are useful for entrapment situations and during transport. More elaborate models are available in accident and emergency units, operating theatres and intensive therapy units. Ventilators should be used only by appropriately trained staff and must be regularly maintained. Obtain the assistance of anaesthetists or intensivists at this point to allow you to attend to surgical priorities.

7. Once ventilation is established, regularly monitor the adequacy of oxygenation using pulse oximetry or arterial blood oxygen levels. Adjust oxygen flow to maintain pulse oximeter saturation readings in excess of 90%, corresponding to arterial oxygen tensions of 11.5–14 kPa (equivalent to 87–105 mmHg). Monitor the effectiveness of ventilation using end-tidal carbon dioxide (CO_2) monitoring or blood CO_2 levels. Acceptable end-tidal CO_2 readings and carbon dioxide tensions range from 4.0–5.5% or kPa (equivalent to 30–42 mmHg).

8. Attempts at spontaneous breathing by the patient may indicate inadequate artificial ventilation due to a leak or incorrect ventilator settings or the presence of excessive secretions. Where ventilation is shown to be adequate a degree of spontaneous breathing is not necessarily harmful providing it does not interfere with ventilator performance. Indeed, modern ventilators are designed to encourage spontaneous breathing during weaning. Generally, however, spontaneous breathing interferes with the performance of simpler ventilators and can be suppressed with small doses of sedative drugs or narcotics. Muscle relaxants may be added judiciously after ensuring that the patient is really unconscious and that adequate monitoring is in progress to warn of disconnection or ventilator malfunction. Carefully time the use of these drugs to avoid conflicting with clinical assessment of conscious level or other neurological tests, and in any event review them once or twice daily during management in ITU.

9. *Secretions*. Tracheobronchial toilet is necessary during artificial ventilation. Sterility is important. Select sterile disposable catheters with a rounded tip and having several side holes in preference to those with a single end aperture. The latter are traumatic, stick to the tracheal wall and are difficult to advance. Choose a suction catheter which is less than half the tracheal tube diameter (12–14F in adults) and use it only once. Insert the catheter using sterile gloves or forceps and apply suction intermittently during its withdrawal, avoiding prolonged suction as this causes hypoxia. Repeat tracheobronchial toilet as often as is indicated by the quantity of secretions aspirated. Remove a sputum-trap specimen for culture initially, and repeat it as necessary. A saline nebulizer or repeated saline instillation of 5–10 ml may be useful when secretions are tenacious.

OXYGEN THERAPY

Appraise

Oxygen is vital for metabolism. In the presence of ineffective ventilation, impaired pulmonary gas transfer or low output states, high inspired concentrations may be required to restore a deficient cellular oxygen supply to normal. Specific indications relevant to surgery include:

1. all acute hypoxaemic states, where inadequate ventilation from central or peripheral causes has occurred, especially intracranial damage, spinal, chest or abdominal injury and abdominal distension, limiting diaphragmatic descent
2. in the immediate postoperative period, especially after thoracic or upper abdominal surgery, where there is pre-existing pulmonary disease or in older subjects
3. In shock of all types, where cardiorespiratory depression leads to impaired pulmonary gas exchange, reduced cardiac output and impaired tissue perfusion; in anaemia, reduced oxygen-carrying capacity of the blood may be partially compensated by oxygen therapy
4. hypermetabolic states, such as hyperthermia, shivering and thyroid crisis, necessitate an increased tissue oxygen requirement
5. decompression sickness, carbon monoxide poisoning or to hasten nitrogen elimination from distended bowel, pneumothorax and pneumoperitoneum

6. hyperbaric oxygen therapy has been used to treat gas gangrene and to improve the viability of skin flaps.

Action

1. For routine oxygen therapy use a disposable transparent plastic face mask of the Hudson design. These are semirigid and perforated. In the event of oxygen failure, the patient is able to breathe air through the holes in the mask. With oxygen flows of 6–10 l/min the final oxygen concentration provided is approximately 30–45% but is not predictable. To provide more precise or long-term oxygen therapy 'fixed performance' masks such as the Vickers Ventimask® are recommended. These use the Venturi principle to provide a high air flow of constant-composition oxygen-enriched air (HAFOE) at flows in excess of the patient's peak inspiratory flow, typically 30 l/min. Patients often complain that the masks are noisy and cause drying; they may not tolerate them as well as other masks. To ensure that the mask delivers flows in excess of the patient's peak flow, the driving oxygen flow must be increased with each higher concentration mask, requiring 2, 4, 6, 10 and 15 l/min oxygen for 24%, 28%, 35%, 40% and 60% masks respectively.

2. Humidification is essential for oxygen therapy lasting more than 3–4 hours, especially where nasal humidification is bypassed during mouth breathing or by intubation. Attempts to humidify the relatively low oxygen flows delivered from the flow meter through small-bore tubes to the mask will prove ineffective. Either air should be humidified before delivery to the mask where oxygen enrichment will occur, or the air and oxygen can be premixed in a humidifier a short distance from the patient and ducted to a Hudson-type mask. In either event large-bore (22 mm) plastic tubes should be used to prevent condensation of the humidified gases. Seek further details of suitable equipment in the books quoted at the end of this chapter or by enquiry of ITU technicians in your hospitals.

3. Nasal oxygen by catheter is still a practicable method for providing oxygen supplementation. Although less predictable than oxygen masks it is well accepted by conscious patients and suitable for long-term use. In the absence of specially designed 'looped' cannulas, an ordinary 10 or 12F disposable suction catheter can be inserted a short distance into the nose. Humidification is not practicable in these devices and the nasal cavity tends to become dry if oxygen flows in excess of 2–3 l/min are attempted.

4. Patients with acute-on-chronic respiratory failure present a special problem. These patients commonly depend upon a certain degree of hypoxic drive for ventilation, and the institution of high oxygen concentrations may lead to progressive underventilation and eventual respiratory arrest. This is unlikely to occur rapidly and the importance of providing adequate oxygenation clearly takes precedence, especially when ventilatory insufficiency is acute and reversible. Start with 28–35% 'fixed performance' HAFOE devices and maintain careful clinical observation of the patient while measuring blood oxygen and carbon dioxide tensions. Change the mask concentration according to need. Aim for arterial oxygen tensions in excess of 11 kPa (83 mmHg) and carbon dioxide tensions below 7 kPa (53 mmHg). Rising carbon dioxide levels indicate impending narcosis and may indicate the need to institute IPPV if oxygenation is still not satisfactory.

5. Conventional oxygen therapy masks for spontaneous ventilation

will not suffice when oxygen concentrations in excess of 60% are required. Such demands are best met using an anaesthetic patient breathing system or high-flow T-piece, with a close-fitting anaesthetic mask or isolated airway and an oxygen flow in excess of 10–15 l/min. The physiological dead space associated with such a severe gas exchange problem is likely to require IPPV anyway.

Dangers

1. Fires and explosions. This risk doubles for each 5% increase in oxygen, although the oxygen concentration does fall rapidly with increasing distance from the mask or circuit valve.

2. Risk of producing respiratory depression in patients with chronic respiratory disease.

3. If a bronchus becomes blocked by secretions or blood, atelectasis may rapidly develop. This is because of the rapid absorption of oxygen in the isolated segment.

Key point

- Adequate humidification, regular tracheobronchial toilet and physiotherapy are vitally important.

---

4. *Oxygen toxicity.* This is never a problem during acute resuscitation and only occurs slowly following exposure to high oxygen concentrations for several days. The clinical picture resembles bronchopneumonia with cough, retrosternal pain, bronchiolar and alveolar exudates. Bronchopulmonary dysplasia may develop, though the condition can resolve if the patient survives the hypoxic episode. In hyperbaric oxygen therapy the condition may evolve within a few hours and convulsions may occur if oxygen levels greater than two atmospheres are used. Neonatal resuscitation with high oxygen concentrations presents a special risk of retrolental fibroplasia, which can develop rapidly. In such unusual situations limit therapy to 40% oxygen unless continuous oximetry or blood oxygen monitoring dictates otherwise.

LOCAL ANAESTHESIA

Appraise

1. Operative procedures under local anaesthesia are regularly undertaken in hospitals, clinics and surgeries. Local anaesthetic techniques are particularly well suited for minor operations such as removal of small non-infected superficial lesions and minor surgery of the hands. It may be useful when general anaesthesia is not readily available or is impracticable (e.g. recent ingestion of food). Local anaesthesia is inexpensive as it does not require the specialized staff and facilities that general anaesthesia demands, is relatively safe, causes less systemic upset than general anaesthesia and enables patients to be discharged soon after surgery.

2. More extensive procedures involving large field blocks may not be as safe as general anaesthesia because of the toxic effect associated with the large volume of local anaesthetic required. Moreover, local anaesthesia does not necessarily block the physiological disturbances such as bradycardia and vomiting which arise from autonomic reflexes during some surgical procedures.

3. Local anaesthetic drugs can be administered in various ways according to the required area of analgesia. These include:

a. *topical anaesthesia*: application of local anaesthetics to the mucous membranes of the conjunctival sac, mouth, nose, tracheobronchial tree and urethra

b. *local infiltration*: direct injection of the anaesthetic into the operative site

c. *field block*: injection of local anaesthetic around the operative site so as to create an analgesic zone

d. *individual peripheral nerve blocks*: e.g. ulnar, pudendal, femoral, common peroneal, etc. The extent of the block varies according to the cutaneous distribution the nerve supplies.

e. *regional block*: injection of local anaesthetic around the individual nerves or nerve trunks supplying the region to be operated upon. Where nerves are grouped together as plexuses then several nerves can be blocked at the same time. The brachial plexus is the best known, but the lumbosacral plexus block is occasionally used. The large volumes required for these blocks approach toxic levels

f. *spinal anaesthesia*: insertion of local anaesthetic drugs directly into the subarachnoid space in small volumes (1.5–3 ml) produces effective sensory and motor block as the nerve roots in this space have negligible covering; low-pressure headache due to cerebrospinal fluid leak is not uncommon following this technique

g. *extradural block*: injection of local anaesthetic into the epidural or caudal space; these blocks require four to 10 times the volumes used in subarachnoid block because of local diffusion and the presence of dural and myelin covering of the nerve roots

h. *regional intravenous anaesthesia*: injection of a large volume of dilute local anaesthetic into the veins of a previously exsanguinated limb.

Agents

1. Various local anaesthetic drugs are available, of which amino amide derivatives are the most commonly used. Most drugs are marketed in the form of their water-soluble salts, usually the hydrochloride. Before they can act in the body they must dissociate to liberate the free base. Dissociation is inhibited in an acid medium, which explains why analgesia may be unpredictable when local anaesthetics are injected into inflamed tissues.

2. The duration of action of some local anaesthetics having a low tissue affinity is increased if they are combined with a vasoconstrictor such as adrenaline. This will also reduce the systemic absorption and toxicity of these agents. For infiltration, concentrations of 1 in 250 000 of adrenaline may be used, by the addition of 1 mg (1 ml of adrenaline tartrate 1/1000) to 250 ml of local anaesthetic solution. There is no advantage in using higher concentrations than this. The total amount of adrenaline injected should not exceed 0.5 mg. Adrenaline may cause tachycardia and hypertension and should be used with caution in patients with cardiovascular disease and those taking cardiac medication (e.g. beta-blockers). Less toxic vasoconstrictors, e.g. felypressin, are available. Injection of vasoconstrictors is *absolutely contraindicated* in areas supplied by end arteries – such as the fingers, toes and penis – as prolonged ischaemia here may lead to tissue necrosis.

a. *Lignocaine*. This is the most widely used local anaesthetic. It is stable, only moderately toxic, produces no vasodilation and has an onset of action within a few minutes and a duration of 60–90 minutes. It is used in concentrations of 4% for topical anaesthesia and concentrations of 0.5–2% for infiltration and nerve blocks. The maximum safe dose is 3 mg/kg body weight when used without adrenaline and 7 mg/kg with adrenaline.

b. *Prilocaine*. Chemically related to lignocaine, prilocaine is less toxic but also less potent. Duration of action is less affected by adrenaline than lignocaine. Prilocaine is used as a 4% solution for topical anaesthesia and in concentrations of 1–3% for nerve blocks. The maximum safe dose is 10 mg/kg. Excessive doses of prilocaine produce methaemoglobinaemia, which may manifest as apparent cyanosis. Hypoxaemia results if more than 15 mg/kg of the agent is administered. Treatment involves the administration of 1% methylene blue, 1–2 mg/kg.

c. *Bupivacaine*. This agent is two to three times as toxic as lignocaine but about four times more potent. It is used in concentrations of 0.25–0.5% and has a maximum safe dose of 2 mg/kg. It is extensively bound in the tissues and hence has the advantage of a long duration of action (3–12 hours). It has a delayed onset compared to lignocaine, although this may be overcome by mixing bupivacaine and lignocaine together (see Methods below).

Toxicity

1. All local anaesthetics exert toxic effects when given in large doses and inadvertent intravascular injection, even in small doses, can cause central nervous and cardiovascular disturbances resulting in restlessness, convulsions, hypotension, bradycardia and, in extreme cases, respiratory and cardiac arrest.

2. Management of these toxic effects includes the use of intra-venous sedatives with anticonvulsant properties (benzodiazepines or thiopentone), oxygen, intravenous fluids and pressor agents (ephedrine or metaraminol). In extreme circumstances tracheal intubation and artificial ventilation may be necessary. The importance of securing intravenous access before local anaesthesia is commenced is obvious.

3. The conduct of thoracic or lumbar spinal and epidural anaesthesia involves blockade of the T1–L1 sympathetic outflow tracts. This results in vasodilation below the block with compensatory vasoconstriction above this level. If the block reaches above T10, hypotension is likely. Compensatory tachycardia may not occur, especially if a high block affects the T1–T4 outflow or the patient is on beta-blockers or has a pacemaker. For this reason good venous access is important; a preload infusion of 300–500 ml crystalloid is recommended before such blocks are commenced. Administer a small subcutaneous or intravenous dose of a vaso- and venoconstrictor such as ephedrine, methoxamine or metaraminol before or during the procedure to protect against hypotension.

4. The risk is particularly high when pre-existing hypovolaemia is present, during supine hypotension syndrome of pregnancy or when unexpected subarachnoid (spinal) anaesthesia occurs. This latter hazard may arise when an epidural technique is complicated by dural puncture or where an existing epidural catheter perforates the sub-arachnoid space. Partial or extensive spinal anaesthesia may also occur from misplaced spinal injection during the conduct of pre- or paravertebral blocks. Profound hypotension, unconsciousness and respiratory paralysis can occur. Emergency management involves oxygenation, intubation, ventilation, intravenous infusion and pharmacological support of the cardiovascular system.

Prepare

1. Check that resuscitation equipment is present and in working order and that competent assistance is available if needed urgently. The minimum equipment required is a self-inflating bag with mask and airways, an oxygen cylinder capable of delivering 8–10 l/min via oxygen mask and resuscitation bag, sedatives to deal with convulsions, intravenous fluids and vasopressors for sudden circulatory failure.

2. Ensure that a quiet environment will be maintained for the duration of surgery. Quiet music may be beneficial but keep casual conversation to a minimum.

3. Take a careful history with particular reference to current therapy, allergies, cardiorespiratory and neurological disease. Examination should include the pulse rate, rhythm and blood pressure. If myocardial disease is suspected have an assistant monitor pulse, blood pressure and electrocardiograph throughout the procedure.

4. Explain to the patient what surgery you are proposing to perform under local anaesthesia, check that the correct site (and side) is being operated on and obtain written consent.

5. Explain the sequence of the events that are going to take place, including the initial preparation of the area, the injection of local anaesthetic and the subsequent surgery. Reassure the patient that the pain from any injection will be temporary and that during surgery there should be no pain, although the sense of touch may remain.

6. Study the landmarks of the area carefully before proceeding.

Place a catheter in a vein well away from the operative site in case resuscitation is required.

7. Choose local anaesthetic drugs with attention to the likely volume required. 0.5% or 1% lignocaine or prilocaine without adrenaline is suitable for most infiltrations or nerve blocks respectively. Calculate the maximum safe dose based on the patient's measured weight. In a 70 kg adult the maximum dose of plain lignocaine is 210 mg (3 mg/kg). As 1% lignocaine contains 10 mg per ml, the maximum safe volume is 21 ml. If larger volumes are required, either reduce these concentrations, add adrenaline or perform part of the block 15–20 minutes later.

Action

1. Exercise full sterile precautions. Wash hands and arms thoroughly before donning gown and gloves. Prepare the skin with 2% iodine in spirit or 0.5% chlorhexidine in 70% alcohol and cover with suitable drapes. Maintain a sterile environment throughout the procedure.

2. Use fine 25SWG needles for initial intradermal injection of local anaesthesia and 22–23SWG needles for infiltration.

3. When performing local infiltration, inject as the needle is being moved. When injecting round specific nerves this is less practicable. Check by aspiration before injecting to minimize the likelihood of intravascular injection.

4. Be on constant lookout for untoward reactions. Drowsiness and slurring of speech are early signs of central nervous system toxicity. If you see these prodromal signs stop injecting local anaesthetic and be prepared to initiate urgent treatment.

5. Wait 10–15 minutes after injection for the local anaesthetic to take full effect. Be careful when testing whether a block is working that the patient does not confuse the sensation of pain with that of touch.

6. Warn the patient that there may be some discomfort when the effects of the block begin to wear off.

Methods

According to the clinical practice and your confidence, the following procedures may be used. Unless otherwise indicated, use the concentrations of local anaesthetics shown in Table 2.1.

Lignocaine and bupivacaine can be mixed to combine the rapid onset of the former with the longer action of the latter. For infiltration anaesthesia equal volumes of 1% lignocaine (with or without adrenaline) and 0.5% bupivacaine may be used, providing the combined dose of drugs does not exceed their cumulative toxic level. Amongst anaesthetists 2% lignocaine and 0.75% bupivacaine have some popularity for use in epidurals to ensure profound sensory and motor block, but such concentrations should not be used routinely.

Table 2.1 Use of local anaesthetics

Method	Anaesthetic
Infiltration	0.5% lignocaine, 0.25% bupivacaine
Nerve blocks	1% lignocaine, 1% prilocaine or 0.5% bupivacaine
Epidural	1.5% lignocaine, 0.5% bupivacaine
Spinal	0.5% heavy bupivacaine

Infiltration anaesthesia

1. Infiltration anaesthesia provides good operating conditions for the removal of small superficial lesions, such as sebaceous cysts and lipomata. Do not use infiltration anaesthesia in infected sites because of the risk of spreading infection and because adequate sensory block is unlikely to be achieved.

2. Follow the general advice on equipment and actions as detailed above. 0.5% lignocaine is generally recommended, avoiding adrenaline where blood supply may be tenuous. Raise a small skin bleb close to the lesion then infiltrate through this bleb, attempting to place the local anaesthetic so that it spreads along tissue planes and the lesion 'floats' in an anaesthetized area.

3. Allow an adequate time for the anaesthetic to take effect before commencing surgery.

Digital nerve blocks

1. Digital nerves to the fingers and toes pass along the anterolateral line of the phalanx. A digital tourniquet may be used but never use adrenaline.

2. Raise a skin bleb over the dorsum of the proximal phalanx using 1 ml of 1% plain lignocaine. Pass a 23SWG needle through this to deposit about 1–2 ml of the agent on either side of the phalanx. Inject the agent close to the web space to avoid undue distension of the tissues. Unlike infiltration analgesia, nerve blocks may require up to 20 minutes to have an effect.

POSTOPERATIVE ANALGESIA

Many doctors consider postoperative pain to be an inevitable consequence of surgery and fail to control it adequately. The review on pain after surgery by the Royal College of Surgeons of England[1] makes compelling reading. In some countries in-hospital 'acute pain teams' are responsible for the management of postoperative pain but these are not a general feature of UK practice at the present time. The financial implications of instituting such a system are considerable, but improvements in pain control can be made within the financial constraints of health service practice. You have an important commitment to minimize postoperative pain and provide leadership to the surgical team (junior staff, anaesthetists, nurses, physiotherapists, etc.) in the way pain control is monitored and managed.

Appraise

1. Failure to relieve pain adequately may have significant repercussions. Pain (real or feared) impairs mobility, and circulation to skin and muscles is reduced. As a consequence healing is slow and pressure sores may develop with frightening rapidity. The risk of thromboembolic disease is significantly increased in immobile patients. Pain is frequently associated with hypertension and tachycardia, which may exacerbate myocardial ischaemia in susceptible individuals. After abdominal and thoracic surgery, pain will limit respiratory function with attendant risk of hypoxia and chest infection. The return of normal gut motility and absorption may be delayed, resulting in dehydration and the need for extended intravenous therapy. Even after straightforward musculoskeletal operations pain profoundly limits activity and full function may be delayed for weeks. In financial terms

alone, unrelieved pain delays healing, prolongs hospital stay and retards the patient's return to taxpayer status.

2. Sex, age and cultural differences may alter pain tolerance but these are irrelevant when considering individual patients. Pain should be controlled according to need and not compared to some arbitrary level of tolerance. Questionnaires and analogue pain scores have limited application for individuals. Pain can best be assessed by a few sympathetic questions and by simple clinical observation, repeated as necessary. Sometimes the severity of the pain can be better appreciated after effective pain control has been established. The improvement in the patient's demeanour will be obvious.

3. Psychological effects of pain should not be ignored. It is easier to control postoperative pain by ensuring that adequate relief is commenced at the end of surgery than to attempt control once the pattern of severe pain is firmly established. The experience of pain may markedly alter a patient's attitude to future surgery. Severe or persistent pain is associated with lack of interest in food or surroundings, depression and withdrawal. This is particularly relevant in children, where expression of pain may be difficult to interpret.

Assess

Formulate a plan for managing postoperative pain in order to provide the most effective control possible.

1. Carefully evaluate the pain with regard to its site, type, severity, and duration. Judge the effect it is having on the patient and the patient's tolerance to the pain. This will enable you to make a decision in respect of the agents to be used, the technique of administration and probable duration of management. The site and characteristics of the pain (continuous or intermittent, constant or varying intensity, sharp, dull or colicky, localizable or diffuse), will provide a clue to the nerve pathways involved. This is particularly relevant when planning regional analgesic techniques.

2. Select an appropriate analgesic. The range of analgesic drugs marketed by the pharmaceutical industry is bewildering. Familiarize yourself with a few agents suitable for the postoperative pain you encounter in your practice. The available drugs include opioids, non-steroidal anti-inflammatory drugs (NSAIDs), local anaesthetic agents or combinations of these.

a. *Opioids*. This term for morphine-like drugs covers both naturally occurring opiate alkaloids and synthetic derivatives. Popular drugs in this group include morphine, diamorphine, pethidine, papaveretum, fentanyl, alfentanil, codeine, dihydrocodeine, methadone, buprenorphine, dextropropoxyphene and tramadol. They appear to exert their effect at specific opioid receptors in the central nervous system and mimic the effect of the naturally occurring enkephalins and endorphins. They are effective against severe pain, especially of visceral origin. Principal side-effects include respiratory depression, drowsiness, nausea and vomiting and dysphoria. Respiratory depression should always be specifically excluded, particularly when opioids are administered by the epidural route. Hypotension, bradycardia, constipation and itching may also occur. Do not let the fear of causing addiction lead to inadequate prescribing of these potent analgesics. The risk of addiction to properly administered opioids is quite low – if pain remains unrelieved, rule out other causes for pain and increase the dose or

frequency of the drug appropriately. Enlist the help of the acute pain management team if practicable.

When comparing opioids, the equipotent doses listed in Table 2.2 may be useful. They are based on typical intramuscular doses used for an adult (70 kg) male.

b. *Non-steroidal anti-inflammatory drugs (NSAIDs)*. Unlike opioids these drugs have a peripheral mode of action and appear to exert their primary effect by inhibition of prostaglandin synthesis, which may explain their anti-inflammatory and antipyretic activity. They are generally administered orally, though some of them can also be administered rectally or by injection. Used alone they are effective against mild postoperative pain, musculoskeletal disorders and inflammatory joint conditions. This diverse group includes aspirin, paracetamol, diclofenac, nefopam, ketorolac, ibuprofen, indomethacin, phenylbutazone, etc. Principal side-effects are haemorrhage from gastric erosions when administered orally and potential kidney damage in patients with incipient or established renal dysfunction. Electrolytes should be carefully monitored and dehydration must be actively treated. Aspirin causes a reduction in platelet adhesiveness, which may interfere with haemostasis. Avoid it in children under 12 years of age because of its association with Reye's syndrome.

Severe postoperative pain may benefit from the synergistic effects of parenterally administered opioids and oral or rectal NSAIDs. Combined oral preparations such as co-proxamol and co-dydramol may suffice subsequently.

c. *Local anaesthetic drugs*. The use of local anaesthetic agents for individual nerve and plexus blocks has already been discussed. Field or regional blocks performed in theatre may continue to provide good analgesia postoperatively for several hours, and may be repeated if required. The insertion of thin catheters during epidural or intrapleural blockade avoids the need to perform repeated blocks and allows intermittent injection or continuous infusions to be continued for several days if necessary. This is particularly useful for patients in whom large dosage of systemic opioids is undesirable. Side-effects of local analgesia include those related to systemic absorption of the drug, numbness and weakness related to blocked nerves, and hypotension from autonomic blockade associated with epidural or spinal analgesia. Opioids combined with local anaesthetic drugs for epidural administration provide smooth control of pain with fewer side-effects than when using either agent alone.

3. Choose the route and frequency of administration. Depending on the drug used it may be best administered by oral, sublingual, transdermal or rectal routes or by subcutaneous, intramuscular, intravenous or epidural injection.

Table 2.2 Equipotent doses of opioids

Drug	Dose
Morphine	15 mg
Diamorphine	7.5–10 mg
Papaveretum	20 mg
Pethidine	100 mg
Codeine phosphate	60 mg
Phenoperidine	2 mg

a. *Oral administration* is simple but may be impracticable if the patient is unable to co-operate, or following gastrointestinal surgery when stasis may persist for some days. First-pass metabolism by the liver may significantly alter the bioavailability of some enteral drugs, with unpredictable results. Some opioids (e.g. buprenorphine) are effective by sublingual absorption, which avoids the problems of first-pass metabolism, though delayed onset significantly limits its usefulness. The rectal route is useful for mild analgesics, e.g. paracetamol and diclofenac, though some patients find rectal administration distressful. For severe pain injectable forms of analgesia (especially opioids) have the advantage of more rapid onset and greater predictability. Oral opioid preparations (including slow-release preparations) may be substituted later and are particularly useful for chronic pain.

b. *Intermittent intramuscular injection* of opioids 'on demand' has remained standard practice for decades. It is simple and inexpensive, though time-consuming for nurses because of the checking procedures and drug documentation required for controlled drugs. After injection there is an inevitable delay in onset pending absorption. Nurses may be too busy to administer injections when the patients require medication, causing further delay in re-establishing effective pain control. Typically given at 4–6-hourly intervals, intramuscular injection results in peaks and troughs of analgesia. Pain may return before the repeat interval has expired and it is important for medical staff to understand that these intervals are not absolute – smaller doses at shorter intervals may be more effective.

c. *Intravenous opioids* have the advantage of predictable uptake and rapid onset, although there is a narrow margin between effective analgesia and potential complications such as respiratory depression. Small bolus doses amounting to 20–30% of the recommended intramuscular doses cited above can be flushed carefully into a vein through a patent cannula. Once the response and duration is known, further supplementary doses can be given as required or a regular infusion commenced using a syringe driver. A typical regime for a 70 kg male would consist of 60 mg morphine in 60 ml saline (1 mg/ml) or 200 mg pethidine in 50 ml saline (4 mg/ml) infused at 3–6 ml/h. Aim for a background level of analgesia that is acceptable to the patient when resting quietly without causing excessive drowsiness or respiratory depression. The rate can be increased when needed for painful procedures such as dressing wounds or physiotherapy.

d. The development of *syringe drivers* and *intravenous pumps* has greatly facilitated pain control methods but staff using them require careful training and strict guidelines for their safe use. The responsibility for filling and administering intravenous infusions varies between hospitals. Your responsibility includes prescribing a safe dose of opioids and ensuring that patent venous access is ensured for their safe delivery. In particular, do not 'piggyback' the catheter upstream of several other infusions. As well as the risk of incompatible drug mixtures, the drug may accumulate in the drip tubing and be inadvertently flushed in later as a large bolus. Subcutaneous infusions have gained some popularity, although the rate of absorption may be unpredictable and the site of the needle or cannula may require frequent resiting.

e. The advent of microprocessor *patient-controlled analgesia devices (PCAs)* has allowed patients to have some control over their own analgesia, although not all patients are capable of using the device, especially soon after surgery. A syringe and connecting catheter are prepared for intravenous or subcutaneous infusion with a known concentration of opioid. The patient can push a button to provide a bolus infusion, which cannot be repeated until the programmed 'lock-out' time has expired. A typical regime would be morphine 1 mg/ml using bolus doses of 1 mg with a lockout of 5 min. Some PCAs can also be programmed to administer a constant background infusion – the cumulative effect of such administrations may be profound. For all automated devices the importance of frequent, regular inspection of patient and machine by nursing staff cannot be exaggerated.

f. *Epidural infusions*. As with intravenous anaesthesia the advent of syringe drivers has facilitated the management of continuous epidural analgesia. The use of a mixture of opioid and local anaesthetic helps avoid the numbness commonly seen when using higher concentrations of local anaesthetics alone while also reducing the risk of respiratory depression noted when using opioids alone. A useful combination is a mixture of 30 ml bupivacaine 0.25%, 30 ml saline and 5 mg powdered diamorphine in a 60 ml syringe, infused into the epidural catheter at 2–6 ml/h.

REFERENCE

1. Commission on the Provision of Surgical Services 1990 Report of the working party on pain after surgery. Royal College of Surgeons of England/College of Anaesthetists, London

FURTHER READING

Aitkenhead AR, Smith G 1995 Textbook of anaesthesia, 3rd edn. Churchill Livingstone, Edinburgh

American College of Surgeons Committee on Trauma 1997 Advanced trauma life support for doctors. American College of Surgeons, Chicago, IL

Eriksson E 1979 Illustrated handbook in local anaesthesia, 2nd edn. Lloyd Luke, London

Evans TR (ed) 1999 ABC of resuscitation, 4th edn. British Medical Journal, London

Hahn MB, McQuillan PM, Sheplock GJ 1996 Regional anesthesia. An atlas of anatomy and techniques of anesthesia. C. V. Mosby, St Louis, MO

The severely injured patient

F. W. Cross and J. Ryan

Contents

INTRODUCTION

This chapter concerns the appraisal of the seriously injured patient and includes definitive management following initial management and resuscitation. However you should be aware that the approach to the injured patient is different from that adopted with other surgical illness, in that potentially life-threatening injuries involving the airway, breathing and circulation are identified and corrected as they are diagnosed. Thus the usual algorithm of taking a detailed history followed by making a detailed clinical examination is largely abandoned. For example, damage control laparotomy is now well described as a resuscitative procedure where the patient fails to respond to transfusion, and is occasionally required almost as an initial procedure, leaving other injuries to be dealt with later.

SURGICAL MANAGEMENT

You should, if necessary, be able to carry out life-saving operations on most parts of the body. One test of judgement is knowing how to modify a standard operation to meet the prevailing requirements. This includes knowing how and when to cut corners safely. The ability to explore a wound successfully is a good test of basic surgical understanding and tissue craft. It is the last stage in diagnosis and at the same time it is the first stage in the treatment of a wound.

In this chapter, it is assumed that the patient has been fully assessed and resuscitated and a decision made to operate. The surgical management of the multiply injured should involve multiple surgical specialists working together. In reality the early management of chest and abdominal wounds, together with complex superficial lacerations, falls to the general surgeon; indeed the management of trauma is truly general surgery. In many countries specialist trauma surgeons trained in general surgery, neurosurgery and orthopaedics have the definitive management of these patients from admission to discharge. This chapter deals with basic procedures in the head and neck, chest, abdomen and pelvis, whether sustained in civilian or military situations. Emergency faciomaxillary, neurosurgical and orthopaedic procedures are dealt with elsewhere in this book.

SOFT TISSUE WOUNDS – GENERAL PRINCIPLES

Exploration of wounds can be a hazardous procedure, especially in the neck. There are situations where, if exploration is indicated, it is better to make a generous incision and achieve control of the major vascular structures as part of the exploration rather than to provoke haemorrhage by disturbing the wound with fingers or instruments.

Appraise

1. This section describes the principles of wound exploration in general terms, which can be applied to most superficial areas of the body, including scalp, face, extremities and superficial wounds of the trunk and perineal area. Specific instructions for particular problems are given later in the chapter or elsewhere in the book where appropriate.

2. Management of the soft tissue wound is a formal procedure consisting of clearly defined stages. This is the part of early management most frequently neglected by surgeons with limited or no experience of trauma and war-wound surgery. With missile injuries the entry and exit wounds give little indication of the damage that may have occurred to deeper structures. The extent of injury can only be detected by full wound exploration. In limb wounds exploration is followed by thorough wound excision after which, with very few exceptions, the wound is left open. Delayed primary closure follows 4–7 days after injury.

Prepare

1. Prepare the wounded area and a large enough surrounding area to allow for unplanned extension of skin incisions. If possible photograph the injured area or make a sketch – this is particularly useful for the receiving doctor if the patient has to be transferred.

2. Clean the skin thoroughly with the antiseptic solution of your choice but be careful to retain pressure dressings over bleeding wounds until the last minute. Wounds are usually contaminated and the presence of such dressings rarely contributes to further overall contamination of the operative area.

3. In the case of penetrating missile injury, preliminary biplanar X-rays are invaluable; they will reveal retained missile fragments and provide clues to the missile track.

Access

1. Identify, by inspection, the extent of visible damage. Knowledge of the force and mechanism of injury and the position of the patient at the time will provide added clues to the extent of the damage.

2. Enlarging the wound is usually necessary for adequate diagnosis and adequate assistance, retraction and lighting are essential. Further enlargement may be necessary later during definitive repair. Do not hesitate to enlarge a wound if you do not have adequate access to damaged structures.

3. Digital exploration may indicate the direction a wound takes but not its depth or eventual extent. The most direct way of doing this may be to incise tissue immediately overlying the track. The site and extent of the resulting wound needs to be considered to a certain extent, particularly if it will need to be extended as part of the definitive procedure or if it crosses major skin creases, but cosmesis is not of primary concern during life-saving surgery.

4. Incise in the long axis of a limb wherever possible, and counter-incisions may be required.

Key point

- It is important to examine preoperatively for nerve injury if this is possible, and to record in the operation notes the nature and extent of the nerve injury as found at surgery. The majority of nerve injuries are neuropraxias and recover spontaneously.

Assess

1. Look carefully into the existing wound and identify its extent, if possible without dissection. An anatomical knowledge of the tissue planes involved is essential.

2. Blood marks the site of injury of tissues and should be followed with retraction and observation. Dissection destroys the natural relationships of the tissues so delay it until absolutely necessary.

3. Explore a wound in layers. Follow any puncture wound through the layers, opening each in turn until no further penetration can be found. Remember that the tissues may no longer be in the same relationship that they were at the time of the injury, and a penetrating wound may seem to take quite a different course from that expected. The tissue layers may thus form a series of baffles. It is for this reason that probing a wound to see if it enters the peritoneal cavity is usually a waste of time.

4. Identify and examine neurovascular bundles in the wound track but nerves need not be dissected out. Nerves considered to be injured and requiring later exploration may have their position marked with a non-absorbable suture.

Action

1. Arrest haemorrhage. This may require temporary manual compression with swabs, proximal and distal control of major vessels with slings, and the application of arterial clamps. The indiscriminate application of artery forceps is dangerous, but small bleeding vessels can be clipped and ligated under direct vision as they are found.

2. Attempts to explore or repair wounds in the presence of bleeding are both futile and dangerous.

3. Once you have done this, start by cleaning the wound. Irrigate with copious quantities of saline followed by aqueous antiseptic. This will remove most superficial foreign material and improve visualization. Deeper contaminants will be removed as exploration progresses.

4. Removal of specific foreign bodies requires good lighting, intelligent retraction and a bloodless field, so arrange all these things before starting. Make sure the anaesthetist is prepared for a prolonged procedure.

5. Radio-opaque objects localized with preoperative films may still be difficult to find and intraoperative screening if available is often helpful. Most glass is radio-opaque.

6. Identifying the layer of tissue in which the object lies is essential; failure to do this often results in failure to localize the object at all. Approach long narrow objects such as glass slivers or needles from the side rather than end-on as they seldom leave discernible tracks.

7. It is not necessary to remove every piece of metal or glass seen on a radiograph. Good clinical judgement is required – for example a small piece of smooth-edged windscreen glass left in the face may not cause much trouble but vegetable material or slivers of wood are a potent source of chronic infection.

8. Identify and rigorously excise dead muscle, which is pale, non-contractile, mushy and does not bleed when incised.

Key points

The four criteria for muscle excision:

- Colour

- Contractility

- Consistency

- Capillary bleeding

---

9. Inspect for tendon damage. Tendon repair need not be performed at the initial procedure. Tattered ends should be trimmed and marked with a non-absorbable suture like nerves – see above.

10. Next, repair any major vessel damage previously diagnosed. Trim damaged vessel ends and carry out a primary anastomosis wherever possible. Avoid tension – this can be done by mobilizing the vessel proximal and distal to the wound. The amount of length that can be added by simple mobilization is often surprising. If this does not work, use an interposition graft. Most surgeons use reversed vein because of problems with infection but the use of synthetic graft material may be unavoidable – put antibiotic powder directly into the wound at the end of the operation and cover any repair with healthy muscle. Always repair interrupted major veins at the same time as arteries. Use a plastic shunt to restore the circulation if immediate repair is not possible – see below. Shunt both the damaged artery and vein if possible since venous engorgement of a limb may compromise its viability. Precise details of vascular repair are covered in Ch. 23.

11. Pay particular attention to comminuted bony injuries. Clean

contaminated bone but do not remove it where it is still attached to viable periosteum or healthy muscle. Discard small unattached bony fragments, which only contribute to postoperative wound infection. Orthopaedic fixation should be carried out after vascular repair. In major long bone fractures, allow therefore for the presence of shortening that will be corrected at orthopaedic repair, particularly when repairing blood vessels.

12. Identify injuries to joints and clean rigorously. Cover exposed cartilage with at least one layer of healthy tissue, ideally with synovium.

13. Irrigate the wound again at the end of the repair procedure. Secure haemostasis before dressing an open contaminated wound or before closing a clean one. Always leave contaminated wounds open. This includes the fascia because damaged muscle deep to fascial layers inevitably swells and this may lead to compartment syndrome. Dress an open wound with lightly fluffed gauze, which allows free drainage. Avoid tight packing. Immobilize the injured soft tissue with cotton wool, conforming bandages and, if necessary, a splint, even in the absence of bony injury. Continue the antibiotic cover started preoperatively.

Checklist

Make sure that all dead tissue has been removed, that an open wound is open enough to drain and that haemostasis is secure. Always check distal limb viability before leaving the operating theatre, particularly in the presence of constrictive dressings.

Closure

Do not close a wound unless you are sure it is recent, clean and healthy. Use delayed primary closure if in doubt. Approximate tissue loosely during closure, never under tension, in its natural layers. It is seldom necessary to repair muscle, but approximate subcutaneous tissue with absorbable sutures, preferably interrupted, to reduce the risk of tissue fluid collecting in dead spaces. Close the skin with interrupted non-absorbable sutures, trimming the edges where required to reduce bevelling. Consider the use of primary split skin grafting in addition to suturing at delayed primary closure, particularly where there has been tissue loss.

Postoperative

Keep the limb or other wounded part immobilized as far as possible. Watch for the signs of sepsis outlined below. Watch also for signs of postoperative limb ischaemia or overt haemorrhage.

🔑 Key points

Signs of sepsis:

- Increasing pain
- Increasing temperature
- Soiling of dressings
- Offensive smell

SPECIFIC SOFT TISSUE SITES – NECK

Appraise

1. Blunt injury to the neck rarely requires operative intervention. The cervical collar provides first-aid immobilization. Institute skull traction to decompress the spinal canal if there are neurological signs. If this fails, neurosurgical intervention is needed to decompress it directly. Partial section of the cervical spinal cord may be treated by early operative decompression and fixation to reduce the amount of residual disability but this is controversial. It is not indicated for complete section. Seek an urgent neurosurgical referral.

2. Penetrating wounds that remain superficial to the platysma need not be explored. If the wound goes deeper, explore it in the presence of brisk bleeding, an expanding haematoma, haemoptysis or haematemesis, neurological injury, surgical emphysema or an obvious air leak. The presence of a pneumothorax in the absence of any of these signs is not an indication for exploration. If none of these are present and arteriography and a thin barium examination of the pharynx are negative, then it is safe to observe the patient. Oesophagoscopy and bronchoscopy are often advised but seldom helpful – any visible lesion is likely to produce one of the above signs in any case.

3. While knife wounds and handgun injuries to the neck may be handled conservatively in the absence of major damage, high-energy-transfer missile wounds often cause extensive disruption and almost always require emergency exploration for the arrest of major haemorrhage.

Action

1. Explore the neck through one of the standard vascular access incisions, either along the clavicle or the anterior border of the sterno-cleidomastoid, so that the carotid and subclavian vessels can be properly controlled in the event of any sudden surprises. Be prepared to remove the middle third of the clavicle with a Gigli or air-driven saw to gain better access. Injuries to the roots of the great vessels may need to be exposed using an additional midline sternotomy.

2. Haemorrhage from one or other of the major vessels can normally be controlled by simple oversewing but if the main arteries are contused use a vein patch or even replace a short section with an artificial graft. Always repair the common or internal carotid unless it is actually clotted, a situation where there is a risk of embolus to the brain if the clot is disturbed. The external carotid may be ligated safely. Haemorrhage from the vertebral artery is usually more difficult to deal with. Obtain access by retracting the carotid sheath medially and developing the prevertebral tissue plane so revealed. Haemostasis can sometimes be achieved with bone wax and pressure but otherwise control the vertebral artery above and below the injury by removing the costal face of the appropriate cervical transverse processes. It is safe to ligate one vessel if the contralateral artery is patent but in an emergency there may be no time for an angiogram. Repair the internal jugular veins whenever possible but all the other neck veins, including the facial veins, which often bleed very briskly, can be safely ligated if necessary. Tilting the patient head-down reduces the risk of an air embolus to the heart but also increases the bleeding; try to clamp the vessel either side of the damage before repair is attempted.

3. The trachea can normally be repaired with a single layer of absorbable material over the endotracheal tube; defects need patching, which is a specialized procedure. The injured pharynx is repaired in two layers and the wound is drained.

? Difficulty?

Sometimes a neck wound is explored for severe haemorrhage and no vascular injury is obvious. Make a thorough search, exploring the wound to its fullest extent. Rebleeding is a real danger if a vascular injury is missed at this stage.

SURGICAL AIRWAY

Appraise
A surgical airway is indicated if the patient's airway is obstructed and it is not possible to perform either an orotracheal or nasotracheal intubation. Severe faciomaxillary injuries are the commonest indication.

Action
1. Cricothyroidotomy is a relatively safe and bloodless method of securing an airway. The procedure is not recommended in children under 12 years of age because the cricoid cartilage is the sole support for the trachea at this level. Instead employ jet insufflation. Insert a 14G intravenous cannula percutaneously through the cricothyroid membrane and connect this to an intermittent oxygen insufflater – a simple oxygen tube with a Y connector cut into it in series such that oxygen only passes through the cannula when the Y connector is digitally occluded. This procedure leads to a certain amount of carbon dioxide retention so use it for no more than 40 minutes. This buys the time to arrange either an expert intubation or a formal tracheostomy. There is no need for special positioning of the patient since the cricothyroid membrane is easily accessible.

2. Check the balloon on the cricothyroidotomy tube before starting. Remove any cervical collar, using an assistant to support the neck rigorously between hands or bent knees. A rigid collar is normally fenestrated and can be replaced after the procedure, passing the airway tube through the fenestration. Identify the cricothyroid membrane between the thyroid and cricoid cartilages and make a 3 cm transverse incision in the skin down on to it. Divide the cricothyroid membrane and enlarge the resulting hole in the trachea with a tracheal dilator or artery forceps. Insert a suitable-sized cuffed adult tracheostomy tube or a purpose-made cricothyroidotomy tube if such is available. Replace the rigid cervical collar.

? Difficulty?

1. Keep the cricothyroidotomy incision small, really no wider than a stab incision with a large blade. Damage to the anterior jugular vein is otherwise a possibility and leads to brisk venous haemorrhage. This can be stopped with pressure but it is probably best to identify, clamp and ligate the cut ends of the vein after the cricothyroidotomy

---

tube is safely secured. Remember that Airway is more urgent than Breathing and, if this mishap occurs, ignore the bleeding until the tube is secure in the trachea.

2. Regard tracheostomy as an elective technique, which is best performed in an anaesthetized, intubated patient. It is also required in children. The only real emergency indication in the adult is for penetrating laryngeal trauma in which the cricothyroid area is damaged. The technique is described in Chapter 39.

3. When there is an open defect in the trachea the tracheostomy tube can often be placed in the trachea directly through the wound. See Chapter 39 for operative details.

SPECIFIC SOFT TISSUE SITES – CHEST

Chest wounds, whether blunt or penetrating, range between trivial and fatal. In war, chest injury is common, with a high immediate mortality, usually from mediastinal disruption, open pneumothorax or massive haemothorax. In blunt injury haemothorax and pneumothorax often accompany falls or other deceleration injuries.

Thoracocentesis

Appraise
Emergency intervention in chest trauma is largely confined to thoracocentesis for tension pneumothorax, haemothorax or a combination of the two. The placing of an intercostal tube drain should be a relatively straightforward, gentle and, with the judicious placement of plenty of local anaesthetic, painless procedure. If there is no urgency, give the local anaesthetic plenty of time to work.

Prepare
The drain is normally placed with the patient sitting upright but this may not be possible in the unconscious patient with multiple injuries. Thoracocentesis is occasionally required as an emergency, in the case of tension pneumothorax, but there is usually time to prepare the patient properly, using an aseptic technique. Use at least a 32Ch gauge fenestrated chest drain. Identify the site of incision in the anterior axillary line just above the nipple line, in order to avoid diaphragmatic or particularly (on the right) hepatic injury. This site will lead you to the fifth or sixth intercostal space, use of which is relatively complication-free. Prepare the chest antiseptic solution. Inject at least 15 ml of 1% lignocaine (preferably with adrenaline 1:200 000) into the skin and deeply and widely into the intercostal muscle.

Action
1. Make a 1 cm transverse incision in the skin and deepen it into the muscle just above the upper border of the rib or you may damage the intercostal vessels. Place two heavy nylon sutures, one as a mattress suture across the hole (not a purse-string) for closing the hole later and the other to the side of the incision to secure the drain.

2. Separate the intercostal muscles using scissors or artery forceps, puncturing the parietal pleura. If possible, sweep a finger around the inside of the hole to exclude or separate lung adhesions.

If there is a tension pneumothorax there will be a brisk gush of air at this point.

3. Select a fenestrated trocar drain, remove the trocar completely and place the drain gently in the pleural cavity about 6 cm deeper than the most proximal fenestration, using an artery forceps to stiffen the tip. There is no need to introduce the drain to the hilt; expansion of the lung will force both air and blood into its lumen whatever its position.

4. Under no circumstances use the pointed trocar to force the drain through the intercostal muscle.

5. Connect the drain to a flutter valve or to an underwater seal drain if available. Secure it with the previously placed suture and apply a light dressing.

❓ Difficulty?

The use of a high interspace in the anterior axillary line is dangerous because of the proximity of hilar structures and the mediastinum, and the application of lengths of 3-inch adhesive plaster to secure the drain is out of date. Avoid the midaxillary line because of the slight but significant occurrence of an accessory mammary artery, which passes down the inside of the chest wall in the midaxillary position. Although this is only present in 2% of cases, one of us has had the misfortune to have to carry out a thoracotomy after referral from a medical team for persistent bleeding after thoracocentesis caused by this problem.

Postoperative

Underwater seal thoracocentesis drains may bubble happily for days without problems, but the persistent drainage of blood is more serious. Carry out thoracotomy if there is immediate drainage of more than 1 litre of blood or the persistent drainage of more than 250 ml per hour.

Pericardiocentesis

Appraise

This procedure is occasionally of some benefit in the management of pericardial tamponade and is recommended in the advanced trauma life support (ATLS) core curriculum as an emergency procedure for the inexperienced doctor working alone.

Prepare

Prepare the skin with antiseptic solution and identify the xiphoid process. Place ECG chest electrodes; if you touch the myocardium with the needle during this procedure you often see ectopics on the monitor.

🔑 Key point

- Call the cardiac surgeons before starting. If the patient requires this procedure to relieve life-threatening tamponade he/she almost certainly needs an emergency thoracotomy.

Action

Introduce a wide-bore needle to the left of the xiphoid, pointing towards the tip of the left scapula. Aspirate using a syringe as the needle is advanced. If blood is obtained, attach a three-way tap and 50 ml syringe to remove larger quantities. Watch the ECG monitor for ectopic activity. The blood is almost always clotted and it is often impossible to remove enough by this technique to relieve the tamponade. Aspiration of blood is not a definitive treatment and the condition will recur. Under these circumstances immediate thoracotomy is the procedure of choice (see Ch. 26).

Thoracotomy

Appraise

Emergency thoracotomy is rarely needed: the procedure is usually required for intractable intrathoracic bleeding, as diagnosed by persistent bleeding into the chest drain. The outcome is far better after penetrating trauma than after blunt because stab wounds usually result in single, small lacerations that can be repaired relatively easily, whereas blunt trauma often leads to widespread contusion and laceration, which is much more difficult to deal with. When possible plan an urgent procedure in theatre. The commonest cause of such bleeding after both blunt or penetrating trauma is damage to the intercostal vessels or lung parenchyma caused either by rib fracture or direct section. Mediastinal trauma is less often a cause of bleeding but, when it is, it is much more serious. Lung resection is seldom required in trauma cases; when it is, try to avoid pneumonectomy, which carries a high mortality, even in previously fit individuals (Fig. 3.1).

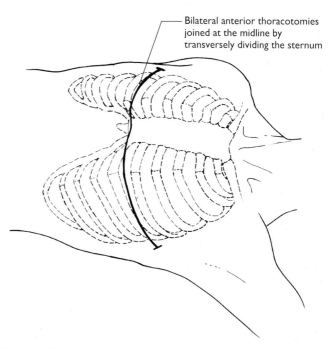

Bilateral anterior thoracotomies joined at the midline by transversely dividing the sternum

Fig. 3.1 The clamshell incision for access to both thoracic cavities and the mediastinum. The internal mammary artery on both sides is cut and should be secured.

'Emergency room thoracotomy' is reserved for penetrating cardiac wounds where tamponade or brisk exsanguination through the entry wound is perceived as an immediate threat to life. The procedure is only indicated in the patient who has vital signs on arrival in the emergency room but who loses them despite the instigation of immediate resuscitative measures. If cardiac output can be maintained the patient should be transferred immediately to the operating theatre. Figures from some centres suggest that the results from this procedure are fairly dismal. There is no indication for this procedure after blunt trauma as the damage is nearly always diffuse, to the mediastinum or aorta.

🔑 Key points

Indications for formal thoracotomy

- More than 1 litre initial blood loss
- Continued loss of more than 250 ml/h
- Cardiac tamponade
- Other mediastinal injuries
- Persistent air leak
- Retained foreign bodies more than 1.5 cm in diameter

Prepare

Give an anaesthetic if the patient is conscious. If there is time, and the anaesthetist is expert, ask to have a double-lumen tube passed so that one lung can be collapsed to facilitate the procedure. This is unlikely to be feasible in a conflict situation. Antiseptic skin preparation is normally applied as this only takes a few seconds.

Access

1. For cardiac injury, use a left anterior approach through the fourth interspace (Fig. 3.2).

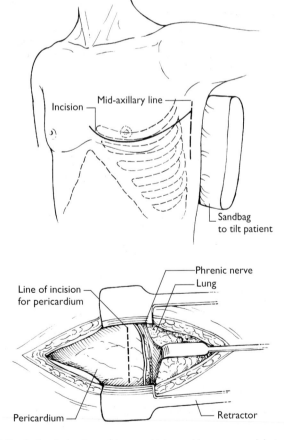

Fig. 3.2 Left anterior thoracotomy, which provides access mainly to the left ventricle and pulmonary conus. Avoid the phrenic nerve.

The entire surface of the heart can be examined through this incision. Even stab wounds to the heart from the right of the sternum can be dealt with satisfactorily through this incision.

2. Use a formal posterolateral incision if time permits since access to the posterior mediastinum is better and the incision seldom needs to be enlarged. This is a better incision for access to the lungs and pleura and should be carried out if there is suspected injury to these structures as well as or instead of mediastinal injury.

3. A midline sternotomy gives the best access to mediastinal structures but there is seldom time to carry out the high-resolution computerized tomography needed to exclude other thoracic injury, making this safely possible, and in any case this investigation may not be available.

4. If a laparotomy will also be required because of penetrating abdominal trauma, use a midline sternotomy. If there is penetrating injury to the abdomen it is best to keep the laparotomy separate from the thoracotomy and the peritoneum isolated from the thoracic cavity because of possible faecal contamination of the chest.

Assess

1. The basic technique for thoracotomy is described in Chapter 26. The description that follows presupposes the use of a posterolateral thoracotomy. Use a large blade to incise through the intercostal muscles to expose the chest cavity and its contents. Insert a rib spreader and examine the thoracic cavity.

2. Evacuate any clot and keep the operative field clear with effective and intelligent retraction and suction.

3. Get the anaesthetist to collapse the lung if a double lumen tube is in place. Otherwise gentle retraction with a lung retractor is required.

4. Examine the chest wall first – the majority of haemothoraces among survivors are associated with injury to the intercostal or internal mammary arteries.

5. Next, examine the lung surfaces for lacerations, which may bleed profusely.

6. Finally turn your attention to the aorta and lung root vessels.

7. Lengthen the thoracotomy wound across the sternum to the contralateral side if access to the other lung is required because of bleeding or an air leak (Fig. 3.1). This is easier with an anterior thoracotomy than with a posterolateral approach since the medial end of the incision is much higher and the choice of incision may well depend on whether unilateral or bilateral injury is suspected.

8. For access to the heart, incise the pericardium, avoiding damage to the phrenic nerve, which runs across the left side of the pericardium

and is usually obvious. Evacuate the pericardial clot and deliver the heart gently, remembering that excessive traction stops the circulation.

Action

1. Control any bleeding from thoracic wall vessels first unless there is massive exsanguination from the pulmonary vessels or aorta, which should otherwise be controlled by direct pressure first. Place a suture around the intercostal bundle or other vessel and tie down, trying to avoid the intercostal nerve, damage to which will otherwise lead to postoperative pain. Minor and moderate tears in the lung parenchyma can be controlled by oversewing or even simple pressure, and often stop bleeding and seal spontaneously when the lung is deflated. A more extensive tear from a penetrating missile injury can be controlled by application of clamps on either side of the track followed by division of the tissue between them and oversewing the bleeding vessels in the exposed wound track (Fig. 3.3).

If this is inappropriate because of major hilar vessel bleeding, consider lobectomy or pneumonectomy.

2. Lobectomy and pneumonectomy in the hands of an inexperienced surgeon have a poor outcome, so summon expert help if at all possible. Tears to the pulmonary arteries often extend into the left atrium and a description of the repair techniques required for this injury are beyond the scope of this chapter. Surgeons working in a conflict situation will be unlikely to see this major injury at emergency thoracotomy, since the mortality is extremely high.

3. Tears or penetrating wounds to the aorta are very difficult to control; occasionally, if the blood pressure has fallen, they may seal spontaneously, in which case oversew using interrupted non-absorbable sutures on a round-bodied needle. Control small tears by the application of a side clamp such as a Brock or Satinsky. Control larger tears or transection by proximal and distal cross-clamping with mobilization, resection of damaged vessel wall and either primary repair or the placing of an interposition tube graft.

4. The superior vena cava is much more difficult to repair since it tends to shred when stitched and the help of an expert is needed. Proximal and distal control is almost always required. In the emergency conflict situation and in a contaminated thoracic wound oversewing the cut ends of the cava is an acceptable alternative.

5. If there is a wound in the heart, place deep sutures in the myocardium using a large, curved, round-bodied needle, carefully identifying and avoiding the coronary arteries. The injured right atrium is thin-walled and floppy and direct apposition of the wound edges using a full-thickness continuous suture is more appropriate (Fig. 3.4).

> **Difficulty?**
>
> 1. Occasionally a penetrating cardiac injury results in a large tear in one of the cardiac chambers and this presents more severe problems. Urgently call for the assistance of the cardiac surgery team if such is available.
>
> 2. Damage to a coronary artery leads to brisk haemorrhage. Such wounds are best repaired formally with magnification and this is a highly skilled procedure.

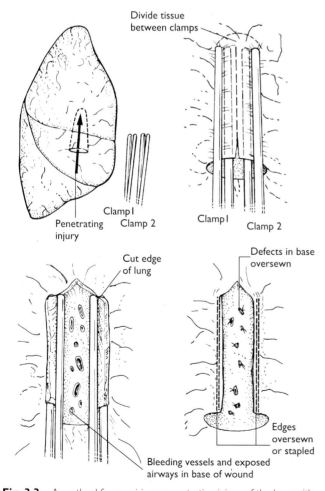

Fig. 3.3 A method for repairing a penetrating injury of the lung with particular emphasis on haemostasis.

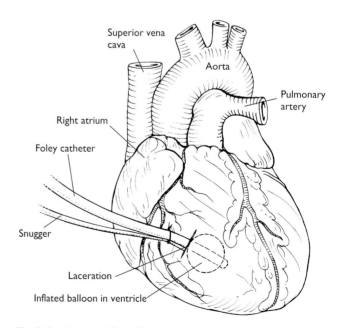

Fig. 3.4 A method for achieving temporary haemostasis in penetrating cardiac trauma using a Foley catheter.

Checklist

Do not close the chest until you have ensured that all major bleeding has been controlled and that the continuity of all damaged structures has been restored.

Closure

The techniques of formal thoracotomy closure in the trauma patient are no different from those used in elective procedures (see Ch. 26). Always use wide-bore (i.e. ≥ 32Ch) fenestrated drains, bearing in mind the possibility of postoperative infection. If the wound is contaminated or infected leave the skin and subcutaneous layers open but you cannot leave the chest cavity open to drain and this is why the drains are important.

🔑 Key points

- Make sure the drains are properly secured with strong (No. 1) nylon stitch material that indents the drain when tied down tightly. If the drains are pulled out inadvertently during transport this is a disaster, particularly if air evacuation is in progress.

- Never clamp drains prior to evacuation by air or road – this can easily lead to an unrecognized tension pneumothorax and death.

Postoperative

Careful observation of the post-thoracotomy patient is essential and is best carried out in a critical care environment. This may be possible even in war and conflict settings with robust, field-tested, modern monitoring devices, the most useful of which is probably the pulse oximeter. If the patient is unable to maintain an adequate oxygen saturation despite the use of oxygen therapy, vigorous physiotherapy or even assisted ventilation may be required. Always carry out a full re-examination to exclude a simple correctable cause such as a pneumothorax or haemothorax, which should be scrupulously sought. Otherwise, such deterioration is nearly always the result of progressive lung infection with atelectasis, which may be followed by the onset of one of the acute lung injury syndromes such as adult respiratory distress syndrome (ARDS).

Complications

1. Complications include bleeding, infection, continuing air leak and cardiac dysrhythmias. Bleeding is only a problem if it is persistent and profuse (i.e. more than 250 ml/h). Postoperative bleeding tends to reduce and stop with time, patience and transfusion. Only reopen the chest if the patient becomes shocked despite adequate resuscitation.

2. Infection of the thoracotomy incision or of such entry and exit wounds as are present is common, particularly if the wound is sustained in a resource-constrained environment. It is treated from first principles, including reopening the wound, draining any pus and giving appropriate antibiotics. Intrathoracic infection usually presents later as an empyema.

3. Continuing air leak is common after lung parenchymal injury and, provided the lung is fully expanded, will stop spontaneously over 24–48 hours. Leaks beyond this point may be associated with previously unrecognized bronchial or even tracheal injury. Consider this if the lung fails to expand despite the presence of two large drains and suction. In the conflict setting, the patient will require evacuation to a specialist centre.

4. The commonest cardiac dysrhythmia following chest injury is atrial fibrillation, which is normally associated with shunting and hypoxia. Ventricular ectopics are associated with post-traumatic myocardial ischaemia. Do not forget that older patients may already have underlying cardiac problems.

Tracheal injuries

Appraise

Injury to the trachea in the neck is open or closed. Open injury is obvious. Closed injury may lead to surgical emphysema in the neck with characteristic crepitus; in penetrating injury the trachea is rarely injured in isolation and the oesophagus must also be investigated (see below). In blunt trauma the diagnosis is more difficult but exploration is mandatory and should be preceded by endoscopy if possible. Injury to the trachea and main bronchi in the chest is unusual but leads to a massive air leak. All that will be found on examination is a tension pneumothorax and when the chest is drained a persistent air leak follows. If the lung does not re-expand after drainage a major airway injury is likely and a second chest drain should be inserted; both should be put on suction.

Prepare

Secure the airway. Because of the likelihood of damage to other structures, including the thyroid and major vessels, expert help should be sought before embarking on a major exploration and repair.

Access

Deal with injuries in the neck locally. Otherwise, carry out a posterolateral thoracotomy.

Assess and Action

1. These two sections are dealt with together because the extent of injury will determine your technique. Closed injuries to the trachea in the neck are oversewn with interrupted absorbable sutures. Open injuries, such as those associated with high-energy-transfer missiles, may be associated with loss of tissue to the extent that direct primary repair is impossible and all you may be able to do is to use the disrupted trachea to insert an endotracheal tube, thus securing the airway and closing the leak at the same time. Expert ENT help will be needed.

2. In the chest, a simple tear of the trachea or main bronchus is oversewn with interrupted non-absorbable material. This is an expert technique: the consequences of a bronchopleural fistula are lethal. More extensive injury will involve the blood vessels and again expert help will be needed. Hilar near-avulsion will probably require pneumonectomy; this injury is unlikely to be encountered in the operating theatre as it is usually quickly fatal.

Oesophageal injury

Appraise

This is usually occult. Clinically, it is diagnosed by finding subcutaneous surgical emphysema in the supraclavicular fossae. Air in the mediastinum on the chest X-ray is also an indicator. The injury is normally associated with other mediastinal injuries, whether blunt or penetrating, and a missed rupture carries the gravest of prognoses, so a high index of suspicion is mandatory. A Gastrografin swallow will confirm the diagnosis.

Prepare

Prepare the patient for a left posterolateral thoracotomy, possibly with a separate neck access incision or a thoracoabdominal extension. Covering antibiotics are essential.

Access

Most of the intrathoracic oesophagus can be reached through the postero-lateral incision. Look out for the phrenic nerve crossing the pericardium, and also the descending thoracic aorta, which may well also be injured.

Assess

A fresh injury will be relatively clean and easy to repair; if there is any delay at all there will be medastinitis with pleural cavity contamination.

Action

1. Dissect the oesophagus free from surrounding structures and sling above and below the site of injury. A fresh injury can be repaired by approximating the mucosa with interrupted absorbable sutures. This is the most important layer; a second muscular suture will add security to the repair. Drain the injury site and close the chest in the usual way.

2. A contaminated ruptured oesophagus is irreparable and has the consistency of wet blotting paper. Management is by drainage and isolation. Drain the site and in addition place a tube gastrostomy in the stomach and via a sternomastoid incision in the neck carry out an open formal pharyngostomy with mucosa to skin as a diversion procedure to keep the saliva out of the mediastinum.

Checklist, closure and postoperative care

As for thoracotomy.

SPECIFIC SOFT TISSUE SITES – ABDOMEN

Laparotomy

1. The conduct of a laparotomy for trauma follows well-worn guidelines that apply irrespective of whether the injury is sustained by blunt or penetrating means. Some techniques may vary depending on the skills and resources available locally.

2. If the patient is stable, diagnostic aid is always required if the patient is unconscious. There is increasing evidence that under these circumstances a CT scan of the abdomen with contrast injection is the single best test, especially when the patient is undergoing a head CT. Remember that if a CT scan of the abdomen is performed very rapidly after injury there may not yet be enough blood in the peritoneal cavity to show unequivocally on the scan. Constant reappraisal of the patient's clinical condition is mandatory. If CT is not available, ultrasound may be useful; if this is not available, then diagnostic peritoneal lavage remains a reliable tool.

3. If the patient is not stable proceed to resuscitative laparotomy without error or delay.

Key points

Laparotomy is indicated:

- when there is unequivocal clinical evidence of peritonitis
- when the patient is difficult to resuscitate as shown by continuing requirements of intravenous fluids and bleeding has been excluded in other areas
- when air is present under the diaphragm or there is evidence of diaphragmatic rupture on the erect chest X-ray
- when there is a positive diagnostic peritoneal lavage or a CT reveals the presence of blood and ruptured solid viscera
- when there is a penetrating or perforating missile wound in a resource-constrained environment.

Appraise

1. The laparotomy is being carried out because either the patient has shown signs of peritonitis or haemorrhage into the peritoneal cavity or a diagnostic test has given a positive result.

2. Penetrating wounds may initially present with few clinical signs but there is always a danger of the patient's condition suddenly deteriorating. Blunt injury giving rise to visceral damage normally leaves tell-tale signs on the abdominal wall such as bruising, abrasion, tyre marks or seatbelt tattooing. Remember always to examine the back.

Prepare

1. There is always time to prepare and drape the abdomen properly before laparotomy.

2. Make sure that rapid transfusion of blood or fluids can be started as soon as the abdomen is opened. The abdominal wall often tamponades bleeding and this is released when the abdomen is opened. Warn the theatre staff to have available necessary equipment such as two powerful suckers, plenty of large packs, and vascular instruments if massive bleeding is likely.

3. Cover as much of the patient as possible with heat-reflective blankets to prevent hypothermia. A warm air blanket is most useful if available. Bleeding patients cool off rapidly, even in hot climates.

Key points – exploration of penetrating wounds

Conventional advice is that all penetrating abdominal wounds should be explored, but this is not necessary provided that:

- the patient is absolutely stable, with no signs of intra-abdominal injury or shock
- you reassess the patient at frequent intervals – every 2 hours if necessary
- at the first sign of deterioration, such as increasing pulse rate, falling blood pressure or increasing abdominal tenderness, you carry out a laparotomy. Treat such an event not as a failure but as a natural resolution of the equivocal physical signs.

4. If the patient has not been given prophylactic antibiotics, give an initial intravenous loading dose of a versatile appropriate antibiotic now.

5. Before surgery, pass a nasogastric tube into the stomach and a urinary catheter into the bladder.

Access

Explore the abdomen through a midline incision, which can be extended in both directions, even into a median sternotomy if indicated.

Assess

Examine all viscera, explore the lesser sac, identify all sources of bleeding and explore all stab wounds to their fullest extent.

Action

1. Control of haemorrhage is the first priority in the abdomen. Major intraperitoneal bleeding can be a daunting prospect. Have two suckers ready as well as a number of large packs.

2. As soon as the peritoneum has been opened try to identify the general area from which the bleeding is coming and clear away as much clot and free blood as possible to identify the specific source.

3. Treat life-threatening exsanguination from abdominal bleeding by opening the left chest and cross-clamping the aorta. The clamp may be left in place for a maximum of 45 minutes while the vascular injury is sought and dealt with.

4. In penetrating trauma explore expanding retroperitoneal haematomata to exclude major vessel injury.

5. In blunt trauma, especially that associated with pelvic fractures, leave the haematomata alone as exploration may lead to uncontrollable venous haemorrhage.

6. Control bleeding from major abdominal vessels with pressure while dissecting around the wound to achieve control above and below the bleeding point. Then repair the vessel with polypropylene sutures. Major damage to the aorta and vena cava requires expert assistance for repair.

7. Oversew smaller bleeding mesenteric vessels. Always examine distal bowel afterwards and resect if there is doubt about viability.

8. Repair damage to the hollow viscera next, thereby limiting contamination of the peritoneum. Examine both surfaces of the stomach. Oversew tears or penetrating injuries. Watch for doubtful viability of the greater curve if there is a longitudinal tear parallel to it. If in doubt, resect.

9. Explore the area of the duodenum if there is retroperitoneal haemorrhage or biliary discoloration in the region of the duodenum. Kocherize the duodenum to examine its posterior surface. Repair rather than resect if possible. Most duodenal tears can either be repaired primarily or patched with a loop of jejunum. Perform a diversionary gastrojejunostomy and place a T-tube in the common bile duct in addition to the repair if there is extensive duodenal damage. Make sure the area is adequately drained after surgery. Duodenal resection may be indicated if there is severe tissue loss and major concurrent pancreatic trauma. The morbidity is formidable.

10. Small-bowel injuries are a little easier to deal with. It is not uncommon for a single stab wound to traverse several loops of small bowel. Carefully oversew all penetrating wounds or tears with absorbable sutures in a single interrupted layer. Consider resection if there are a large number of tears in a short length of bowel, or if there is doubt about viability.

11. Large bowel injury is more likely to require resection. If there is only a small penetrating wound less than 6 hours old, particularly on the right side of the colon, oversewing is the treatment of choice. A grossly contaminated wound of the right side of the colon can be treated with right hemicolectomy and primary anastomosis. Grossly contaminated left-sided colonic injury is best treated with resection, anastomosis and covering colostomy unless there is generalized established faecal peritonitis, where a Hartmann's procedure may be safer. Conservative surgery of large bowel perforation is possible but controversial, and such decisions should be made at a senior level.

12. Hepatic tears are often mild and may have stopped bleeding by the time the laparotomy is performed. Suture more major tears with a liver needle. Use care to prevent the needle moving laterally in the parenchyma and making the tear worse. If there is substantial haemorrhage from the liver use the Pringle manoeuvre. Place a soft clamp over the portal triad with one blade through the foramen of Winslow into the lesser sac. This compresses the hepatic artery and portal vein while the liver damage is assessed and repaired. Continued haemorrhage after clamping is coming from the hepatic veins or inferior vena cava (IVC). The clamp should not be left in place for more than 20 minutes.

13. Major hepatic injury may require lobectomy. Damage to the retrohepatic inferior vena cava can be a severe injury with access and control problems; in some cases it may be necessary to control the IVC in the chest via a midline sternotomy and pass a bypass tube from the right atrium to the infrarenal IVC, isolating the hepatic veins and retrohepatic cava for repair. Summon expert help. Survival rates from this injury are extremely disappointing.

14. Pack otherwise uncontrollable haemorrhage and re-operate at 24 hours to remove the packs and reassess the position. Repack if the bleeding restarts. There is increasing evidence that a conservative approach to hepatic trauma may be of benefit in up to 20% of cases. Again, these decisions are best taken at a senior level.

15. Splenectomy is the safest approach to the ruptured spleen. Sweep the hand between the diaphragm and the spleen to break down any adhesions and deliver the spleen forwards into the wound. Clamp the gastrosplenic and lienorenal ligaments, avoiding the tail of the pancreas, resect the spleen and double tie the pedicles with heavy absorbable suture material. Oozing from disrupted adhesions can be controlled by packing and it normally stops without further attention; if it doesn't, use diathermy. Splenic salvage surgery involves the application of haemostatic agents such as microfibrillar collagen or polyglactin 910 mesh bags, together with diathermy and oversewing of the defect. There is increasing evidence that conservative management of the ruptured spleen may be successful in up to a quarter of patients. This may be a course to pursue in children who are haemodynamically stable; children are far more likely to develop overwhelming postsplenectomy infections (OPSI) than adults. Active conservative management is the key to success. Don't forget to arrange for immunization against pneumococcus and long-term antibiotics if the spleen does have to be resected.

16. Avoid surgery for blunt renal trauma unless there is intractable parenchymal bleeding, signified by gross haemodynamically significant haematuria for more than 24 hours, or a urinary

leak, or an expanding perirenal haematoma found at laparotomy. Penetrating trauma is less often possible to manage conservatively but this can usually be done with confidence by employing the intravenous urogram (IVU) and CT to exclude blood or urine leaks. The IVU will show you whether both kidneys are functioning before considering a nephrectomy. Always approach the damaged kidney via a midline laparotomy. Other viscera may be damaged and cannot be dealt with through a loin incision. Oversew contused or penetrated bleeding areas with deep liver sutures. Conserve as much kidney as possible, bearing in mind the end-artery anatomy of this organ. Repair injury to the ureters and bladder primarily using absorbable suture material: single layer to the ureter over a double J stent, double layer to the bladder over a suprapubic catheter. Repair of injury to the urethra is described elsewhere.

17. Pancreatic injury can be problematic. If the injury is slight and the ducts are intact, stop all bleeding. Do not try to repair the injury but leave a drain down to the injured part. Treat distal injuries involving the duct by distal resection. Injuries to the head of the pancreas involving the duct are more difficult to deal with. Repair the duct or anastomose it to a jejunal loop. These are specialized procedures so call for experienced assistance if possible.

18. Retroperitoneal access for bleeding can be difficult. Access to the inferior vena cava on the right of the abdomen is achieved by dividing the congenital adhesions in the right paracolic gutter and sweeping the entire right colon together with the duodenum to the left. The cava can then be controlled proximally and distally. Injuries to the retrohepatic cava high up at the level of the hepatic veins are particularly difficult to deal with and may require the insertion of an excluding shunt within the cava (see above under hepatic injuries). These injuries are nearly always fatal. Injuries to the aorta are exposed similarly by dividing the congenital adhesions in the left paracolic gutter and swinging the entire left colon, including if necessary the spleen and left kidney, to the right. In this way suprarenal and coeliac level injuries to the aorta may be visualized and controlled.

Checklist

1. Haemostasis must be secure and the peritoneal cavity well washed out, even in cases of recent injury, before you can even think about closing the abdomen. Also, confirm visceral viability once the viscera have been returned to the abdomen and are not under tension.

2. Check that adequate drains have been properly placed and secured to the abdominal wall, and that stoma bags are placed or that stomata are covered with dressings before closure to avoid wound contamination.

Closure

1. Close the laparotomy using the mass closure technique, using a single layer of loop size 1 nylon.

2. Leave open a grossly contaminated abdomen or one with major retroperitoneal oedema. Cover the wound with wet gauze swabs or, alternatively and probably more appropriately, use a Bogota Bag. This is a technique using the inner sterile surface of an intravenous fluid bag which has been opened up, shaped and then sutured loosely to the skin edges with a continuous nylon suture. It is a crude but highly effective technique that allows both continuous inspection of abdominal contents and their drainage, and is particularly useful if there are worries concerning abdominal compartment syndrome or bowel viability. Its use is particularly appropriate in a resource-constrained environment.

3. Leave open associated missile entrance and exit wounds in the abdominal wall. Excise these and leave them for delayed primary closure.

Postoperative

1. Major abdominal surgery may lead to surprisingly few postoperative problems provided adequate preparation has been carried out beforehand. This is seldom possible in the trauma patient and the immediate postoperative management is crucial. This should take place in a critical care environment and details are beyond the scope of this chapter.

2. Where a resuscitative 'damage control' laparotomy has been carried out a subsequent 'second look' laparotomy is nearly always necessary in order to check tissue viability and to search for and correct injuries missed during resuscitation.

Complications

1. Bleeding is the most important postoperative complication and demands relaparotomy. Its control is either simple or extremely difficult – there is seldom anything in between. Remember that bleeding may be due to clotting deficiency and may thus not be surgically correctable. This situation may be avoided to a certain extent by giving 1 unit of fresh frozen plasma to every 4 units of transfused stored blood, together with calcium gluconate injections to reverse the EDTA in the blood. Platelets will be needed once the total transfused volume exceeds 10 units; they must be given even if the platelet count appears relatively normal, as many of these platelets will be non-functional. A low body temperature wrecks the clotting system completely and the patient must be kept warm.

Key points

The fatal triad of

- Hypothermia

- Metabolic acidosis

- Coagulopathy

is particularly lethal in the trauma patient.

---

2. Sepsis is a potent cause of collapse at the 48–72-hour point. An immediate postoperative temperature increase is nearly always respiratory and should be actively treated with physiotherapy and appropriate antibiotics, with suction if the patient is on a ventilator. Progressive abdominal sepsis is relentless in its course and will lead to multisystem failure, including renal, respiratory and hepatic collapse, unless dealt with surgically by drainage and under these circumstances a re-look laparotomy is both mandatory and urgent.

3. Anastomotic leaks are more likely to occur after trauma surgery than after elective surgery and the judicious drainage of such is

essential to provide early warning of trouble. They should be treated conservatively. Low-output fistulae will normally respond to a few days of nil by mouth with nasogastric aspiration. High-output fistulae will need parenteral nutrition and the administration of somatostatin or similar agents, in a critical care environment.

4. The specific management of multiorgan failure is a complex subject dealt with elsewhere.

FURTHER READING

American College of Surgeons 1989 Advanced trauma life support course for physicians. American College of Surgeons, Chicago, IL

Hollands MJ, Little JM 1991 Non-operative management of blunt liver injuries. British Journal of Surgery 78: 968–972

Jeffries DJ 1991 Zidovudine after occupational exposure to HIV. British Medical Journal 302: 1349–1351

Jennet B, Teasdale G, Braakman R et al 1976 Predicting outcome in individual patients after severe head injury. Lancet 1: 1031–1034

Khoury HI, Peschiera JL, Welling RE 1991 Non-operative management of blunt splenic trauma a 10 year experience. Injury 22: 349–352

Knottenbelt JD 1991 University of Cape Town trauma handbook. UCT Press, Cape Town, p. 46

Krige JEJ, Bornman PC, Terblanche J 1992 Therapeutic packing in complex liver trauma. British Journal of Surgery 79: 43–46

Mattox KL, Moore WS, Feliciano D 1991 Trauma, 3rd edn. Appleton & Lange, New York

Norrell H 1980 The early management of spinal injuries. Clinical Neurosurgery 27: 385–391

Royal College of Surgeons of England 1988 Commission on the Provision of Surgical Services. Report of the working party on the management of patients with major injuries. Royal College of Surgeons of England, London

Skinner D, Driscoll P, Earlam RJ (eds) 1991 ABC of major trauma. British Medical Journal, London

Trunkey DD 1989 Report to the Council of the Association of Surgeons of Great Britain and Ireland. British Medical Journal 299: 31–33

Trunkey DD 1991 Initial treatment of patients with extensive trauma. New England Journal of Medicine 324: 1259–1263

Wood PR, Peel WJ, Foley MA, Lawler PG 1990 Junior medical staff and the assessment of trauma. Annals of the Royal College of Surgeons of England 72: 196–198

Laparotomy: elective and emergency

R. M. Kirk and R. C. N. Williamson

Contents

INTRODUCTION

1. Surgeons' attitudes to laparotomy have undergone a marked change within a very few years. This change has brought great benefits but also potential dangers. Formerly, good surgeons took great care to make abdominal incisions sufficiently long to allow full exploration in order to confirm the diagnosis and exclude others, and also to carry out the correct procedure through an adequate exposure. In contrast, many operations are now carried out through restricted incisions. Indeed, certain procedures are routinely performed by the technique of 'minimal access' (see Ch. 5). The change has come about for two reasons. Improvements in imaging and laboratory tests have had a beneficial effect on diagnosis. In addition, the technical facilities have developed dramatically. It is very difficult to predict the future; we are presently seeing the usual enthusiasm for exploring the limits of minimal access procedures in competition with radiological and other indirect manipulations. Laparoscopy is, of course, available not only as a therapeutic but also as a diagnostic tool, particularly for the acute abdomen. However, never forget that most diseases of the gastrointestinal tract primarily affect the mucosa; examining the hollow viscera from within the abdomen laparoscopically or at laparotomy does not replace endoscopic examination where this is possible.

2. An increasing number of conditions previously treated by operation can now be managed by alternative methods. Uncomplicated chronic peptic ulcer is usually amenable to medical treatment. Selected patients with perforated peptic ulcer can be managed conservatively. Gastrointestinal bleeding can often be successfully treated by endoscopic or radiological methods. Strictures can be dilated effectively with single or repeated balloon dilatation with additional stenting if necessary.

> 🔑 **Key point**
>
> • A continuing danger is the fallacious belief that abdominal exploration will reveal the truth, making preoperative investigation seem unnecessary once laparotomy has been decided upon.

3. Not only may intra-abdominal examination of hollow viscera fail to reveal intraluminal disease but you may also miss disease processes that are deeply placed in solid organs. However, intraoperative use of high-frequency, high-resolution ultrasound promises to be a valuable diagnostic tool. Vascular blockage or constriction from atheroma is often difficult or impossible to detect in mesenteric vessels at laparotomy because of pulsatile backflow from patent vessels. Undoubtedly, the best time to make the diagnosis is before operation; this knowledge allows you to plan the best treatment. In some cases adequate preoperative investigation may spare the patient the need for operation, for example by showing advanced neoplasia for which surgical management would be ineffective.

4. Do not place too much reliance on tests. Results expressed numerically have a sometimes spurious appearance of objectivity. Imaging techniques are operator-dependent and generally have an accuracy of no more than 85%. The most certain method of making a diagnosis remains the taking of a good history, carrying out a careful, thorough examination, followed by carefully selected and interpreted investigations. If these methods fail, the next step is not necessarily exploratory laparotomy. Whenever possible, it is better to repeat the diagnostic process from the start, after an interval. Alternatively, ask a trusted colleague to take a completely fresh view of the problem. Computer-aided diagnosis has improved accuracy in dealing with the acute abdomen. Perhaps the general application of this technique will be valuable in elective surgery to prevent inappropriate laparotomy.

AVOIDING ADHESIONS

Appraise

1. There have been a number of studies of postoperative adhesions, and particularly of their consequences.[1] Well-known technical factors are extensive trauma, bleeding, infection, foreign material, intraperitoneal chemotherapeutic agents and, especially, ischaemic tissue. In

Britain there are 12 000–14 400 admissions each year resulting from abdominal adhesions and in the USA they account for approximately 950 000 patient-days in hospital.

2. One of the most frequently identified causes is the use of starch glove powder. Swedish hospitals admit at least 4700 patients each year with adhesive small-bowel obstruction and of these 2200 were operated on in order to relieve it. Only a quarter of the responders to a questionnaire used powder-free gloves and less than half of them ever washed their gloves. Those who did wash their gloves used ineffective methods. The Swedish authors also indicted suturing of the peritoneum as a probable cause of adhesion formation.

3. Prefer powderless gloves. If you use starch-powdered gloves, wash off the powder by the effective method of Fraser.[2] Put on the gloves and carry out a 10-minute surgical scrub using 10 ml of povidone-iodine 7.5% in a non-toxic detergent base, which combines with the starch. Now rinse in 500 ml of sterile water during 30 seconds.

4. It is likely that the increasing use of minimal access techniques will reduce the incidence of adhesions, although the technique has not abolished the problem.

5. Liberal irrigation of the peritoneal cavity with Ringer's lactate solution, before abdominal closure, is said to reduce adhesion formation. In the last few years adhesion-prevention barriers have been developed that prevent the formation of fibrin bridges.

REFERENCES

1. Ellis H 1997 The clinical significance of adhesions: focus on intestinal obstruction. European Journal of Surgery Supplement 577: 7–9
2. Fraser I 1982 Simple and effective method of removing starch powder from surgical gloves. British Journal of Surgery 284: 1835

OPENING THE ABDOMEN

Preparation

1. Preferably see the patient in the ward before the premedication is given, or in the anaesthetic room while he or she is still awake. Check that this is the correct patient by visual identification and inspection of the identity bracelet.

2. Inspect the case notes and make sure that any relevant X-rays are available in theatre. If the lesion is unilateral, be quite certain that the operation will be carried out on the correct side (this should have been marked beforehand). It is inexcusable to neglect these elementary precautions.

3. If the bowel will be opened, or if necrotic or infected tissues are likely to be encountered, ensure that a prophylactic injection of an appropriate antibiotic is given at this stage. The choice depends on the nature of expected organisms. Remember that in seriously ill patients facultative organisms must be considered.[1-3]

4. Carefully palpate the relaxed abdomen of the anaesthetized patient before making the incision.

5. Make sure that the anaesthetist is prepared for the operation to start. Laparotomy is nearly always performed under general anaesthesia, with endotracheal intubation and an intravenous cannula in situ.

6. Cleanse the skin of the operation area with an antiseptic solution applied on gauze held in long sponge-holding forceps. Appropriate solutions include chlorhexidine 1:5000, povidone-iodine 10% in alcoholic solution, cetrimide 1% and 95% white spirit. Apply the solution along the line of the incision and continue to apply it in a centrifugal manner of increasingly wide circles over a wide area. Do not use an inflammable agent, such as white spirit, if you intend to employ diathermy to the skin or immediate subcutaneous tissues.

7. Apply sterile sheets or drapes and secure them to the skin with towel clips (unless local anaesthetic is being used). Leave exposed a limited extent of the abdomen on either side of the proposed line of incision. Alternatively, clip the drapes to each other, or apply an adhesive plastic sheet over the area, which seals off the skin over the proposed incision, extending over and securing the drapes. The incision will be made through the sheet.

Types of incision (Figs 4.1, 4.2)

1. Plan the incision with care to give:

a. good exposure of the target area and versatility; it may be necessary to extend it
b. minimal damage to intervening structures
c. sound, cosmetically acceptable repair.

2. *Midline* incisions transgress the linea alba, the tough and relatively avascular cord that unites the anterior and posterior rectus sheaths. They therefore have the advantages of being relatively quick

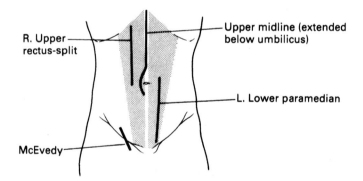

Fig. 4.1   Some vertical laparotomy incisions.

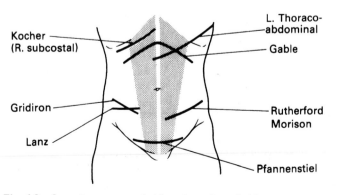

Fig. 4.2   Some transverse and oblique laparotomy incisions.

to make and to close and of provoking less bleeding than incisions that divide muscle fibres. Midline incisions can provide access to most abdominal viscera (Table 4.1).

In the upper abdomen you can avoid the falciform ligament by keeping just to one or other side of the midline when entering the peritoneal cavity. In the lower abdomen remember that the linea alba is less well developed, so take corresponding care to close the wound securely. When necessary, bypass the umbilicus by curving the skin incision and bevelling the underlying cut to regain the midline of the aponeurosis below it

3. *Paramedian* incisions provide very similar access to the upper, central or lower abdomen. All layers are divided in the line of the vertical skin incision, placed 2 cm to the right or left of the midline, except that the rectus muscle is dissected free and is drawn laterally, thus remaining intact. At the end of the operation allow the rectus muscle to fall medially, covering the line of closure of the peritoneum and, in the upper abdomen, the posterior rectus sheath.

4. *Rectus-splitting* incisions are made 3–4 cm lateral to the midline and divide all the tissues in this line (splitting the rectus muscle and its intersections). They avoid the time-consuming dissection required to free the muscle belly. In theory the medial part of the rectus muscle

Table 4.1 Incisions to expose the abdominal viscera

Midline	Upper	Hiatus, oesophagus, stomach, duodenum, spleen, liver, pancreas, biliary tract
	Central	Small bowel, colon
	Lower	Sigmoid, rectum, ovary/tube/uterus, bladder and prostate (extraperitoneal)
	Throughout	Aorta
Paramedian (incl. rectus split)	Upper	Biliary tract (right), spleen (left), etc.
	Central	Small bowel, colon
	Lower	Pelvic viscera, lower ureter (extraperitoneal)
Oblique	Subcostal	Liver and biliary tract (right), spleen (left)
	Gable	Pancreas, liver, adrenals
	Gridiron	Caecum–appendix (right)
	Rutherford Morison	Caecum–appendix (right), sigmoid (left), ureter and external iliac vessels (extraperitoneal)
	Posterolateral	Kidney and adrenal (extraperitoneal)
Transverse	Right upper quadrant	Gallbladder, infant pylorus, colostomy
	Mid-abdominal	Small bowel, colon, kidney, lumbar sympathetic chain, vena cava (right)
	Lanz	Caecum–appendix (right)
	Pfannenstiel	Ovary/tube/uterus, prostate (extraperitoneal)
Thoraco-abdominal	Right	Liver and portal vein
	Left	Gastro-oesophageal junction, enormous spleen

is denervated and thus rendered atrophic, but in practice the wounds heal strongly. A right upper rectus split provides good access to the gallbladder.

5. *Oblique* incisions can sometimes provide good access. Kocher's incision extends 2 cm below the right costal margin from the midline to the lateral edge of the rectus muscle and exposes the gallbladder. The equivalent left subcostal incision can be used to approach the spleen. In the lower abdomen, Rutherford Morison's incision starts just above the anterior superior iliac spine and divides all tissues in the line of the external oblique muscle and aponeurosis. The gridiron incision splits each of the three muscle layers of the abdominal wall in the line of its fibres; it therefore seldom gives rise to an incisional hernia. It provides an excellent approach to the appendix and can be enlarged by extending the skin incision in either direction and by dividing the internal oblique and transversus muscles (i.e. conversion into a Rutherford Morison incision).

6. *Transverse* incisions usually leave the best cosmetic scars and provide adequate exposure, provided they are made long enough. They are therefore best suited for limited exposure in a planned procedure. Ramstedt's pyloromyotomy or transverse colostomy may be performed through a short transverse incision. Transverse laparotomy is useful in children, in certain obese patients and in the upper abdomen when the costal angle is broad. The Lanz incision is a horizontal modification of the gridiron incision for appendicectomy and provides the least obtrusive scar at the expense of slightly inferior access. Pfannenstiel's incision runs transversely above the pubis but just below the hairline. The aponeurosis is divided transversely and reflected above and below, allowing the rectus muscles to be separated vertically in the midline. Gynaecologists then open the peritoneum to gain access to the female reproductive organs, whereas urologists stay in the extraperitoneal plane for retropubic approach to the bladder and prostate.

7. *Angled* incisions provide not a mere slit that can be pulled into an ellipse but a space in the abdominal wall. Combined right and left subcostal incisions joining at the xiphisternum (the 'high gable' incision) enable a large flap to be turned down and provide excellent access for hepatectomy, pancreatectomy and bilateral adrenalectomy. A vertical incision with a T-shaped transverse extension (or vice versa) allows two flaps to be turned back. These incisions take longer to make and repair but can be invaluable for difficult or very extensive operations.

8. *Thoracoabdominal* incisions usually follow the line of a rib and extend obliquely into the upper abdomen. They make light of the cartilaginous cage protecting the upper abdomen. Alternatively, a vertical upper abdominal incision is sometimes converted into a thoracoabdominal approach by extending a thoracic incision in the line of a rib across the costal margin, to join it. Radial incision of the diaphragm towards the oesophageal hiatus (left) or vena cava (right) throws the abdomen and thorax into one cavity and provides unparalleled access for oesophagogastrectomy and right hepatic lobectomy. Thoracolaparotomy may be indicated for removal of an enormous tumour of the kidney, adrenal or spleen.

9. *Posterolateral* incisions for approach to the kidney, adrenal and upper ureter are described in the relevant chapters.

Making the incision
1. Incise the skin with the belly of the knife. Cut cleanly down to the aponeurosis or muscle. Discard the knife.

2. Stop the bleeding. Firmly press each bleeding site with a swab, then remove the swab quickly and pick up the vessel with the minimum surrounding tissue. Use fine-toothed or non-toothed dissecting forceps, which are touched with the diathermy electrode to coagulate the vessel. Alternatively, use diathermy forceps. Bipolar diathermy ensures that current passes only between the two tips of the grasping forceps. In either case, be careful not to burn the skin when coagulating superficial vessels. Capture larger vessels with artery forceps and ligate them with fine absorbable suture material. As you tighten the first half-hitch, have your assistant smoothly release the forceps, removing them when he or she is confident that you have safely secured the vessel. Complete a reef knot. Have the ligature cut 2–3 mm beyond the knot for small vessels and 4–5 mm beyond, when tying larger vessels.

3. Apply wound towels to the skin edges, if these are to be used. Fix the towels with clips or stitches. Wound towels help to prevent contamination of the wound by the fluid contents of abdominal viscera. If you use them, make sure that if they become contaminated, they are immediately removed and replaced with fresh sterile towels.

4. Incise the aponeurosis with a clean knife in the line of the skin incision.

5. Cut, split or displace the muscles of the abdominal wall.

a. Cut the muscles with a knife or diathermy blade. When cutting the rectus muscle transversely, it helps to insinuate a pair of curved artery forceps beneath the muscle and then divide the fibres on to the forceps. Your assistant picks up vessels running vertically so that they can be ligated or coagulated.

b. Split the muscles if the fibres run in the line of the incision or in the gridiron and Lanz incisions.

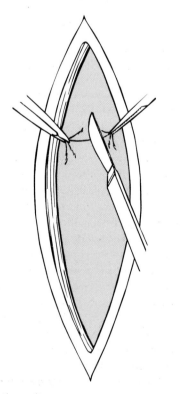

Fig. 4.3 Incising the peritoneum.

c. In a paramedian approach displace the rectus muscle laterally within its sheath. Cut the tendinous intersection free from the medial part of the sheath and draw the muscle belly laterally.

6. Stop the bleeding with diathermy coagulation or fine ligatures. Control persistent muscle bleeding by inserting a 2/0 absorbable stitch on a round-bodied needle, tying it just tightly enough to stop the bleeding and not so tight that it cuts through the muscle.

7. Open the peritoneum (Fig. 4.3).

Pick it up with toothed dissecting forceps and grip the tented portion with artery forceps. Release the artery forceps and reapply to the peritoneum. The change of grip allows the viscera to escape if they are caught by the first application of the forceps. Incise the peritoneum with the belly of the knife. Air enters the abdomen and the viscera fall clear. Insert the blades of non-toothed dissecting forceps and use them to lift the peritoneum clear of viscera. Complete the peritoneal opening with scissors with the deep blade protected between the blades of the dissecting forceps, taking care not to injure the abdominal contents.

REOPENING THE ABDOMEN

Appraise

1. Does the previous incision coincide with the site you would have chosen for present access? If so, reopen it. If not, ignore it and make a new incision in the correct site.

2. Remember that you may require a longer incision than would be necessary for an initial operation.

> **Key points**
>
> • If the previous incision is convenient there is little advantage in creating a fresh incision. As a rule you will need to dissect off adhesions from within. From a fresh incision you will see them only from one side. Moreover, if the new incision is parallel to the first, there is an intervening denervated panel.

Access through the old incision

1. Make an incision down the centre of the old scar. If the scar is ugly or stretched, excise it as an elongated ellipse.

2. Do not attempt to dissect out a previous paramedian incision, but cut through all the tissues in the line of the skin wound. Do not cut too boldly, because the deeper layers may be defective, so that you may quickly enter the cavity or even the contents of the abdomen.

3. When opening the peritoneum in the line of the previous incision, remember that viscera may be adherent to its undersurface. Entering the abdomen is greatly facilitated if you extend the wound at one end, so that unscarred peritoneum can be incised first. Alternatively incise the peritoneum slightly to one side of the old incision line.

4. Once the abdomen is opened, carefully extend the incision little by little. Ensure that you identify every structure you cut.

5. Ensure that you leave the abdominal wall and, if possible, the peritoneal lining intact so that you can achieve a satisfactory closure.

1. Do not inexorably separate firmly fixed structures through an incomplete incision. Either skirt around them so that they now remain attached to one side of the wound, or open the other end of the wound and approach them from a different direction.

2. Have the wound edge lifted with tissue-holding forceps and encircle the adherent structures to estimate the degree of fixity and the plane of cleavage between them and the original parietal peritoneum. At intervals in the dissection allow the structures to relax, assess progress and start again, possibly from a new approach. Use a scalpel or scissors, remembering never to cut what cannot be seen.

3. If you damage a structure, assess and repair the damage now. Check the repair at the end of the operation.

Access through a new incision

🔑 Key points

- Although this approach may be initially easier, remember that after a previous operation, viscera may be adherent to the parietal peritoneum anywhere.

Once the abdomen is opened at a distance from the previous incision, have the intervening abdominal wall lifted with retractors. Arrange for the light to be directed towards any structures attached to the previous scar. If necessary roll the patient slightly to one or other side, to improve access. Dissect adherent viscera from the undersurface of the old scar, frequently feeling around the other side.

Division of adhesions

1. Separation of adherent viscera from the wound edge has already been described. It can be an arduous and hazardous task, and the small bowel is particularly vulnerable to injury. If you enter the small-bowel lumen inadvertently, close the defect with two layers of fine absorbable sutures immediately, pausing only to free the damaged loop of bowel to facilitate closure. Try and limit contamination of the wound with intestinal contents by prompt use of the sucker and gauze swabs. If contamination occurs nevertheless, consider lavage of the wound and peritoneal cavity with warm saline.

2. It is not necessary to divide every single adhesion between viscera during every laparotomy; indeed such a policy would often be counterproductive. On the other hand, when the viscera are tangled together it can be difficult to progress with the operation until the normal anatomical relationships have been restored. Learn to recognize thick, fleshy band adhesions that could distort the small bowel and give rise to future symptoms. When operating for adhesion obstruction, it is usually best to take down the adhesions completely and replace the small bowel in an orderly fashion.

3. When dividing intra-abdominal adhesions, vary the point of attack but do not become aimless. Keep in mind the objects of the dissection:

a. to allow adequate exploration
b. to permit safe closure without fear of damaging the viscera
c. to prevent subsequent kinking or herniation of the bowel.

EXPLORATORY LAPAROTOMY

Appraise

1. Full exploration of the abdomen was in the past considered a normal part of most operations, provided that it did not result in the spread of infection or malignant disease. If a standard procedure was to be performed, then careful surgeons routinely explored the whole abdomen to ensure that the diagnosed condition was really the cause of symptoms and to exclude incidental conditions that might be noted or demand treatment. The improvement of diagnostic capability, in particular endoscopy and imaging methods, has eroded this principle. In procedures deliberately planned to be carried out through restricted access, wide exploration is impossible. For example, confidently diagnosed acute appendicitis, perforated peptic ulcer, the creation of a colostomy, the drainage of a localized abscess and the relief of biliary obstruction in patients with advanced pancreatic carcinoma are normally performed through limited incisions.

🔑 Key points

- In general, carefully explore the abdomen whenever possible. However, intraoperative use of high-frequency, high-resolution ultrasound promises to be a valuable diagnostic tool, even if the exploration has to be limited. In this way you will acquire a familiarity with the feel of normal structures. One of the most testing clinical decisions is to state that something is normal, so you must know what is the range of normality.

- Once an operation has been carried out, if symptoms continue or fresh features emerge, it is reassuring to know that other serious disease has been excluded.

2. In dealing with emergencies, a clearcut preoperative diagnosis may not be made and the decision is limited to the need for operation. In this case, exploration may be required to determine the cause of the presenting clinical features.

3. In patients who have extensive carcinoma, adhesions that are unlikely to cause obstruction or a localized abscess that has been adequately drained, obsessive exploration is detrimental.

4. Intraoperative ultrasound scanning promises to be a valuable diagnostic tool. Solid organs may contain lesions that are impalpable. Those lesions that have been detected by preoperative tests may not be located at operation. Intraoperative ultrasound scanning aids the display or biopsy of such lesions. Within diseased tissues it may be difficult to identify vital structures by conventional means.

5. Exploration of the abdomen is still occasionally carried out as an elective 'final' diagnostic procedure when patients have had inexplicable distressing or sinister symptoms. Improvement in diagnostic techniques has drastically reduced the indications but occasionally they are equivocal.

6. As previously emphasized, access to the abdominal cavity does not provide direct access to the site of most disease processes, such as

the lumen of the bowel, visceral ducts or blood vessels. For this reason do not try to replace careful endoscopy, radiology and other imaging techniques with laparotomy. A few diseases affect the peritoneal surfaces and some of these can be studied by peritoneal tap or diagnostic laparoscopy.

7. Sadly, patients are still occasionally explored for pain that is referred or which arises in the abdominal wall. Make sure that you have excluded sources of referred pain. If you suspect that the pain arises in the abdominal wall, try the effect of testing for tenderness with the abdominal wall relaxed and then tensed. The tensed muscles protect an internal source of pain from pressure. Tenderness remaining, or even increased, when the muscles are tensed strongly suggests an abdominal wall cause. The diagnosis is strengthened if the injection of local anaesthetic into the tender site gives relief – but warn the patient that the relief will be short-lived.

8. In the presence of unrevealed but clinically suspected intra-abdominal sepsis, time spent waiting for a series of increasingly complex list of investigations is often wasteful.

Key points

- In emergency circumstances, if you are in doubt, use the time during which you are resuscitating the patient to repeat the taking of the history and examination. The features may change!
- When in doubt, trust your clinical acumen rather than 'suggestive' results of investigations, or the results of investigations that are at odds with your clinical findings.

Access

Choice of incision

1. Never forget that the prime function of an incision is to provide safe access. Although important, unsightliness, liability to herniation and discomfort are side issues. Remember that incisions heal from the sides and not the ends.

2. Open the abdomen over the site of the suspected lesion, so far as the costal margin and iliac crest allow. Use one of the established types of laparotomy incision. Remember that the incision may need to be extended, particularly if you do not have a confident pre-operative diagnosis.

3. The choice of incision for a particular operation is listed in Table 4.1 and discussed in the chapter devoted to the relevant organ. The choice may vary according to circumstances. For example, some surgeons perform elective cholecystectomy through a transverse incision, which leaves an excellent scar, but prefer the greater flexibility of a vertical incision when tackling the gallbladder in an emergency or in the presence of obstructive jaundice. In emergency colonic surgery, bear in mind the possible need for an intestinal stoma when selecting the laparotomy incision.

4. In emergency laparotomy for unexplained peritonitis or abdominal trauma, use either a right paramedian incision or a midline incision that skirts the umbilicus. Place the incision more above or more below the umbilicus, depending on the probable site of disease or damage. Incisions that extend on either side of the umbilicus can readily be extended in either direction once the pathology is revealed.

5. Midline incisions are quicker to create (and close) than paramedian incisions, so prefer them in cases of rapid bleeding, such as ruptured spleen or leaking aortic aneurysm.

6. Be prepared to use a previous laparotomy incision if it is conveniently placed or can readily be extended to allow appropriate access. The technique of abdominal re-entry is described in the preceding section of this chapter.

Access within the abdomen

1. If, on entering the peritoneal cavity you find that the incision is likely to provide inadequate exposure, do not hesitate to extend it. If the incision proves to be inappropriate (e.g. a right Lanz incision for perforated peptic ulcer), close it and start again. Never be too proud to perform one or other of these manoeuvres. Disasters tend to occur when inexperienced surgeons struggle to complete an operation through the wrong incision.

2. Figure 4.4 illustrates ways in which certain common incisions can be extended to deal with unexpected lesions or intraoperative difficulties.

3. Remember that the position of the patient on the operating table can greatly affect exposure, particularly of organs at either end of the abdominal cavity. To approach the pelvic viscera ask the anaesthetist to tilt the table head-down (Trendelenburg position). Have the patient tilted head-up (reversed Trendelenburg) for access to the lower oesophagus and diaphragmatic hiatus. Rotating the table away from yourself facilitates an extraperitoneal approach to the ureter or lumbar sympathetic chain on your side. Rotation towards yourself when operating from the patient's right may improve access to the spleen. If you anticipate steep tilts in any direction, secure the patient adequately beforehand, using a pelvic strap and/or a support beneath the heels.

4. Nearly every laparotomy requires some retraction of the abdominal wall and adjacent viscera to expose the organ(s) in question. Retraction of the wound edge will assist the initial

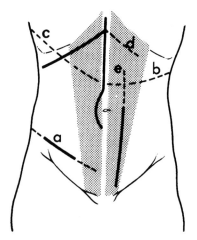

Fig. 4.4 Methods of extending certain abdominal incisions: (a) gridiron incision extended laterally and (to a greater extent) medially; (b) midline incision with T extension into left upper quadrant to deal with profuse splenic haemorrhage; (c) midline incision with T extension into the right chest for ruptured liver; (d) Kocher incision with left subcostal extension for major hepatic procedures; (e) left lower paramedian incision extended upwards for mobilization of left colic flexure.

exploratory laparotomy. When you have assessed the abdominal viscera and determined your operative strategy, insert retractor(s) and instruct your assistant(s) how to hold them. Pack away 'unwanted' organs, principally small-bowel loops, using large gauze swabs to which metal rings have been sewn, or large artery forceps attached, to minimize the risk of their being left in the abdomen during closure. The rings or forceps are attached to the packs by tapes, so that they can always hang outside the wound. These packs should be wrung out in warm physiological saline, and they are more effective at restraining the bowel if they are not completely unfolded.

5. Marshal the forces at your disposal carefully. Use of a self-retaining retractor may release an assistant to provide more direct help. Instruments of the De Bakey pattern have an optional third blade, which may help to keep the small bowel out of the pelvis. A sternal retractor is invaluable in operations on the abdominal oesophagus and upper stomach. The instrument hooks under the xiphisternum and is connected to a gantry over the patient's head.

6. Specific manoeuvres are either essential or extremely helpful in the exposure of certain organs. For access to the oesophagus and hiatus, mobilize the left lobe of liver by dividing its peritoneal attachment to the diaphragm. To examine fully the back wall of the stomach and the body of pancreas, you must enter the lesser sac, usually by dividing part of the gastrocolic or the gastrohepatic (lesser) omentum. For thorough examination of the duodenum, divide the peritoneum along the convexity of its loop (Kocher's manoeuvre). Displace the small bowel into the upper abdomen to approach the pelvic viscera and out of the abdominal cavity into a plastic bag for operations on the aorta.

Assess

1. If you are not wearing powder-free gloves, wash off the starch powder. Wash blood from the gloves. Deal with established adhesions.

2. Make sure that there are no instruments near the wound except for a retractor for your assistant and a sucker tube available for yourself. It is helpful to have someone in attendance to adjust the theatre light as necessary.

3. Carry out a methodical examination of the abdomen and its contents by feel and, whenever possible, by sight. Always follow the same sequence (Fig. 4.5):

a. right lobe of liver, gallbladder, left lobe of liver, spleen
b. diaphragmatic hiatus, abdominal oesophagus and stomach: cardia, body, lesser curve, antrum, pylorus and then duodenal bulb
c. bile ducts, right kidney, duodenal loop, head of pancreas; now draw the transverse colon out of the wound towards the patient's head
d. body and tail of pancreas, left kidney
e. root of mesentery, superior mesenteric and middle colic vessels, aorta, inferior mesenteric artery and vein, small bowel and mesentery from ligament of Treitz to ileocaecal valve
f. appendix, caecum, the rest of the colon, rectum
g. pelvic peritoneum, uterus, tubes and ovaries in the female, bladder
h. hernial orifices and main iliac vessels on each side. The ureters can sometimes be seen in thin patients, or if they are dilated.

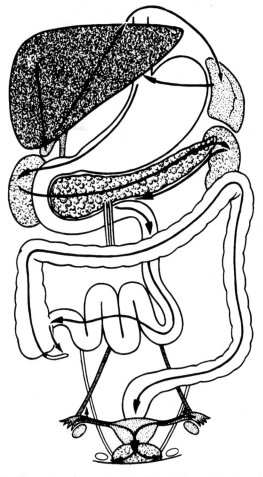

Fig. 4.5 The order of examining the abdominal contents at exploratory laparotomy.

4. Aim to carry out a thorough examination (as above) in most *elective* cases, and record your findings carefully and in detail. These principles are particularly important when laparotomy is the last of a series of investigations to identify the cause of symptoms. Sometimes the incision chosen precludes a complete exploration, for example in interval appendicectomy or pyloromyotomy in infancy. Sometimes the condition found makes further exploration pointless, for example in carcinomatosis peritonei. In this circumstance make a gentle search for the primary tumour, obtain a biopsy from one of the deposits, make sure no palliative procedure (e.g. intestinal bypass) is required and close the abdomen. As a general rule do not touch a malignant tumour more than is essential, for fear of dissemination.

5. In *emergency* laparotomy immediate action may be required, for example to stop bleeding or close a perforation. Thereafter, proceed to a methodical examination of the other viscera as before, unless the patient's general condition is poor or there is localized infection. Drainage of an abscess should usually be treated as a local condition. Do not forget to note the nature and amount of any free fluid, collecting some for chemical, cytological and microbiological examination. Obtain swabs for bacteriological culture of any potentially infected collection.

Action

1. In deciding the definitive procedure now to be undertaken, you will be guided by your preoperative knowledge of the patient, the extent of disease as revealed at laparotomy and the patient's age and general condition. Options include partial or total resection of an organ, bypass, drainage, exteriorization, closure of perforation, removal of foreign body, biopsy or perhaps no active procedure. In elderly or sick patients, control of the emergency or major elective condition should take precedence over the complete eradication of disease. Once you have formulated a plan of campaign, discuss your intentions with the anaesthetist and intimate how long you are likely to take to carry them out.

2. Be wary of tackling incidental procedures, such as prophylactic appendicectomy, without a clear indication. The chance finding of conditions such as gallstones, diverticula, fibroids or ovarian cysts does not automatically call for action unless they pose an immediate threat to health or offer a better explanation for symptoms than the condition originally diagnosed. By contrast, an unsuspected neoplasm should ordinarily be removed, if necessary through a separate incision, provided the patient's condition allows. Whatever course you adopt, be sure to record all your findings in the operation notes.

3. Remember that the interior of the distal small bowel and the entire large bowel is unsterile. Contents of hollow viscera that are normally sterile (e.g. bile, urine, gastric juice) may also become infected as a result of inflammation and obstruction. Before opening the bowel or other potentially contaminated viscera, isolate them from contact with the wound and other organs. Consider using non-crushing clamps to occlude the lumen, and make sure that you have an efficient suction apparatus to remove any contents that spill. Pack away other structures before opening the viscus and discard the packs once it is closed. Remember that all the instruments used on opened bowel become unsterile, therefore they must be isolated and subsequently discarded. Likewise, change your gloves before closing the abdomen.

4. The danger of infection is one of degree. Healthy tissues can normally cope with a small number of organisms but are overwhelmed by heavy contamination or re-infection. 'It should be axiomatic that reducing bacterial contamination reduces infection.'[1] In patients with impaired local host defences be sure to obtain culture specimens because they may be growing facultative organisms, particularly if they have had previous antibiotics. *Enterococcus* and *Candida* may be pathogens.[2] Generally, wounds are more susceptible to infection than the peritoneal cavity itself. If there has been gross spillage of infected visceral contents, wash out the abdominal cavity with warm saline and start broad-spectrum antibiotic therapy but be guided by the microbiologist in case of doubt.[3]

5. Intestinal clamps are of two types: crushing and non-crushing. *Crushing* clamps are applied to seal the bowel when it is cut. Payr's powerful double-action clamps are most frequently used, but Lang Stevenson devised a similar clamp with narrow blades. Cope's triple clamps allow the middle clamp to be removed, so that the bowel can be divided through the crushed area, leaving its ends sealed. *Non-crushing* clamps have longitudinal ridges and control the leakage of bowel contents without causing irreversible damage to the gut. Lane's twin clamps, which can be locked together, allow two pieces of gut to be occluded and held in apposition for anastomosis. Pringle's clamps hold cut ends of bowel securely, and the crushed segment is so narrow that it can safely be incorporated in the anastomosis.

6. The danger of leaving articles in the abdominal cavity is ever-present, but to do so in inexcusable. Unfortunately, there is no single routine that will entirely guard against this mishap. Always use the minimum number of instruments and the largest swabs, which remain attached to a large instrument lying outside the abdominal wound. Make sure they are never out of sight. As far as possible, use long-handled instruments for long-term holding, so that the handles protrude from the wound. Involve all your team in guarding against leaving an instrument or swab, even though you must accept the responsibility personally. If the scrub nurse reports a missing swab or instrument while you are closing the abdomen, check the peritoneal cavity once again. If all else fails, obtain an abdominal X-ray before letting the patient wake from the anaesthetic.

> #### 🔑 Key point
>
> - If this is an exploration for undiagnosed acute or chronic symptoms, or if the expected diagnosis is not confirmed and no cause is found, do not carry out any procedure. Resist the desire to 'do something'. You may give yourself a false sense of security, cause further complications or confuse the diagnosis. Having made sure you have overlooked nothing, close the abdomen and determine to record all your findings.

REFERENCES

1. Raahave D 1998 Wound contamination and post-operative infection. A review. Danish Medical Bulletin 38: 481–485
2. Farber MS, Abrams JH 1997 Antibiotics for the acute abdomen. Surgical Clinics of North America 77: 1395–1417
3. Bartlett JG 1995 Intra-abdominal sepsis. Medical Clinics of North America 79: 599–617

CLOSING THE ABDOMEN

Assess

1. Before starting to close, make sure that the swab and instrument counts are both correct. Check for haemostasis. Decide whether you need to drain the abdomen (see below). Remove any odds and ends of suture material and replace the viscera in their correct anatomical position.

> #### 🔑 Key point
>
> - Many needle-stick injuries are sustained during abdominal wall closure. Avoid using hand needles. However, even when using curved needles held in a needle holder, there is a danger of injury. A valuable development is the introduction of blunt tipped (often called 'Taper-point') needles, which nevertheless pass through the tissues but penetrate gloves and skin only if pressed fairly hard against them. Protect yourself. Do not risk acquiring a transmitted viral disease.

2. There are several different techniques for abdominal closure and three are described below. The choice depends upon the type of

incision, the extent of the operation, the patient's general condition and your preference. If you are a trainee, as you assist different surgeons you will learn various technical modifications and develop your own methods of closing the abdomen under differing circumstances. It is a common error among surgical trainees to sew up the abdomen too tightly, for fear it will fall apart. Remember that wounds swell during the first 3–4 postoperative days, oedema will make the sutures even tighter and there is a risk of tissue necrosis and subsequent dehiscence.

3. The most popular method of closure is now a continuous, spiralled, unlocked mass closure of the abdominal wall except for the skin and superficial fascia. The length of suture material used for the aponeurotic layer(s) should be at least four times the length of the incision, although this does not seem critical for lateral paramedian incisions. Place each suture 1 cm from the edge of the wound and 1 cm away from the previous 'bite'.

4. Select a strong non-absorbable suture material for closing the deeper (aponeurotic) layers of the abdominal wall; 1 monofilament nylon on a taper-point, round-bodied needle is very satisfactory in adults. Some surgeons use a doubled length of finer material (e.g. 0 nylon) and run the first stitch through the loop to avoid having a knot at the end of the wound. Synthetic polyglactin 910, polydioxanone or glycomer 631 (which are absorbable) have many adherents because they are less likely to produce chronic sinuses than non-absorbable nylon. With a long wound or an obese patient it may be more convenient to use two lengths of suture, starting at each end and meeting in the middle.

5. There is strong disagreement about the use of tension sutures. Proponents use them if the abdomen is distended or obese, if the wound is infected or likely to become so, if the patient is malnourished, jaundiced, suffering from advanced cancer or has a chronic cough – in short, in any situation where wound healing is prejudiced. It is likely that they have gained a poor reputation because the term 'tension' is often transferred to the tightness of the stitches; the suture is designed to withstand tension not to create it.

6. Remember that the abdominal wound is the only part of the operation that the patient can see, so take care to produce a neat result. Bury the knots used to tie off the deep sutures, especially in a thin patient. In an uncontaminated wound, aim for close apposition of the skin and a fine linear scar; therefore, consider using subcuticular sutures.

Action

Layered closure

1. Some surgeons do not bother to close the peritoneum, especially in a midline incision. There is a view that suturing the peritoneum encourages adhesions in response to the foreign material. Certainly there is little strength to this layer, and a new mesothelial lining develops to cover the defect from within. Where the posterior rectus sheath exists as a separate layer, as in paramedian, transverse and oblique incisions in the upper abdomen, the peritoneum can also be incorporated in the deepest layer of sutures. Use a continuous, unlocked spiral stitch so that the tension can be evenly distributed along the whole suture line.

2. Pick up the edges of the peritoneum and posterior rectus sheath, and apply one pair of artery forceps to these combined layers on each side of the wound and at each end. Make sure that the bowel is not caught. Have the assistant hold up the artery forceps, so that the peritoneum is lifted clear of the viscera as you insert each suture.

3. Starting at one or other end of the incision, take a bite on each side close to the apex and tie the knot securely. Make sure that the needle does not pick up bowel or omentum. Take generous bites with each stitch and pull up snugly but not tightly, passing it to your assistant to maintain the tension while the next stitch is inserted. Repeatedly tightening and loosening the suture has a sawing effect on the tissues and also tends to fray the stitch. After placing four or five stitches and gently and evenly tightening them, insert a finger to confirm that the bowel is free. Tie the knots securely, and do not have the ends shorter than 5 mm.

4. When muscles have been cut or split, unite them with interrupted 2/0 polyglactin 910, polydioxanone or lactomer 9-1 sutures. Tie the sutures just tightly enough to appose the edges. When the rectus muscle is cut transversely, it is not necessary to repair it with sutures because the tendinous intersections limit retraction. Similarly, in a paramedian incision, the rectus muscle falls back into place after closing the peritoneum and no sutures are required. If the muscle does not cover the posterior suture line, draw it medially by inserting stitches through the fibrous intersections and through the medial edge of the rectus sheath.

5. Repair the aponeurosis of external oblique or the anterior rectus sheath using slowly absorbed synthetic or non-absorbable suture such as polyamide. After tying the knot at the end of the incision, cut the end of suture material short and take the next bite from within to without; this manoeuvre will help to bury the knot. Once again, have the assistant maintain an even tension on the thread and avoid pulling up each suture so tightly that you strangle tissue.

6. Ensure that there is no oozing of blood in the superficial layers. Ligate or coagulate any residual bleeding vessels. If the subcutaneous tissues are deep, consider using a few interrupted fine 4/0 absorbable sutures to appose them.

7. Appose the skin edges, using one of several standard techniques. Interrupted sutures are preferable in a contaminated or irregular wound. Mattress sutures help to evert the skin edges slightly and bring together the deeper layers. Suitable suture materials include 2/0 black silk, 2/0 or 3/0 monofilament polyamide or polypropylene; skin clips and adhesive skin strips are alternatives. Some surgeons use a continuous over-and-over or continuous mattress suture routinely.

8. In a clean and straightforward wound, a very acceptable scar results following subcuticular suture, using 2/0 polypropylene. Insert the needle in the line of the incision about 1 cm away from its apex and bring it out through the apex in the subcuticular plane. Now continue along the incision taking small and frequent bites of the subcutis; avoid piercing the skin. When you reach the other end, bring the needle out through the skin about 1 cm beyond the apex of the incision. Tighten the suture material to close the wound and make sure that it runs freely. Fix the suture at each end with tiny lead weights, or tie the ends in a slack loop.

Mass closure

1. This simple, rapid technique can be used routinely or reserved for difficult cases. It is particularly useful when closing an incision through a previous scar, when the layers are often partly fused. The

peritoneum and rectus sheaths are closed together, or the linea alba may be closed in one layer without suturing the peritoneum.

2. Insert a continuous running stitch of 1 monofilament nylon mounted on a taper-pointed needle. Place the stitches 1–2 cm from the edges, 1–2 cm apart, catching all the included layers. Monofilament synthetic, slowly absorbable sutures may be successfully used.

3. Gently tighten the stitches as you proceed, checking that the bowel is free beneath. Do not let the stitch slip afterwards by getting your assistant to follow-up, but avoid undue tension. Make doubly sure the bowel is free before tightening and tying the last stitch. Cut the bristly ends of nylon short.

4. Close the skin as for layered closure.

Closure with tension sutures (Fig. 4.6)
1. Tension sutures usually pass through all layers of the abdominal wall, including the skin, so they can be removed subsequently. Alternatively they may be placed subcutaneously, where they remain permanently. Insert all the interrupted through-and-through sutures and tie them at the end. Use them to supplement a standard closure in poor-risk patients.

2. Use a strong non-absorbable suture material, such as 1 monofilament nylon, swaged to a curved taper-point needle. Take deep bites about 3 cm away from the edge of the wound, incorporating all layers. Be very careful neither to prick the bowel when inserting the stitches nor to trap it when tightening them. If possible always interpose the greater omentum between the wound and the small intestine to lessen this risk.

3. After inserting each deep tension suture, leave artery forceps attached to both ends of the suture while closing the deeper layers of the abdominal wall. Then tie the tension sutures to appose the skin and subcutaneous tissues. If skin is included, thread each suture over a length of polyethylene or rubber tubing to prevent it cutting in, and be particularly careful not to tie it too tightly. Complete the closure with a limited number of interrupted skin sutures.

4. If healing proceeds satisfactorily, remove the skin sutures 7–10 days postoperatively but leave the tension sutures for a further 2–4 days.

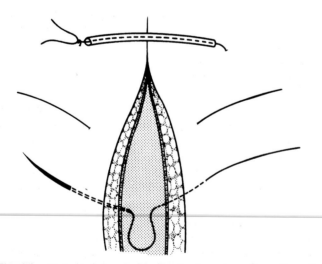

Fig. 4.6 Abdominal closure with deep tension sutures. Strong through-and-through sutures are placed 2–3 cm apart and tied over a protective polyethylene bar (after all sutures have been inserted).

Delayed closure
1. If the abdominal cavity is grossly contaminated, as in faecal peritonitis, some degree of wound sepsis is almost inevitable. One option is to close the superficial tissues lightly around a drain. Another is delayed primary suture, leaving the skin and subcutaneous tissue widely open. In either case give parenteral antibiotics and drain the peritoneal cavity. Consider also the possibility of postoperative lavage (see below).

2. Close the musculoaponeurotic layers of the abdominal wall with a continuous monofilament nylon suture. Be particularly careful not to draw the edges together too tightly, because considerable swelling can be anticipated. Superficial to this layer, loosely pack the wound with gauze swabs wrung out in saline.

3. Change the packs and inspect the wound daily. Delayed primary suture can be performed when the patient's condition improves and any wound sepsis has abated.

4. If peritonitis is particularly severe, for example after a major colonic perforation or resulting from infected pancreatic necrosis, it may be appropriate to leave the abdomen completely open as a

'laparostomy'. Make no attempt to close the abdominal wall. Cover the exposed viscera with moist gauze swabs and change them every 24–48 hours. In patients who survive the wound will shrink with time.

5. An alternative to attempted coverage with skin is to apply a clear, sterile plastic sheet after drawing down the omentum, if possible. Over this are laid sump drains. The whole is covered by a double layer of iodophor-impregnated adhesive sheet. It has been successfully used following trauma.

6. Yet another method is to use a zipper, with daily irrigations.

ABDOMINAL COMPARTMENT SYNDROME

Key point

- Compartment syndrome is a rise in intra-abdominal pressure from a wide variety of causes. It is a potentially fatal condition unless it is correctly diagnosed and managed.

Appraise

1. Peritonitis, intra-abdominal abscess, intestinal obstruction or paralytic ileus, tension pneumoperitoneum, mesenteric venous thrombosis, acute gastric dilatation, intra-abdominal haemorrhage, ascites, large neoplasm, peritoneal dialysis, laparoscopic procedure or abdominal wound closure under tension may provoke changes labelled 'abdominal compartment syndrome'. Other causes are massive visceral oedema, retroperitoneal haematoma and the need to pack the abdomen as a haemostatic measure.[1]

2. The physiological consequences are a rise in pulse rate and inferior vena cava pressure, with a fall in cardiac output, venous return and glomerular filtration rate. Blood pressure is not usually affected.

Action

1. Do not attempt to close the abdomen formally, or be prepared to reopen it if features develop of rising intra-abdominal pressure.

2. If possible, close the skin after drawing the greater omentum down over the viscera.

3. An alternative is to leave the fascia and skin open and cover the viscera with an absorbable or non-absorbable sheet. One such method is to use a Velcro®-like closure (HIDIH® Surgical, Doerrebach, Germany).

4. If the underlying condition can be corrected, the abdomen may be formally closed in 2–14 days

5. A longer delay may result in a defect requiring reconstruction, e.g. by bilateral advancement of the rectus muscles and fascia and by skin relaxing incisions to complete the closure.

REFERENCE

1. Schein M, Whittmann DH, Aprahamian CC, Condon RE 1995 The abdominal compartment syndrome; the physiological and clinical consequences of elevated intra-abdominal pressure. Journal of the American College of Surgeons 185: 745–753

DRAINS AND DRESSINGS

1. Tubular or corrugated drains of plastic or rubber may be inserted either through the end of the wound or through a separate stab hole in the abdominal wall. The inner end of the drain is placed in the region of the operation site to evacuate blood and any other fluid contents from the peritoneal cavity. Fine-bore polyethylene tube drains are now available, which can be screwed to a special trocar for insertion through the abdominal wall. They have many tiny drainage holes, all of which should be placed within the peritoneum, and they can be connected to a vacuum bottle or bag to maintain suction down the tube.

2. Other tube drains can be used to drain certain viscera to the exterior during the postoperative period. Again, insert these through a separate stab incision. Examples are a T-tube into the bile duct, a gastrostomy or suprapubic cystostomy catheter and a feeding jejunostomy tube.

3. Stitch the drain to the skin. When possible, insert a large safety pin through the drain to prevent any possibility of it being lost within the abdomen. If a drainage tube is attached to a closed bag or suction apparatus, tie the stitch securely around the tube.

4. Apply dressings to seal the main wound, with separate dressings over the drain wound. The drain may then be re-dressed, shortened and removed without disturbing the main wound.

5. Opinions differ widely concerning the use of drains following laparotomy. Drains rarely do harm when properly inserted, provided they are removed after about 48 hours if there is no discharge. A closed drainage system should not introduce infection. Insertion of a drainage tube is no substitute for good operative technique, however. Some generally accepted indications for draining the peritoneal cavity are as follows:

a. after operations on the gallbladder, bile duct or pancreas, in case there is leakage of bile or pancreatic juice
b. when there is a localized abscess
c. after suture of a perforated viscus, such as stomach, duodenum or colonic diverticulum, when the tissues are friable. Consider if another operative manoeuvre would give greater safety
d. when there is a large raw area from which oozing can occur. Do not make insertion of a drain an excuse for failure to control bleeding, however
e. sometimes after operations for general peritonitis, even if you have removed the cause.

6. Wound drains are occasionally indicated in very obese patients or grossly contaminated wounds. A thin corrugated drain or a tube suction drain is inserted deep to the skin and subcutaneous tissues and removed after 2–3 days or when it ceases to discharge.

7. Dressings are also controversial. From a bacteriological standpoint it probably makes little difference whether the wound is occluded by a dressing or left open to the atmosphere. Transparent adhesive dressings have the advantage of allowing the surgeon to inspect the wound repeatedly without disturbing the dressing. If a good deal of discharge is anticipated, use dressing gauze and wool. Remember that some patients are sensitive to adhesive strapping.

8. If primary closure of the superficial layers is not possible, or is inadvisable because of tension, skin loss or contamination, avoid

applying hydrocolloid dressings if the wound could be contaminated with anaerobic organisms.

Lavage

1. The peritoneal cavity has a remarkable ability to combat sepsis. None the less, spillage of contaminated contents, such as faeces or infected bile, may lead to early septicaemia and late abdominal abscess.

2. Where local peritonitis is marked, scrupulously remove all pus and debris from that part of the abdomen. Consider washing out the area with aliquots of warm saline (c. 500 ml in toto), sucking out the fluid and inserting a drain. The theoretical risk of disseminating the infection through the peritoneal cavity does not appear to hold true in practice.

3. In generalized peritonitis, thoroughly clean the abdomen with warm saline (1–2 litres) at the end of the operation. In very severe cases (e.g. pancreatic necrosis, faecal peritonitis), consider inserting one or two delivery tubes and one or two drainage tubes for postoperative lavage. One drainage tube is placed in the abscess cavity and one in the pelvis; soft, wide-bore, silicone tubes or sump drains are appropriate. Use warmed (37°C) peritoneal dialysis fluid (Dialaflex 61) with added potassium for lavage, irrigating between 50 and 200 ml per hour, depending on the extent of sepsis. Try and obtain a water-tight closure of the abdominal wound and start with small amounts of dialysate (50 ml/h) overnight, until the peritoneum seals the defects. Postoperative lavage is well tolerated and does not seem to interfere with intestinal motility. Continue the treatment for up to 2 weeks and remove the drains when the return fluid becomes clear.

4. As an alternative to abdominal closure with lavage, the laparotomy incision can be left open in patients with necrotizing pancreatitis or severe faecal peritonitis.

BURST ABDOMEN

Appraise

1. Wound dehiscence results from poor healing, excessive strain on the wound or poor closure technique. Septicaemia, abdominal wound contamination, haematoma or seroma, advanced neoplasia, diabetes, uraemia, jaundice, hypoproteinaemia, steroid or cytotoxic therapy can all impair healing. Abdominal distension from intestinal obstruction, intraperitoneal ascites, unresectable tumour or following loss of abdominal wall may place an excessive strain on the wound closure. However, the remarkably low rate of wound dehiscence reported by some surgeons tends to discount the importance of impaired healing or excess strain. Indict technical failure. The suture material may be incorrectly selected, damaged by crushing or abrasion, imperfectly inserted, overtightened, improperly knotted or trimmed too short at the knots. Layered closure appears to be associated with a higher incidence of burst abdomen than mass closure.

2. Suspect impending wound dehiscence if the patient's abdomen remains silent in the absence of an obvious cause, often accompanied by a low-grade unexplained pyrexia. A premonitory sign is the discharge of slightly bloodstained serous fluid from the wound.

3. Dehiscence usually declares itself 7–14 days postoperatively following straining or the removal of the sutures. The patient feels something 'give' and may partially eviscerate. Burst abdomen is rarely painful; the patient is apprehensive but seldom shocked. The skin may remain healed, but as the patient strains the wound bulges.

If the patient is managed conservatively, the skin may remain healed, leaving an incisional hernia.

Prepare

1. Reassure the patient; explain that the wound has given way.

2. Cover the wound with large sterile packs held in place with an encircling bandage or corset or using adhesive, elastic strips.

3. For most patients immediate reoperation is indicated, in which case give the premedication now and pass a nasogastric tube to aspirate the stomach.

Action

1. Dissect the skin and subcutaneous tissues from the aponeurotic layer on each side to clear 2 cm of aponeurosis (or muscle). Similarly, free the omentum and bowel for a short distance on the deep aspect of the wound on each side.

2. Insert deep tension sutures, as described in the previous section. Pass each suture through all layers of the abdominal wall, including the skin. Allow 3–4 cm between tension sutures.

3. Now proceed with mass closure of the peritoneum and rectus sheath or the linea alba. Some surgeons prefer to use interrupted stitches of a strong nonabsorbable material. Be certain to take deep bites of tissue, using plenty of suture material, and again avoid tension on the wound. Although recurrent burst abdomen is rare, pulling too tightly on strong thread passed through damaged tissue provokes stitches to cut out.

4. Whether continuous or interrupted sutures are employed, take great care not to incorporate the viscera in any of the stitches. If possible, draw the omentum down over the abdominal contents.

5. Now loosely tie the deep tension sutures, once more remembering that they are there to resist tension, not to cause it.

6. Close the skin fairly loosely and consider using a superficial wound drain. In the presence of gross wound sepsis, leave the skin unsutured and place sterile packs on the deep wound closure. Carry out delayed suture when the wound is clean, graft the area, or allow the wound to heal by granulation.

7. A many-tailed bandage or an elastic corset provides extra support.

LAPAROTOMY FOR ABDOMINAL TRAUMA

See Chapter 3.

LAPAROTOMY FOR GENERAL PERITONITIS

Appraise

1. The parietal peritoneum is locally irritated by contact with inflamed organs such as the appendix, gallbladder, colon with a segment of diverticulitis, or uterine salpinx. It is irritated by chemical contact from gastric acid, urine, bile, activated pancreatic enzymes, bowel content, blood or foreign materials such as talc and starch. It becomes intensely inflamed by contact with pus or material infected with microorganisms such as infected bile, faecal leakage and bowel content exuding from gangrenous bowel.

2. If the patient becomes septicaemic the temperature may fall

and multisystem failure can develop. Features often change rapidly, so be prepared to repeat the assessment at intervals in case of doubt.

3. Immunocompromised patients such as those suffering from AIDS present particular diagnostic problems including toxic megacolon, which may perforate, or appendicitis caused by cytomegalovirus (CMV). Atypical mycobacterial infection is also reported.

4. Very occasionally generalized peritonitis develops in the absence of any overt visceral disease. Primary peritonitis can occur spontaneously in children and seems to be commoner in patients with ascites or nephrotic syndrome. The pneumococcus is one of the commoner infecting organisms.

Decide

In the past many surgeons made only one decision – whether or not to operate on the acute abdomen. We frequently still have to fall back on the aphorism, 'It's better to look and see than wait and see'. There are times when delay is vacillation and others when precipitate action offers an excuse for not thinking the problem through.

Prepare

1. Restore the patient's fluid, electrolyte and acid/base balance intravenously.

2. Pass a nasogastric tube and aspirate the stomach.

3. As far as possible, assess and correct incidental medical conditions, in particular cardiorespiratory disease.

4. Start parenteral antibiotic therapy with a third generation cephalosporin together with an aminoglycoside and metronidazole. The organisms found within the abdomen are often not those expected, particularly in critically ill patients. *Candida albicans*, *Enterococcus* sp. and *Staphylococcus epidermidis* are more common than most surgeons suspect, so the antibiotic range may need to be broadened.

Access

If there are no localizing signs, use a midline or right paramedian incision placed half above and half below the umbilicus. Be prepared to extend it in either direction once the lesion is revealed. Examination of the abdomen under anaesthetic may reveal an unsuspected mass, which helps you to site the incision correctly in the first place.

Assess

1. Note any free fluid or pus and save a specimen for laboratory examination.

2. After a rapid preliminary examination of the abdomen, carry out a methodical exploration.

Action

> **Key point**
>
> • In all emergency operations and operations carried out on ill patients, never lose sight of the object of the procedure. You are operating for a specific reason. Do not indulge in unnecessary 'heroic' procedures – it is not you who is being heroic. It is the patient who will need to be courageous afterwards. Nevertheless, remember that you must assiduously and fully correct the cause of the condition, though by the simplest and most effective means.

1. Make sure that the incision, the assistance and the instruments available are adequate for the proposed procedure.

2. Resect an inflamed appendix, gallbladder, segment of gangrenous or damaged bowel, perforated neoplasm or Meckel's diverticulum.

3. Repair ruptured small bowel or a leaking suture line from a previous operation. Close a perforated peptic ulcer. Consider definitive procedures such as proximal gastric vagotomy only in appropriate patients with a long history of indigestion who are fit and would merit elective surgical treatment before the perforation occurred. Such patients are now rare.

4. Resect a specimen of perforated colon, but be very cautious about restoring intestinal continuity without a proximal diverting colostomy. Resection with exteriorization of the bowel ends is an even safer option. Closure of a perforated sigmoid diverticulum with or without transverse colostomy may be appropriate in selected cases, but perforated carcinomas should be resected if possible.

5. Make sure no dead or ischaemic tissue remains.

6. Remove any foreign bodies from the peritoneal cavity. Consider saline lavage and postoperative drainage if there is gross infection or contamination with intestinal contents. Drain an abscess.

7. Normally take no definitive action if you encounter acute pancreatitis, acute salpingitis, uncomplicated ileitis or primary peritonitis. Consider whether a biopsy (e.g. of a lymph node in Crohn's disease) or bacteriological culture swab (e.g. of the uterine tube) might provide useful information.

8. If there has been extensive contamination, carefully wash out the peritoneal cavity using sterile normal saline at body temperature, repeating this until the aspirate is clear.

9. Some surgeons continue lavage after operation by inserting an inflow catheter and a pelvic sump drain. If you use this method, carefully chart and monitor fluid balance.

10. Drains usually drain for a few hours to drain exudate, although they occasionally drain for much longer.

LAPAROTOMY FOR INTESTINAL OBSTRUCTION

Appraise

1. The diagnosis of intestinal obstruction is not always easy to make, nor is it an automatic indication for operation. The features may be indefinite and sometimes fleeting, so that a once-for-all history-taking and examination are often misleading. Classically there are four cardinal features – colic, distension, vomiting and constipation – but the prominence of each of these is affected by the site and type of obstruction.

> **Key point**
>
> • Intestinal obstruction is not a once-for-all diagnosis. Examine the patient generally, locally and rectally at intervals to identify localizing features and indications that there may be strangulation, sepsis, perforation or other associated conditions in what appeared to be straightforward mechanical obstruction.

2. Classically, it is possible to distinguish strangulation from simple obstruction because there is residual pain between bouts of

colic. Of course there may also be tenderness but this is often detectable at the site of simple obstruction. There may also be guarding and rigidity but this is frequently a late sign as are increasing tachycardia, pyrexia, hypovolaemic shock and a rising white cell count. These features may also be produced by perforation and infection. Do not delay. Carry out a rapid assessment of the likely cause, correct the patient's fluid, electrolyte and acid/base balance, administer versatile antibiotics intravenously and proceed with exploratory laparotomy.

3. Perhaps the most difficult diagnostic problem is postoperative obstruction following abdominal surgery. The history and physical signs are atypical because they are added to the expected postoperative delay in function, discomfort, wound pain, tenderness and tensely held abdominal wall.

🔑 Key point

- It is often said that early obstruction is usually less significant than later obstruction. Too often the more serious late obstruction is the continuing missed early obstruction.

Prepare

It is rarely beneficial to embark on immediate operation. Some conditions respond to conservative treatment, some require further assessment. The condition of the patient must be restored as much as possible, both from the effects of the obstruction and from any underlying disease.

Access

Make a midline incision half above and half below the umbilicus and at least 15 cm long, unless the site of obstruction is known. Alternatively, use a right paramedian incision of similar length.

Assess

1. Aspirate any free fluid after obtaining a bacteriological specimen.

2. Insert your hand and gently explore the abdomen. Identify the caecum; if it is collapsed, the obstruction lies within the small bowel.

Action

Small bowel obstruction

1. Release the obstruction if possible. Divide adhesions and bands. Reduce an internal hernia or overlooked external hernia or volvulus of the small bowel. If the bowel is grossly distended, empty it before closing the abdomen.

2. Pause if strangulated bowel has been released. When the blood vessels are constricted the low pressure veins are occluded first; as arterial blood pumps in, the small vessels distend with blood that stagnates, losing its oxygen. If the constriction is released now, the dark, congested bowel rapidly improves in colour. If constriction continues, however, the distended small vessels rupture and blood leaks into the interstitial tissues, including the subserosa. Do not then expect the colour to improve greatly when the vascular occlusion is released; it will take days for the extravasated blood to be removed. The bowel may still appear purple or black. Provided it retains its sheen and the supplying blood vessels pulsate, it usually survives, although the most metabolically active layer, the mucosa, may ulcerate and possibly form a stricture when it heals. The critical site to examine is the bowel wall where it has been included in the constricting band or ring. It is usually white from ischaemia, but if it soon regains its colour it may safely be left. Any small doubtful area can be invaginated with a few seromuscular stitches. If the colour of the constriction rings fails to improve at all, or if they are green or purple in colour, excise the segment, ensure the remaining bowel ends are well supplied with blood and carry out an anastomosis.

3. Sometimes a knuckle of small bowel that has been trapped in an internal or external hernia will spontaneously reduce itself. If you observe constriction rings, look for the possible site of hernia and try to close the defect. Constriction rings that remain slightly ischaemic may be invaginated by Lembert sutures.

4. Resect the obstructed bowel if there is a neoplasm or if the bowel or its blood supply are damaged. Massive resection may be necessary if the main vessels are blocked; consider embolectomy in selected patients.

5. Bypass the obstruction if it cannot be removed.

6. Break up, push on or remove intraluminal obstruction such as a food bolus, gallstone or collection of worms.

7. Reduce an intussusception. Resect a polyp or other pathological lesion at the apex of the intussusception (usually in adults).

8. Stricture resulting from Crohn's disease is conventionally treated by resection and anastomosis. In recent years a much more conservative policy has become popular, supported by the fact that what appear to be unaffected healthy segments of bowel are already histologically diseased. For this reason resection of strictures is kept as short as possible, transgressing macroscopically diseased but unstrictured bowel. For short segments, strictureplasty seems to be satisfactory. The operation is performed after the fashion of a Heineke–Mikulicz pyloroplasty; the bowel is incised longitudinally throughout the length of the stricture and opened out so that the incision can be closed to produce a horizontal suture line.

9. If no other relief can be given, be prepared on occasion to create a proximal stoma as a terminal palliative measure, rather than leave a patient obstructed and vomiting without relief.

Large bowel obstruction

1. Release an external cause of obstruction. Sometimes a loop of small bowel is adherent to an inflammatory diverticular mass and requires release.

2. A diverticular mass may totally obstruct the sigmoid colon. The conventional method of overcoming this is to perform loop transverse colostomy with subsequent resection of the diseased segment electively and, at a third stage, close the colostomy. If a resection is performed, a temporary terminal iliac colostomy can be formed, and the lower cut end is closed over and dropped back into the pelvis (Hartmann's procedure).

3. Resect an obstructing carcinoma of the caecum, ascending colon or transverse colon, and restore continuity by end-to-end ileocolostomy.

4. Traditionally, obstructing carcinoma of the sigmoid colon and rectum is treated in three stages, the first stage being transverse colostomy. Subsequently elective colectomy is performed and finally the colostomy is closed. Occasionally this is still the best choice. However, many patients are elderly and some have a short life expectation. The three-stage procedure erodes their remaining life, and there is a high failure rate to complete the full restoration to normal function.

5. If the obstruction is not gross it is sometimes feasible to carry out primary resection and anastomosis.

6. In gross obstruction, always carefully inspect the caecum, since if it is overdistended it may perforate or develop gangrene and subsequently burst. In case of doubt perform a caecostomy.

7. Bypass an irresectable carcinoma of the right colon by ileotransverse colostomy. Bypass an irresectable carcinoma of the left colon by colocolostomy if possible. Relieve unresectable obstructing carcinoma of the distal colon or rectum by means of a transverse loop colostomy or left iliac colostomy. If you carry out a terminal left iliac colostomy, bring the lower cut end to the surface as a mucous fistula. If you close it, you have left a closed loop above the obstructing carcinoma.

8. Always obtain a biopsy specimen if you do not resect the carcinoma.

9. Untwist a volvulus. Have a rectal tube in place so that the distended bowel can be deflated.

10. Move on, break up or remove intraluminal obstruction such as a faecolith.

11. Ischaemic colitis that obstructs is best resected and the ends brought to the surface, because it is difficult to be sure how much of the colon will survive.

12. Never forget the purpose of this emergency operation. Do not perform any procedure that does not fulfil this purpose.

Closure

This can be difficult if the abdomen is distended. Take care to avoid injuring dilated loops of small bowel. Consider inserting tension sutures if abdominal distension is gross.

Difficulty?

1. In the presence of grossly distended bowel, do not flounder within the abdomen through an inadequate incision. Extend the incision and gently deliver the entire small bowel. Consider decompressing the small bowel by means of a special sucker. Decompress the upper small bowel by milking contents back up to within reach of the nasogastric tube, and try to manoeuvre this tube through the pylorus into the duodenum or jejunum.

2. Sometimes adhesions prevent easy delivery of the small bowel or produce an apparently inextricable tangle. Such cases can be very testing. Settle down to a prolonged dissection. Make sure that the incision is adequate for you to visualize the restraining bands, which should then be divided. Patiently disentangle all adherent loops and run the whole small bowel through your hands to make sure it is unravelled.

LAPAROTOMY FOR GASTROINTESTINAL BLEEDING

Appraise

1. Ideally, manage patients with gastrointestinal bleeding jointly with a gastroenterological physician with whom you have an agreed policy.

2. Never fail to carry out a thorough examination including rectal examination, proctoscopy and sigmoidoscopy. The availability of more complex methods of investigation sometimes beguiles clinicians into forgetting basic manoeuvres. Consider the possibility that the condition may result from a bleeding or clotting disorder, parasitic infestation, Peutz–Jeghers syndrome or drug therapy. Order appropriate tests. Consider the possibility of the patient suffering from AIDS.

3. The availability of superb flexible endoscopes has dramatically improved diagnostic ability.

There is a wide choice of endoscopic methods for controlling bleeding.

Prepare

1. As you assess the patient, initiate appropriate resuscitation. Do not place too much reliance on the initial haemoglobin and haematocrit results because they are affected by physiological blood dilution.

2. Operations for the control of severe gastrointestinal bleeding require to be performed by experienced surgeons backed by expert anaesthetists and a trained team of assistants. If you are not experienced in this very demanding field, urgently seek help.

3. Never take a patient to the operating theatre without having available fibreoptic endoscopes.

Access

Make a midline or right paramedian incision, sited in the upper or lower abdomen according to the preoperative diagnosis or midway if this is uncertain (see p. 93).

Assess

1. Blood in the lumen can be recognized from without owing to the bluish-black coloration of the gut. The distribution of blood in the stomach, small bowel and colon may roughly localize the site of bleeding, but remember that blood can travel for a considerable distance proximal as well as distal to the lesion.

2. Inspect and palpate the alimentary canal from oesophagus to rectum.

Action

1. If there is evidence of *upper* gastrointestinal bleeding, concentrate on the stomach, duodenum and jejunum.

2. If there is evidence of *lower* gastrointestinal bleeding, concentrate on the colon and ileum. The site of bleeding can be difficult to identify in the intestine.

Key point

- Never forget the purpose of the operation. It is to control life-threatening bleeding and prevent it from recurring. Do not perform any procedure outside this purpose. Do not, for example, carry out a definitive operation for peptic ulcer, unless it is vital to accomplish your purpose. Chronic peptic ulcer is amenable to non-operative treatment.

FURTHER READING

Adams ID, Chan M, Clifford PC et al 1986 Computer-aided diagnosis of acute abdominal pain: a multicentre study. British Medical Journal 293: 800–804

Ausobsky JR, Evans M, Pollock AV 1985 Does mass closure of midline laparotomies stand the test of time? A random control trial. Annals of the Royal College of Surgeons of England 67: 159–161

Bucknall TE 1983 Factors influencing wound complications. A clinical and experimental study. Annals of the Royal College of Surgeons of England 65: 71–77

Couch NP, Tilney NL, Rayner AA, Moore FD 1981 The high cost of low frequency events. The anatomy and economics of surgical mishaps. New England Journal of Medicine 304: 634–637

De Dombal FT, Leaper DJ, Horrocks JC et al 1974 Human and computer-aided diagnosis of abdominal pain: further report with emphasis on performance of clinicians. British Medical Journal i: 376–380

Editorial 1980 Peritonitis today. British Medical Journal 280: 1095–1096

Irvin TT 1989 Abdominal pain: a surgical audit of 1190 emergency admissions. British Journal of Surgery 76: 1121–1125

Jenkins TRN 1976 The burst abdominal wound: a mechanical approach. British Journal of Surgery 63: 873–876

Jones PF, Krukowski ZH, Young GG 1998 Emergency abdominal surgery, 3rd edn. Chapman and Hall, London

Kirk RM 1990 Chronic and recurring abdominal pain. Transactions of the Medical Society of London 105: 1–4

Kirk RM 1990 Reoperation for early intra-abdominal complications following abdominal and abdominothoracic operations. Hospital Update 16: 303–310

Paterson-Brown S 1991 Strategies for reducing inappropriate laparotomy rate in the acute abdomen. British Medical Journal 303: 1115–1118

Sawyer RG, Rosenlof LK, Adams RB et al 1992 Peritonitis into the 1990s: changing pathogens and changing strategies in the critically ill. American Surgeon 58: 82–87

Williamson RCN, Cooper MJ (eds) 1990 Emergency abdominal surgery. Churchill Livingstone, Edinburgh

Principles of minimal access surgery

A. Darzi and P. A. Paraskeva

GENERAL PRINCIPLES OF LAPAROSCOPY

1. Minimal access surgery (MAS) is surgery is intended to cause the least anatomical, physiological and psychological trauma to the patient. The rapid advancements in this type of surgery since the late 1980s have seen the dawning of an age of surgical technological innovation. It would not have been possible without the simultaneous development of improved methods of imaging to replace the traditional 'hands in' method of open surgery assessment.

2. Along with these developments it has been recognized that adequate education and training in minimal access techniques combined with well considered pre- and postoperative care are essential for successful application of these new approaches.

3. Many surgical and gynaecological procedures are regularly performed using a minimal access approach. Table 5.1 shows examples of the uses of therapeutic laparoscopy. The majority of the discussion in this chapter will be related to laparoscopy.

4. Minimal access surgery has had implications for the economics of hospitals offering surgical services. Capital equipment is expensive and requires regular servicing to ensure good working standards. Consumables are particularly expensive, and reusing equipment may prejudice performance. Theatre times are increased initially, although they decrease as the surgeons gain experience. Short-stay and 5-day wards with rapid turnover reduce 'hotel' costs, freeing main ward beds and helping to reduce waiting lists.

5. All members of the surgical team need adequate training in the techniques and care of the equipment. This has led to the establishment of minimal access therapy training units (MATTUs) offering basic and higher training courses with availability to senior surgeons trained in open surgery.

Appraise

Advantages

a. Allows operations to be performed through small incisions in body cavities
b. Procedures are less disabling by causing less postoperative pain and discomfort
c. Decreased wound-related pathology, e.g. wound infection
d. Decreased tissue trauma
e. Decreased physiological insult to the patient when compared to open surgery
f. Earlier return to full activity
g. Significantly reduced stay in hospital postoperation, leading to cost-effectiveness
h. Cosmetic acceptability
i. Decreased direct surgeon contact with pathogens such as

Table 5.1 Examples of minimal access surgery

General surgery
Diagnostic laparoscopy
Cholecystectomy
Choledochoscopy
Hernia repair
Adhesiolysis
Nissen's fundoplication
Repair of perforated duodenal ulcer
Appendicectomy
Excision of Meckel's diverticulum
Rectopexy
Splenectomy
Vagotomy
Colectomy

Gynaecology
Oophorectomy
Treatment of ectopic pregnancy
Hysterectomy
Diagnosis and ablation of endometriosis
Ovarian cystectomy
Myomectomy
Tubal surgery
Infertility treatment

Others
Arthroscopy
Ureteroscopy
Cystoscopy

human immunodeficiency virus (HIV) and hepatitis B virus (HBV)
j. The use of video records aids in the art of communication between doctors and with patients and their families. It may also help improve clinical decision-making.

Disadvantages

a. Lack of tactile feedback from tissues, which is taken for granted in open surgery, is lost. You must rely completely on hand–eye co-ordination
b. Bleeding is difficult to control, because of the confined working environment and blood obscuring the view obtained through the endoscope

c. Procedures take longer, especially on the initial slope of the surgical learning curve

d. Technical expertise, advice and specialist equipment is required for minimal access surgery, all of which increase the cost of the procedures. Additional training and equipment costs have to be placed against the benefits of reduced hospital stay and quicker return to activity

e. Iatrogenic damage has been a greater problem following minimal access surgery than following traditional open techniques, for example bile duct injuries during laparoscopic cholecystectomy

f. There is concern about the reported incidence of metastases at laparoscopic port sites after operations for malignant disease.

Absolute contraindications

a. Generalized peritonitis
b. Intestinal obstruction
c. Clotting abnormalities
d. Liver cirrhosis
e. Failure to tolerate general anaesthesia
f. Uncontrolled shock
g. Patient refusal.

Relative contraindications

a. Gross obesity. Simple overweight is no contraindication; such patients suffer less from postoperative respiratory complications than they would following open surgery
b. Pregnancy
c. Multiple abdominal adhesions. Provided the first instrument port is inserted by an open technique, laparoscopy can be safely performed on patients with moderate adhesions following, for example, previous surgery
d. Organomegaly (enlarged liver or spleen)
e. Abdominal aortic aneurysm.

Prepare

1. Admit patients before or on the day of planned surgery. Preoperative evaluation and investigations can be performed in a preadmission clinic. The patient's fitness may be graded using the ASA (American Association of Anesthesiologists) assessment. Those in grades 1 and 2 are fit for day surgery; grade 3 patients require anaesthetic evaluation.

2. Obtain informed consent, including permission to convert to open operation if necessary. Warn patients that they may experience postoperative shoulder tip pain and also surgical emphysema.

3. In the absence of contraindications give antithrombotic prophylaxis such as low-dose heparin and compression stockings. Give prophylactic antibiotics if organs such as the gallbladder are to be removed. Bowel preparation is not necessary.

4. Some anaesthetists prefer nonsteroidal anti-inflammatory drugs rather than opiates as premedication, if necessary with the addition of short-acting benzodiazepines.

5. *Equipment*:

a. The monitors should be large, with good-quality high-resolution screens, mounted on a mobile trolley also containing the light source, insufflator and camera. Position the monitors on either side of the patient, allowing you and your assistants to view them (Fig. 5.1).

You should be able to see the light source, usually xenon or halogen, and monitor the light intensity. Ensure that the patient is not at risk of burning. Have the rapid-flow insufflator, which supplies carbon dioxide to create and maintain the pneumoperitoneum, placed so you can see the display of the intra-abdominal pressure and gas flow in response to preset pressure values. It may also incorporate a gas warmer.

b. The video camera head, either a single microchip or a superior three-chip instrument, is attached to the laparoscope to form an electrical/optic interface. The camera is connected by cable to a video processor which interprets and modifies the signal and transmits it to the monitors. Most systems incorporate a 'white balance' function, which can be calibrated to represent the colours accurately.

c. The laparoscope transmits the image using a rod-lens system while the field is illuminated through fibreoptics running alongside the lens. They are usually 10 mm (or less often 5 mm) in diameter with fields of view of 0° or 30°. For cholecystectomy a 10 mm, 0° laparoscope is usually employed. Check the function. It should be warmed to prevent fogging of the lens. For the same reason do not insufflate cold carbon dioxide through the same port as the camera. Ensure that the camera operator will follow your movements and keep the area of interest in the centre of the field of view.

d. Suction and irrigation are carried out through a probe connected to a pressurized reservoir and a suction source, controlled by buttons.

e. The ports for insertion of instruments can be disposable or reusable. More expensive disposable ports have the advantage of being sharp, radiolucent and sterile. They may have blunt ends for

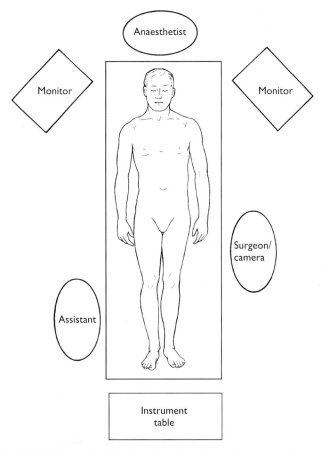

Fig. 5.1 Diagram showing the positioning of the patient, surgeon, assistant and video monitors for a laparoscopic cholecystectomy.

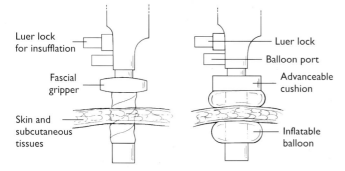

Fig. 5.2 Diagram of two types of laparoscopic port, one with a screw collar and the second with inflatable balloons; both help to prevent gas leaks around the ports.

open induction of pneumoperitoneum, or be fitted with a sharp, spring-loaded trocar with a plastic guard that projects beyond the point as soon as the trocar enters the peritoneal cavity. They are of a range of sizes to accommodate various instruments but large ports can be fitted with sizers to reduce the lumen. All have attachments to allow insufflation and valves to prevent gas leaks. Some have collars, allowing them to be secured in position (Fig. 5.2).

f. In the closed method of insufflation a Veress needle is inserted. This incorporates a spring-loaded obturator that covers the sharp needle tip as soon as it enters the peritoneal cavity. It incorporates an attachment to the gas supply (Fig. 5.3).

g. A large range of graspers, staplers, dissectors, scissors and diathermy applicators have been developed, either reusable or disposable.

6. The theatre team needs to be trained and efficient, with knowledge of how the equipment functions.

7. General anaesthesia is usually accompanied by muscle relaxation, intubation and ventilation so that pneumoperitoneum can be induced without causing cardiorespiratory embarrassment. The anaesthetist monitors abdominal distension and its effect on blood pressure and airways pressure throughout.

Access

1. Induce a pneumoperitoneum. The initial penetration of the abdominal cavity to produce a pneumoperitoneum can be a hazardous task in laparoscopic surgery.

> 🔑 **Key point**
>
> • Careless insertion of instruments can lead to injury to underlying viscera such as bowel or bladder, or even deeper structures such as the aorta and the vena cava.

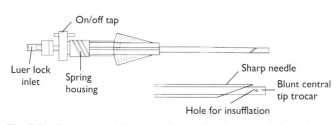

Fig. 5.3 Diagram of a Veress needle showing the device in its entirety and the spring-loaded tip.

Once the first port is established you can insert additional ports in relative safety. There are open and closed methods of producing a pneumoperitoneum:

a. Choose the safe, open (Hasson) method of port insertion especially if there has been previous surgery. Make a 1–2 cm infra-umbilical incision, deepening it down to the linea alba. Incise the linea alba between two stay sutures and open the peritoneum under direct vision. Insert a finger to sweep away any adhesions around the insertion site before inserting a blunt tipped trocar. Connect the gas supply and establish a pneumoperitoneum. The main disadvantage of this method is the increased incidence of gas leaks around the port; special ports with sealing balloons have been developed to prevent this.

b. The closed (Veress needle) technique is most commonly used. As before make an infra-umbilical skin incision. Apply 20–30° Trendelenburg tilt to the patient. Together with your assistant grasp the anterior abdominal wall and lift it up. Insert a Veress needle (Fig. 5.4) perpendicular to the abdominal wall until it penetrates the linea alba and the peritoneum. As soon as a 'give' is felt as the needle enters the peritoneal cavity, direct the needle downwards towards the pelvis to avoid damaging the great vessels.

> 🔑 **Key points**
>
> The position of the Veress needle tip can be checked by the following points:
>
> • The needle is freely mobile
>
> • A drop of saline placed on the Luer connector of the Veress needle should fall freely into the abdomen, where the pressure is subatmospheric
>
> • Aspirate to check that you do not obtain bowel content or blood
>
> • Inject 5 ml of saline, which should flow freely through the needle
>
> • Insufflate gas slowly; this should not produce a significant rise in the pressure reading if the needle is in the peritoneal cavity.

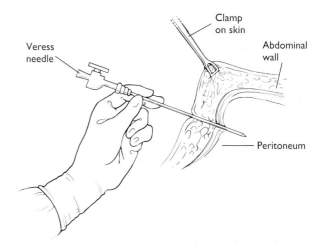
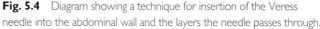

Fig. 5.4 Diagram showing a technique for insertion of the Veress needle into the abdominal wall and the layers the needle passes through.

2. Insufflate (Latin *sufflare* = to blow) the abdomen once you are certain that the port or Veress needle is in the correct position. Preset the insufflator to 13–15 mmHg and gas flow at high rate – the machine will deliver 3–4 litres of carbon dioxide and thereafter automatically delivers more gas if the pressure falls below the set pressure.

? Difficulty?

If the intra-abdominal pressure rises above the preset level, an alarm usually sounds:

● Stop insufflation

● Check port/needle positioning

● Check gas tubing is not obstructed and control taps are on

● If there has been too much gas introduced into the abdomen, let some gas out via one of the ports

● Liaise with the anaesthetist in case there has been a loss of muscle relaxation.

---

3. When the abdomen is fully distended and tympanitic to percussion, withdraw the Veress needle and enlarge the superficial part of the incision to accommodate the cannula. Insert a 10 mm trocar and cannula, aiming the tip anterior to the sacral promontory, parallel to the aorta. Use a drilling action from the wrist while lifting the abdominal wall below the insertion site. Withdraw the trocar, insert the laparoscope and connect it to the insufflator. Observe the view as you insert it to ensure the viscera are not at risk. Inspect the abdomen to identify structures that could be potentially damaged when the other ports are inserted. Secure the port either using a threaded collar or with stay sutures.

4. Insert additional ports under direct vision. You may first infiltrate the tissues with local anaesthetic prior to incision. The sites, size and number are determined by the intended procedure. Each trocar and cannula is inserted while your assistant moves the camera to provide a view so you do not spear the viscera or vessels. Secure the ports with threaded collars or stay sutures.

Assess

1. Now survey the abdomen prior to performing the procedure. Be systematic in identifying landmarks and inspecting the relevant area. Locate the ligamentum teres and falciform ligament. In the right upper quadrant visualize the liver, gallbladder and the underside of the right hemidiaphragm. Now manipulate the laparoscope under the ligamentum teres to look at the left lobe of the liver and the spleen. Change the patient's position to aid visualization by moving the bowel. Inspect both the left and right paracolic gutters, facilitating the exposure by inserting a probe or grasper to manipulate the bowel if necessary.

2. Place the patient in the Trendelenburg position to locate the caecum and appendix. Insert an endoscopic grasper to manoeuvre the bowel while you examine it from distal to proximal. While the patient is in the head-down position examine the pelvis; this is especially important in female patients when they have lower abdominal pain of unknown cause. You can directly visualize the ovaries, uterus and vermiform appendix.

In order to inspect organs such as the pancreas, additional manipulation and dissection may be necessary. Diseases such as Hodgkin's can be staged, and masses biopsied.

Diathermy

1. Carefully identify the correct structure. The commonest injury results from misidentification and hence burning the wrong structure.

🔑 Key point

● Diathermy used during laparoscopic surgery along with sutures and clips to achieve haemostasis can cause unrecognized, inadvertent, even fatal injury.

---

2. Inadvertent activation of the diathermy pedal risks damaging other structures in the abdominal cavity, especially when the electrode is outside the field of view.

3. Faulty insulation, especially in old instruments subjected to abrasive cleaning, allows a conducting surface other than the electrode to come into contact with a viscus. If burning does not directly cause a perforation, it may lead to autodigestion and perforation at a later date.

4. Current may flow from the active electrode to a contiguous conducting instrument – this is an example of direct coupling. The result is poor function at the active electrode and an unnoticed burn from the second instrument.

5. After use, diathermy electrodes can remain sufficiently hot to cause burns. After use, withdraw the electrode or keep it in view.

6. As in open surgery, diathermy of a pedicle concentrates the current density and so can lead to inadvertent perforation of structures, such as the common bile duct during a laparoscopic cholecystectomy.

7. Alternating currents can pass through insulating materials, as occurs in devices called capacitors. During laparoscopy a capacitor may be inadvertently formed so current induced in a metal port then flows into neighbouring bowel and causes a burn. Avoid capacitative coupling by using a non-conducting electrode. If you are using a metal port ensure that it makes good contact with the abdominal wall. Avoid open circuit activation, and high-voltage diathermy, e.g. fulguration.

Closure

1. Before removing the ports ensure that haemostasis is complete and that there are no free bodies in the abdomen such as spilt gallstones. Remove all laparoscopic instruments and ports under direct vision while checking for port site bleeding. Make sure no intra-abdominal structures have become trapped in the ports or port sites. Remove the final port slowly, with the laparoscope still inside to finally check.

2. Palpate the abdomen, helping to expel any remaining carbon dioxide, then close the port holes. Identify and grasp the fascia with toothed forceps. Use interrupted absorbable synthetic sutures such as polyglactin 910 or polydiaxonone (PDS). Take care not to pick up bowel with the stitch. Close the skin either with absorbable or non-absorbable sutures.

Postoperative

1. Monitor all patients as following an open laparotomy, with regular observations. Remind them of referred shoulder tip pain from stretching of the peritoneum lining the hemidiaphragms following pneumoperitoneum. Mobilize patients early and encourage them to eat and drink.

2. Most patients can be discharged within 24 hours of laparoscopy: the length of stay increases with more extensive procedures. Some surgeons now perform day-case laparoscopic cholecystectomy.

Complications

1. Since laparoscopic surgery usually requires a general anaesthetic, patients are susceptible to the usual complications related to this.

2. Complications common to laparoscopy and pneumoperitoneum include:

a. damage to viscus or vessels from Veress needle
b. misplacement of the needle, e.g. in extraperitoneal space
c. insufflation of the bowel lumen
d. CO_2 embolus and metabolic acidosis may complicate pneumoperitoneum
e. over-insufflation of the peritoneal cavity may cause cardiorespiratory problems.

3. During insertion of the ports the trocar may:

a. damage underlying structures, cause bleeding from the port site, subsequent herniation or wound infection
b. be poorly placed, requiring replacement.

4. Some complications are related to the type of surgery but some are common to all:

a. diathermy-related injuries
b. inadvertent organ ligation or division
c. unrecognized haemorrhage.

Patient related complications

a. Obesity – makes operation more difficult, increasing operating time, and may require special instruments
b. Ascites causes oozing from port sites, increasing the risk of port site damage
c. Organomegaly increases the risk of organ damage
d. Clotting problems may result in haemorrhage, or conversely in deep vein thrombosis
e. Following operation for malignant disease, cancer cells may be transferred to the port site, resulting in metastases.

FURTHER READING

Cuschieri A 1989 The laparoscopic revolution: walk carefully before we can run. Journal of the Royal College of Surgeons of Edinburgh 34: 295

Darzi A, Fowler C 1999 Minimal access surgery. In: Kirk RM, Mansfield AO, Cochrane J (ed) Clinical surgery in general, 4th edn. Churchill Livingstone, Edinburgh, Chapter 18.

Darzi A, Monson JRT 1994 Laparoscopic inguinal hernia repair. ISIS Medical Media, Oxford

Darzi A, Talamini M, Dunn DC 1997 Atlas of laparoscopic surgical technique. WB Saunders, London

Hall F 1994 Minimal access surgery for operating room and theatre personnel. Radcliffe Medical Press, Oxford

Hasson HM 1971 Modified instrument method for laparoscopy. American Journal of Obstetrics and Gynecology 110: 886–887

Abdominal wall and groin

D. F. L. Watkin and R. M. Kirk

Contents

GENERAL ISSUES IN HERNIA SURGERY

1. Consider whether there is another cause for the patient's symptoms. Groin pain may be due to osteoarthrosis of the hip rather than the obvious inguinal hernia. Epigastric pain may be biliary colic or a symptom of peptic ulcer and not a consequence of the epigastric hernia.

2. Make sure that patients who come for operation on the day of admission are thoroughly checked beforehand, know what is involved, have consented to operation and understand the circumstances under which it will be performed. They must also know about discharge arrangements.

3. The hernia may not be evident in the anaesthetized patient so it is essential that the site (and side) are marked preoperatively.

4. When prosthetic mesh is to be used for the repair, many surgeons give a prophylactic dose of antibiotic at induction. This *must* be administered in operations for strangulated hernia, because the wound may be subject to contamination.

5. Local anaesthesia is suitable for the repair of many groin hernias and some other hernias but is less well tolerated in young adults, who may require the addition of sedation. There are economic benefits in its use and it is particularly advantageous in the day-case setting and in the elderly. However it is not devoid of risk and the following general considerations apply.

a. The blood pressure, pulse rate and oxygen saturation should be monitored.

b. Make sure you know the appropriate procedures for resuscitation in case the patient develops an adverse reaction.

c. For effective anaesthesia a sufficient *volume* is needed so my preference is for 0.5% lignocaine with adrenaline (epinephrine) 1:100000. Alternatively, bupivacaine (0.25%) may be used but it acts more slowly. Some surgeons use a mixture of lignocaine and bupivacaine.

d. Decide which local anaesthetic you are going to use for hernia operations and stick to it to avoid confusion.

e. Do not exceed the safe dose of local anaesthetic; for lignocaine with adrenaline this is 500 mg, equivalent to 100 ml of a 0.5% solution.

f. Clearly record the dose of local anaesthetic and other drugs in the notes.

6. Non-absorbable sutures on curved, round-bodied, eyeless needles should always be used for the repair. Monofilament materials minimize the risk of persistence of a wound infection, polyamide (nylon) and polypropylene being the most popular. Remember that monofilament sutures require extra knots for security. Steel wire is now rarely used because it is difficult to handle.

7. Handle the synthetic monofilament suture material with great care. Do not hold it with instruments, or jerk it when tying knots, or you will seriously weaken it.

8. Do not drag the fine suture through the tissues, since it will cut them, enlarging the holes.

9. Do not tie the sutures too tightly. They will either cut out now or strangulate the tissues and weaken them later.

10. Do not take even bites of the tissues. Although this looks neat, evenly inserted stitches tend to detach a strip of aponeurosis. Therefore take successive bites at differing distances from the edge.

11. Two materials are in common use for mesh repairs. Polypropylene mesh is stiff enough to lie flat between tissue layers, needing only tacking sutures to stabilize it if there is no tension. Polypropylene is also the material for the preformed plugs or 'umbrellas' now being introduced for groin hernias. It is rapidly incorporated into fibrous tissue, giving a strong repair, but, as a corollary, must not be exposed to the intestines as obstructive adhesions may result. Polyester mesh is softer and so needs to be fully sutured into position. There is less fibrotic response so the strength of the repair is more dependent upon the sutures, but, by the same token, it may be placed at peritoneal level with negligible risk of adhesions. Expanded PTFE is also being used for incisional hernias.

12. Skin closure may be with sutures, clips, staples or adhesive strips. However a continuous subcuticular absorbable stitch (e.g. polyglactin 910) provides a very neat result and avoids the discomfort and cost of suture removal.

13. Postoperative analgesia is particularly important in day case work, but also for in-patients discharged the following morning. For patients in whom there is no contraindication, discuss with your anaesthetist the administration of rectal diclofenac in theatre but remember that the patient's prior consent is needed. Postoperatively a regular oral dose of diclofenac 50 mg TDS for 2 days, plus co-codamol as required, provides good pain control.

14. Outpatient follow-up provides valuable information on wound infections and other local complications such as numbness or pain. It is not feasible to offer the long-term surveillance necessary to monitor recurrence rates.

INGUINAL HERNIA

Appraise

1. In the past indirect hernias were usually repaired; diffuse direct hernias were treated with a truss. Now it is customary to operate on most inguinal hernias. The only reasons not to operate are trivial direct hernias in elderly, inactive or terminally ill patients and those who will not consent. The few who do not have an operation are generally best left without a truss, which is uncomfortable and difficult to manage.

2. In a very obese patient with a large, diffuse direct hernia, defer operation until the patient has lost weight.

3. In Britain, surgical repair of inguinal hernias was usually performed under general anaesthesia but, in patients with cardiovascular or respiratory disease, epidural or local anaesthesia can be used. At the Shouldice Clinic in Toronto, the vast majority of hernias are repaired under local anaesthesia. There are economic pressures for hernia repairs to be carried out on a day-case or short-stay basis. Local anaesthesia is therefore increasingly used.

4. Bilateral hernias may be repaired at the same time. It has been said that the results are not quite so good as when they are repaired separately, but this has to be set against the economic advantage to the patient and the service. Do not hesitate to repair a severe hernia on one side, deferring repair of a minor hernia on the other side until later.

5. If this is a recurrent hernia and repair will be difficult, will it be necessary, in a male patient, to remove the testis? If so, discuss it with the patient and obtain written consent.

6. Many surgeons accept the challenge of repairing recurrent diffuse hernias in obese patients with stretched, fat-infiltrated tissues or with chronic coughs. We are reluctant to do so. These patients are not at risk of strangulation and recurrence is likely following repair. As a trainee, do not embark on these operations.

7. There seem to be almost as many techniques for repairing hernias as there are surgeons.[1] If you watch two surgeons performing what they claim to be a particular method, you will observe numerous departures from the described technique, variously called 'My little modification', 'A little trick I learned' or, more assertively, 'My improvement on the method'. For example a purist could say that only those using stainless-steel wire are following the Shouldice technique, although most of those claiming to use the method employ polyamide or polypropylene. Surgeons often attribute their excellent results to particular details of technique but the common factor that produces their success is the perfection with which the procedure is accomplished. For this reason, do not attempt to acquire mastery of all the techniques but become familiar with a small range that will deal with most demands.

8. Individual surgeons have achieved low recurrence rates using sutured methods of repair of the posterior wall of the inguinal canal, bringing the conjoint tendon to the inguinal ligament, with or without a relaxing incision in the rectus sheath (Tanner's slide), or overlapping the transversalis fascia (Shouldice repair). Indeed, the Shouldice Clinic in Toronto has the lowest recorded recurrence rate – less than 1%. Others employed a darn to reinforce the posterior wall. The development of laparoscopic repair of groin hernias in the early 1990s prompted a reappraisal of open technique and overall recurrence rates were found to be approaching 10%. The widely used darn repair has generally been abandoned. The Shouldice method has a relatively long learning curve, so the Lichtenstein mesh repair has been adopted by the majority of surgeons, particularly for training, as it has a similarly low recurrence rate and is simpler. The latter two techniques will be described in detail.

9. Laparoscopic repair of groin hernias is currently in competition with the open or 'anterior' approach and at this stage there is no clear winner.[2]

Inspect

1. The diagnosis of groin swellings is notoriously difficult. Experienced as well as inexperienced surgeons make frequent mistakes. Do not accept the diagnosis of the referring doctor. Indeed, it is sometimes valuable to defer reading the accompanying letter until after examining the patient. Take a fresh history and carry out a complete examination, however obvious the diagnosis seems to be. Palpation is not the only, or even the most important, method of examination. Look with the patient standing and again with the patient supine. Ask the patient to cough but remember that a cough impulse is not always present over a hernia. Apart from obstructed and strangulated hernia, a cough impulse is often absent, especially over a femoral hernia in which a small sac is covered by much fatty extraperitoneal tissue. Conversely, a cough impulse is present over Malgaigne's bulgings, which do not merit the title of hernia, and also over a saphena varix.

2. If you see a lump, ask yourself 'Where is it?' If it is reducible, where does it first reappear on coughing or straining?

3. Never fail to examine the scrotum and its contents in male patients. If there is a swelling, ask yourself the fundamental question, 'Can I get above it?'

4. Finally, carefully and gently examine and palpate the hernial orifices. Remember that the presence of one hernia does not preclude others, nor does the presence of a hernia exclude other pathology. It is not disastrous to confuse indirect or direct inguinal and femoral hernias, since they can all be satisfactorily dealt with through standard approaches, but it is inexcusable to submit a patient to a hernia operation only to find another cause of the swelling that might require further investigation, or non-operative treatment.

Prepare

1. Many operations can be performed on a day-case basis in fit people who have good home circumstances. Bilateral procedures and operations in unfit or elderly patients or those who live alone require overnight or 48-hour stay.

2. Observe General issues 1–4.

Local anaesthesia for inguinal hernia repair[3]

1. Follow the instructions for local anaesthesia in paragraph 5 of General issues. Remember the maximum dose, e.g. 100 ml of lignocaine 0.5% with adrenaline.

2. Inject 20 ml along the line of the proposed incision using a fine needle to raise a continuous bleb within the epidermis.

3. Replace the needle with a larger one to inject deeply and along the same line superficial to the anterior wall of the canal.

4. Blunt the needle to improve the 'feel' of passage through the aponeurosis and inject 5 ml of fluid 3 cm above and medial to the anterior superior iliac spine deep to the external oblique to block the iliohypogastric and ilioinguinal nerves.

5. Reserve about half the anaesthetic to inject under the external oblique, around the neck of the sac and into other sensitive areas during the operation.

Access

1. Make an incision 2 cm above the medial two-thirds of the inguinal ligament, after identifying the pubic tubercle and anterior superior iliac spine. Cut through the fascia to expose the external oblique aponeurosis, ligating and dividing two or three large veins that cross the line of the incision. Avoid cutting into the hernial sac and spermatic cord at the medial end of the incision.

2. Expose the glistening fibres of the external oblique aponeurosis and identify the external inguinal ring, which confirms the line of the inguinal canal.

3. Make a short split with a knife in the line of the fibres of the external oblique aponeurosis over the inguinal canal. Enlarge the split medially and laterally by pushing the half-closed blades of the scissors in the line of the fibres. At the medial end of the split, the external inguinal ring will be opened – be sure to enter the external ring and do not allow the curved blades of the scissors to skirt around outside its crura.

4. Apply artery forceps to the edges of the aponeurosis and gently elevate each side. As the upper leaf is turned back, look for the arching lower border of internal oblique muscle, with the cord below it. As the lower leaf is everted, sweep loose tissue from the deep surface of the inguinal ligament.

5. Preserve the ilioinguinal nerve lying on the anterior aspect of the cord, to minimize the risk of postoperative numbness and pain.

Assess (Fig. 6.1)

1. Start to mobilize the cord by incising, just above and lateral to the pubic tubercle, the 'mesentery' of fascia and fibres of cremasteric muscle that extends downwards from the medial part of the conjoint tendon to envelop the cord. Deepen this small incision behind the cord, while drawing the latter downwards, to develop a plane to encircle it where it crosses the pubic tubercle, and apply a hernia ring.

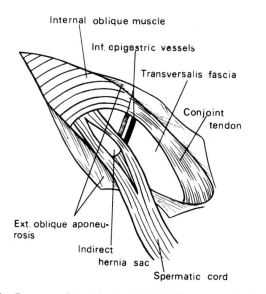

Fig. 6.1 Exposure of the right inguinal canal. The cremasteric fascia of the cord is split to show an indirect hernial sac.

Key point

- Do not rely on preoperative diagnosis of the type of inguinal hernia; determine this during mobilization.

2. The cord is then dislocated laterally and downwards by incision of the coverings along a line just above it. This will expose a direct hernia, which can be freed from the cord.

3. Carefully divide the fibres of cremaster just distal to the internal ring, ensuring haemostasis.

4. Examine the cord, even though a direct hernia is evident. Normally it is about the thickness of a pencil. It is markedly distended by an unreduced, sometimes adherent, or sliding, hernia. A thickened sac results from a longstanding indirect hernia. Cord lipomas produce thickening, as does an encysted hydrocele of the cord. In females, the processus vaginalis may become isolated as a hydrocele of the canal of Nuck. To *exclude* an indirect sac, open the spermatic fascia covering the cord and identify the edge of the peritoneum deep to the internal ring.

5. Identify the lower arching fibres of the internal oblique muscle, becoming tendinous at the conjoint tendon, and examine the posterior wall below this. A direct hernia may be a large bulge, a diffuse weakness of the whole posterior wall or, less often, a funicular hernia through a small localized defect (Ogilvie's hernia). If you are in real doubt, ask the anaesthetist to temporarily increase intra-abdominal pressure while you watch for distension and bulging.

6. If there is concern that a femoral hernia may be present, incise the transversalis fascia (as in a Shouldice repair) to expose the upper aspect of the femoral canal. If a femoral sac is present it is then dealt with as a Lothiesen procedure (see p. 62).

7. The cremasteric vessels pass medially from the inferior epigastric vessels adjacent to the cord. Do not tear them but carefully identify, isolate, ligate and then divide them to facilitate a snug repair at the internal ring. If they are damaged more medially ligate them at the pubic tubercle and excise the intervening portion.

Hernial sac

Indirect sac

1. With the left thumb in front, gently stretch the previously mobilized cord over the left index finger, which is placed behind the cord. Make a short split with a knife, in the line of the cord, through the cremasteric and internal spermatic fascial layers. Continue the split in the fascial layers proximally to the internal ring using scissors, first with their blades on the flat, separating fascia from deeper layers, then splitting the fascia.

2. Look for the sac. A white curved edge may be seen if the hernial sac is small (Fig. 6.1); if it is large it will be obvious as the fascial layers are separated. Using the point of the scalpel, gently incise the fibres crossing the fundus or the lateral edge of the sac. Unless it is very adherent it will then be possible to peel the sac out of the cord, with the aid of a few further stokes of the blade. The sac is then dissected back to the level of the abdominal peritoneum, using a combination of wiping with a gauze swab and snipping firm attachments with scissors. Keep the dissection close to the sac and avoid damaging other structures in the cord.

3. Pick up the sac with two artery forceps and open it between the forceps with a knife. Note any contents of the sac and return them to the peritoneal cavity.

4. Pass the little finger through the neck if it will slip through easily; ensure that the finger reaches the main peritoneal cavity and can be moved in all directions. Feel the posterior wall of the inguinal canal from inside the abdomen.

5. While the empty sac is held vertically by means of the artery forceps, transfix its neck with a suture of chromic catgut or synthetic absorbable material. Tie the ends of the suture-ligature into a half hitch, completely encircle the neck of the sac and tie a triple throw knot to ligate the neck of the sac. If contents tend to bulge into the sac, gently hold them back using non-toothed dissecting forceps, sliding them out as the ligature is tightened.

6. Do not let your assistant cut the ends of the ligature. First excise the sac 1 cm distal to the ligature. Examine the cut end to ensure that only sac is seen, then cut the ligature yourself. The stump of the sac should retract through the internal ring.

Large sac

1. Complete hernias, or scrotal funicular hernias, have no distal edge to the sac as seen at the level of the pubic tubercle. Attempts to dissect out the whole sac cause the scrotal part of the sac and the testis to be drawn into the wound. Excessive scrotal dissection of an indirect sac with damage to the pampiniform venous plexus may result in ischaemic orchitis.

2. The sac should be purposefully divided straight across within the inguinal canal. Isolate the proximal portion up to the internal ring, and leave the distal portion open. In this way the dissection is kept to a minimum.

3. If the sac is adherent, open the sac in front and place artery forceps at intervals round the inside as markers. Lift up two forceps, stretch the portion of sac between them, separate the sac from the cord and cut it distal to the forceps. Take the next two forceps and repeat the manoeuvre. Continue in this manner until the proximal circumference of the sac is completely sectioned, with the edges still held in the forceps.

4. After stripping the proximal part of the sac to the inguinal ring, transfix and ligate the neck.

5. Leave the distal part of the sac open.

Sliding hernia

1. In some hernias, abdominal retroperitoneal structures slide down to form part of the sac wall. The caecum, sigmoid colon or bladder are most commonly found. Always be on the look-out for sliding hernia.

2. The organ lying outside the sac is discovered when an attempt is made to empty and free the sac.

3. If the sac is intact, do not open it. You will need to close it again if you do, and it may be difficult to find a satisfactory strong edge all the way round the defect you have made.

4. If the sac has been opened, mark the fringe of peritoneum on the viscus with artery forceps and close the sac. Ensure that closure is complete.

5. Before replacing the viscus and closed sac inside the abdomen, make sure that neither the organ nor its blood supply was damaged before the true situation was recognized. If the bladder was damaged,

repair the wall and remember to insert an indwelling urethral catheter at the end of the operation.

6. The entire hernia sac and sliding viscus must be fully mobilized from the cord and replaced in the abdomen.

7. Carry out the best possible repair of the posterior wall of the inguinal canal.

Hernia in infants

1. Infants' tissues are not suitable for handling by impatient or rough surgeons.

2. Exposure is difficult if the pubic fat is thick. Make an incision in the skin crease just above the superficial inguinal ring. The well-developed deep fascia is easily mistaken for the external oblique aponeurosis.

3. The internal and external rings are almost superimposed at this age and it is therefore unnecessary to split the external oblique aponeurosis.

4. Isolate the cord just distal to the external ring, open the external fascial layers of the cord longitudinally and look for the sac. Pick up each layer with two pairs of fine artery forceps and open it between the forceps in the line of the cord. A short sac can be recognized by the white curved distal edge. The easy movement of the slippery internal surfaces of a large sac helps in identifying it. Make sure you are in the correct layer. When the sac is opened, the inner wall is shiny and slippery and the tips of the forceps can be passed into the peritoneal cavity.

5. Take great care in dissecting the fragile sac proximally – avoid tearing or splitting it. Avoid damaging the inconspicuous and adherent vas deferens. The sight of extraperitoneal fat confirms that the neck has been reached. If the hernia is complete, i.e. it extends down to the testis, do not dissect it distally. Carefully free it circumferentially just distal to the external ring, either from the outside if it is unopened or from within if it is open. Transect the sac, leave the distal end open and dissect the proximal sac. At the external ring, transfix, ligate and divide the neck of the sac. Do not twist the sac, because the vas may be inadvertently twisted with it and damaged.

6. If the external ring has been stretched by a large hernia narrow it with one or two chromic catgut or absorbable synthetic stitches. No other repair is necessary in an infant.

7. Close the subcutaneous layers with fine absorbable sutures. Close the skin with a fine absorbable subcuticular suture.

Hernia in women

1. The approach is similar to that employed in men.

2. The round ligament of the uterus lies in the position of the male spermatic cord. Ligate and excise it at the level of the internal ring to allow closure of the latter.

3. Recognize and isolate the sac, then transfix, ligate and divide it at its neck.

4. If the hernial sac is small, herniotomy is sufficient, combined with closure of the internal ring. For a larger hernia repair the posterior wall as in a male.

Direct hernia

1. Always look for an indirect sac first.

2. If the direct sac is funicular, resulting from a localized defect in

the posterior wall, isolate it, empty it, if necessary after opening it, then transfix, ligate and divide it at the neck. Define the margins of the posterior wall defect. If the hole is small and it can be closed without tension, suture it now, with non-absorbable material on a fine, curved, round-bodied needle.

3. More often the sac is diffuse and associated with a general weakness of the posterior wall; do not open it. If a Lichtenstein repair is to be employed, push it inwards and maintain the invagination by a running suture, of 2/0 polypropylene or polyglactin 910, carried across the stretched transversalis fascia so as to flatten the bulge without tension. The sutures must not bite deeply or the bowel or bladder may be damaged. If a Shouldice repair is to be used excise any excess of transversalis fascia when preparing the flaps for overlapping.

4. Carry out a suitable repair of the posterior wall of the canal.

Combined direct and indirect hernia

1. Such hernias protrude on either side of the inferior epigastric vessels. They are sometimes likened to the legs of pantaloons.

2. In a few cases a direct funicular sac can be manoeuvred laterally so both sacs emerge lateral to the vessels and can be dealt with together.

3. Do not struggle and distort the anatomy to achieve this, especially if the neck of the direct sac neck is wide. Deal with each sac separately.

> ### ❓ Difficulty?
>
> 1. If you cannot find the sac or recognize the tissues, first find the vas deferens, which can be felt as a string-like structure towards the back of the cord. The testicular vessels lie near the vas and, once these are separated, the rest of the cord may be cautiously divided, starting at the front, while keeping in mind that abdominal organs may be encountered. If a structure seems to be the sac, cautiously open it after tenting a portion between two artery forceps. Look for a glistening inner surface and insert a finger to determine if the sac communicates with the peritoneal cavity.
>
> 2. *Torn neck of sac?* Carefully free peritoneum from the abdomen to form a new neck.
>
> 3. Sometimes large, lipomatous masses of extraperitoneal fat are found. Isolate them and divide them with care, ligating the proximal ends. Ensure that there is no peritoneal sac in any of them.

Repair

1. In an infant, child or adolescent with a small indirect hernia, herniotomy is all that is required.

2. If the margins of the internal ring have been stretched by an indirect hernia, narrow the gap in the posterior wall using a non-absorbable suture, such as monofilament polypropylene or nylon. Approximate the attenuated margins of the transversalis fascia medial to the cord. (This is one of the effects of a Shouldice repair)

3. Further repairs to the posterior wall in general use are of two types.

a. Tissues are brought in from the margins to strengthen the posterior wall. In the Bassini repair, the lower fibres of the internal oblique and transversus abdominis muscles, with their medial aponeurosis, are sutured to the inguinal ligament behind the cord. The Shouldice repair

is a development of this theme. Other methods, such as Halsted's, which placed the external oblique aponeurosis behind the cord, are now of interest only when found at operation for recurrence.

b. Natural or artificial material may be inserted as a sheet to bridge the defect. The insert must be large, so as to overlap normal tissue and form a strong fibrous union with it, otherwise the repair will fail. This is exemplified by the Lichtenstein repair.[4] Additionally or alternatively a mesh 'plug' may be inserted into the defect.[5] The use of a darn of nylon or polypropylene to reinforce the posterior wall has largely been abandoned because of a high overall recurrence rate.

Shouldice repair (Fig. 6.2)[3]

1. The results obtained at the Shouldice Clinic in Toronto are so outstanding that the method has been widely used elsewhere. Hernia repairs alone are carried out at the clinic and many thousands of patients have been operated upon, usually under local anaesthesia, as short-stay patients. The same technique is used for all types of inguinal hernia and the recurrence rate for primary repairs is well below 1%.

2. Of course much credit must go to the operators, who have refined their technique in a vast experience. However, other surgeons achieve comparable results using the Shouldice method.

Action

1. Expose the inguinal canal and mobilize the cord. If there is an oblique sac deal with it as described above.

2. Carefully incise the cremasteric muscle and fascia, contributed by the internal oblique muscle, circumferentially around the cord at the level of the internal inguinal ring, securing haemostasis by ligation or diathermy, taking care not to damage the pampiniform venous plexus. It is not necessary to excise the coverings of the cord, as originally described, which may cause bleeding. If there are any large extraperitoneal lipomata, carefully isolate, ligate and divide them but do not try to dissect out all the fatty tissue.

3. The internal inguinal ring is not a hole, since the transversalis fascia continues on to the cord as the thinned internal spermatic fascia. Identify this and carefully incise the fascia circumferentially around the cord to leave it free within the internal ring.

4. Look again for any protrusion of peritoneum between the vas deferens and the ring. If one is present, however small, isolate and empty it, ligate its neck and excise it.

5. If there is not a large direct hernia, gently insinuate the closed tips of non-toothed dissecting forceps under the medial edge of the internal ring and pass them medially towards the pubic tubercle, separating the transversalis fascia from the inferior (deep) epigastric vessels. Allow the blades of the forceps to separate by a small amount and insert the deep blade of slightly opened scissors beneath the medial edge of the internal ring, between the forceps blades. Divide the medial edge of the internal ring and continue medially, to split the transversalis fascia as far as the pubic tubercle, halfway between the conjoint tendon and the inguinal ligament (Fig. 6.2a). Bleeding from small vessels in the fascia often requires diathermy.

6. If there is a large direct hernia, make a spindle-shaped incision in the transversalis fascia, judged so as to preserve suitable-sized upper and lower flaps. The intervening, excess, portion of the fascia is then inverted with the hernia.

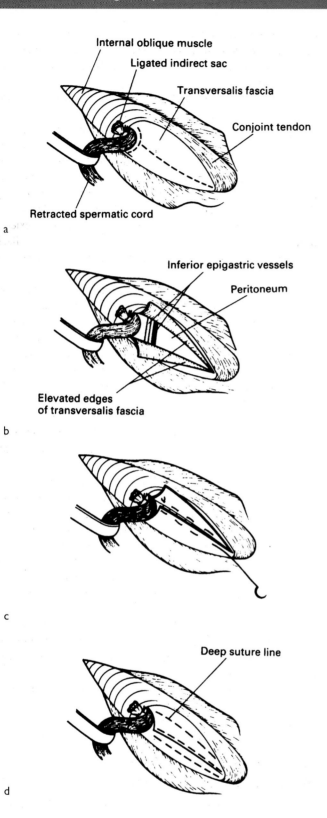

Internal oblique muscle
Ligated indirect sac
Transversalis fascia
Conjoint tendon
Retracted spermatic cord

a

Inferior epigastric vessels
Peritoneum
Elevated edges
of transversalis fascia

b

c

Deep suture line

d

Fig. 6.2 Shouldice repair: (a) the broken line is the incision in transversalis fascia and around the internal ring; (b) the upper and lower flaps have been elevated; (c) the lower flap is sutured to the undersurface of the upper flap; (d) the upper flap is sutured over the lower flap.

7. Elevate the upper flap of transversalis fascia from the underlying extraperitoneal tissue, brushing the fat away to expose its shiny white deep surface at the level of the conjoint tendon.

8. If you have not already isolated, ligated and divided the cremasteric vessels close to their origin from the inferior (deep) epigastric vessels when you mobilized the cord, do so now.

9. Separate the lower flap of transversalis fascia down to the inguinal ligament where it continues inferiorly as the femoral sheath (Fig. 6.2b). Take the opportunity to check that there is no femoral hernia.

10. The transversalis fascia will be repaired by overlapping the upper and lower flaps. This is made difficult if the extraperitoneal tissues bulge into the wound. It can be prevented by inserting a small dry gauze swab into the extraperitoneal space, removing it just before the first suture line is completed (removal is your responsibility!). Alternatively, a flat retractor or closed sponge-holding forceps can be used to push back the extraperitoneal tissues, being gradually withdrawn as the repair is completed.

11. Lift the upper flap of transversalis fascia and bring to its under-surface the edge of the lower leaf (Fig. 6.2c). Start at the medial end, using a continuous 2/0 (3 metric) monofilament nylon or polypropylene suture. Insert the sutures approximately 3 mm apart, at irregular distances from the lower flap edge. On the upper flap, pick up the more robust white transversalis fascia thickened at the level of the conjoint tendon. As you reach the lateral end, refashion the internal ring snugly around the thinned, emerging cord, taking exceptional care that a ligated indirect sac stump does not slip out.

12. Now fold down the upper flap of fascia transversalis and suture it into the lower flap where it thickens (the iliopubic tract) as it passes under the inguinal ligament (Fig. 6.2d). Suture it securely medially and, at the lateral end, carefully suture it around the medial aspect of the internal ring to reinforce the snug fit around the emerging cord.

13. Further strengthen the posterior wall by suturing the conjoint tendon down to the inguinal ligament. Start medially at the pubic tubercle and work laterally, everting the internal oblique muscle in order to catch the tendinous portion. Take great care, when you reach the internal ring, to snugly enclose it.

14. Lay the cord back into place.

Closure

1. Close the external oblique aponeurosis with a synthetic absorbable suture, starting laterally and ending medially to re-form the external ring snugly but not tightly around the emerging cord. Once again, take care to take bites at unequal distances from the edges, otherwise you will pull from the cut edges a strip of aponeurosis.

2. If the patient is a woman the internal ring and external oblique aponeurosis may be completely closed.

3. Appose the subcutaneous fascia with fine absorbable stitches.

4. Close the skin wound with stitches, clips or adhesive strips. However, a subcuticular absorbable suture spares the cost and discomfort of stitch removal.

Lichtenstein repair[4]

1. The Lichtenstein repair employs a sheet of polypropylene mesh covering the posterior wall of the inguinal canal and extending, for

security, over adjacent structures, with a hole to transmit the cord. It is also described as a 'tension free repair'.

2. Expose the inguinal canal and mobilize the cord. If there is an indirect sac deal with it as described above. If there is a substantial direct bulge this may be plicated so as to invert the excess, but the suture line should be placed so as not to create tension.

3. The mesh should have overall dimensions of 11×6 cm. To accommodate this, the external oblique aponeurosis must be separated from the deeper layers superiorly and medially and from the muscular part of internal oblique laterally to create an adequate pocket to receive the mesh.

4. Prepare the polypropylene mesh as indicated in Fig. 6.3a.

The lower medial corner is slightly rounded, the upper medial corner rather more so. The mesh is then incised from its lateral margin, placing the cut one-third of the distance from the lower edge. The cut extends for approximately half the length of the mesh, depending upon the size of the patient; it may need to be extended when the mesh is in place (Step 7). In small patients the upper edge may need to be trimmed slightly.

5. Take a 2/0 (metric 3) polypropylene suture on a 30 mm curved needle, pass the needle through the mesh, near its lower medial

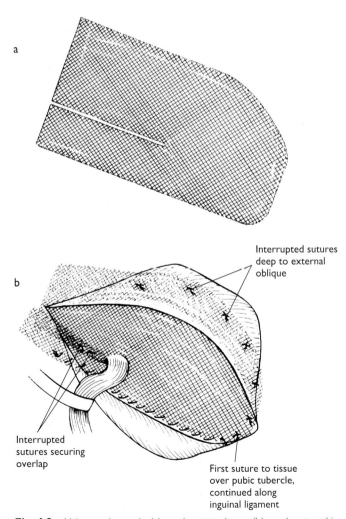

Interrupted sutures deep to external oblique

Interrupted sutures securing overlap

First suture to tissue over pubic tubercle, continued along inguinal ligament

Fig. 6.3 Lichtenstein repair: (a) mesh cut to shape; (b) mesh sutured in place.

corner, take bite of the tissue overlying the pubic tubercle and pass the needle back through the mesh. Tie the knot so as to fix the corner of the mesh, cut the short end of the suture but retain the long end with the needle.

6. Before inserting any further sutures place the mesh in its final position (Fig. 6.3b). Lift the cord and bring the narrow lower tail through under it, below the internal ring. Then tuck the lateral end under the external oblique; the lower edge of the mesh now lies along the inguinal ligament. Now insert the upper two-thirds of the mesh so that it lies under the external oblique aponeurosis superiorly and medially, ensuring that there is a good overlap on the rectus sheath medially. Tuck the wide upper tail under the external oblique laterally, with its lower edge over the lower tail. Insert your fingers under external oblique superiorly and laterally to ensure that the mesh lies quite flat in the peripheral part of the pocket, though there may be a slight bulge centrally.

7. Use the already attached polypropylene to form a continuous suture between the lower edge of the mesh and the inguinal ligament, working from medial to lateral, extending to at least 2cm lateral to the internal ring. Take irregular bites of the inguinal ligament to avoid splitting it and do not allow the lower leaf of external oblique to roll in and be included in the sutures; if this happens then there will be no external oblique left to close. For the medial part of this suture line it is best to retract the cord downwards. Then as the suture approaches the internal ring, move the cord cephalad and pass the needle through under it to continue laterally. When suturing immediately in front of the femoral vessels be careful to take only the ligament and not a bite of a major vessel!

8. If the slit in the mesh is too short it should be extended so that the cord passes directly from the internal ring to the opening in the mesh. A bulky cord may be accommodated by making a small cut in the mesh at right angles to the slit. If too long a cut has been made, all is not lost; simply shorten the slit with one or two sutures.

9. Secure the overlap of the tails of the mesh with two interrupted sutures lateral to the cord, bringing the edge of the upper portion over the lower tail by about 1 cm. The resulting opening in the mesh should be a snug, but not a tight, fit around the cord.

10. The medial and upper margins of the mesh are then secured with about six interrupted sutures (Fig. 6.3b). These are most conveniently placed 0.5 cm away from the edge, so that the mesh lies flat on the underlying aponeurosis or muscle. The medial sutures are particularly important as there is less overlapping of the mesh there, making it a potential site for recurrence.

11. The mesh repair is now completed. It appears slightly redundant centrally but that does not matter.

> **Key point**
>
> - Provided there is a good area of overlap medially, superiorly and laterally, with a good suture line inferiorly, the fibrosis induced by the polypropylene mesh will produce a sound result.

12. Replace the cord in the inguinal canal.

13. Close the external oblique aponeurosis and the wound as described for the Shouldice operation.

Recurrent inguinal hernia

It is advisable, where appropriate, to obtain written permission from the patient to divide the cord and excise the testis if necessary.

Access

1. Incise or excise the previous skin scar.

2. Deepen the incision at a higher level than the previous approach, so that unscarred external oblique aponeurosis is encountered first.

3. Display the external oblique aponeurosis downwards to the inguinal ligament.

4. Reopen the inguinal canal through the scar in the external oblique aponeurosis. Avoid damaging the contents of the canal, which may be adherent.

5. Elevate the upper and lower leaves of the external oblique aponeurosis until you reach unscarred tissue.

6. Isolate the spermatic cord below the pubic tubercle and follow it up to the internal ring. It may lie in an unusual place or be adherent and the vas may have been separated from the vessels.

Action

Hernial sac

1. Look for an indirect recurrence. If a sac is found isolate it, empty it, then transfix, ligate and divide it at the neck.

2. Look for a direct recurrence. If the recurrence is funicular, isolate it, empty it, then transfix, ligate and divide it at the neck. If it is a diffuse bulge, invert the sac and suture the wide neck to maintain the invagination.

Repair

1. Dissect the edges of the posterior wall of the canal until you reach firm tissue. Make a decision regarding the form of repair. A small direct defect may be protected by insertion of a small piece of polypropylene mesh extraperitoneally, either as an underlay or a 'plug'. For all other inguinal recurrences the Lichtenstein method is the best open repair.

2. For the underlay repair of a small, well-defined direct defect, take a piece of polypropylene mesh 2 cm larger in diameter than the defect. At each quadrant insert a 2/0 polypropylene suture through the intact tissue about 8 mm from the edge of the defect, pick up a small bite of the mesh and pass the needle back out through the intact tissue of the posterior wall, close to the point of entry. Hold the suture with an artery forceps and repeat the manoeuvre at each quadrant of the defect. Then parachute the mesh through the defect into the extraperitoneal space and tie the four sutures. Additionally, suture the edge of the defect to the surface of the mesh with continuous polypropylene.

3. In the 'plug' repair of a small defect, insert a bunched-up piece of polypropylene mesh into the extraperitoneal space and secure it with a few sutures across the open defect.

Postoperative

1. Following repair of inguinal hernia under local anaesthesia, the patient may leave the operating theatre on foot, which is good for confidence.

2. Patients should mobilize immediately after recovery from general anaesthesia. Inpatients generally go home the next day.

3. Light activities should be limited only by the patient's comfort. A sedentary job may be resumed at 1–2 weeks (though some patients will choose to wait longer). After a Lichtenstein repair a physically demanding job or active sports may be resumed at 4 weeks.

4. Many patients ask what is the likelihood of recurrence and what can they do to avoid the possibility. There is only one way in which they can prejudice the repair and that is to put on weight, especially if this is done rapidly.

5. Numbness in the distribution of the ilioinguinal nerve is common postoperatively and sometimes persists. A few patients have continuing pain at the operation site, requiring referral to a pain specialist.

6. Persistence of infection with sinus formation was a troublesome complication when catgut, silk or braided materials were used. Monofilament synthetic fibres seem to be very well tolerated. A wound infection (which should be uncommon) usually heals after drainage of any collection and only rarely is it necessary to explore the wound to remove sutures or a mesh.

? Difficulty?

1. The dissection described for a recurrent hernia assumes that the anatomical relationships have not been altered by previous operations. There are several findings that may perplex you.

2. In the Halsted method, the posterior wall was reinforced by closing the external oblique aponeurosis behind the cord, bringing the cord through the external oblique laterally, thus superimposing the internal and external rings. Attempts to reopen the canal are difficult because the posterior wall and the external oblique aponeurosis tend to fuse. A recurrence may appear alongside the cord, leaving the rest of the repair sound. Isolate the sac, empty it, then transfix, ligate and divide it at the neck. Define the edges of the stretched ring. This is one circumstance in which it may be best, with the patient's prior permission, to divide the cord so that the ring may be closed, but there will be a 15% risk of ischaemic orchitis.

3. The previous use of a tantalum gauze or plastic mesh insert may result in a recurrent hernia in which the tissues are matted together, making dissection difficult. Where this is known it is best to arrange for a laparoscopic repair.

4. Recurrences following darns with non-absorbable material or fascia lata are usually local defects, suitable for the underlay mesh repair. Leave the sound parts undisturbed.

5. Operation for recurrence after open repair may be much more straightforward laparoscopically. Conversely a recurrence after laparoscopic repair may be treated by open operation.

REFERENCES

1. Kirk RM 1983 Which inguinal hernia repair? British Medical Journal 287: 4–5

2. Stoker DL, Spiegelhalter DJ, Singh R, Wellwood JM 1994 Laparoscopic versus open inguinal hernia repair: randomised prospective trial. Lancet 343: 1243–1245

3. Glassow F 1984 Inguinal hernia repair using local anaesthesia. Annals of the Royal College of Surgeons of England 66: 382–387

4. Lichtenstein IL, Shulman AG, Amid PK 1989 Tension-free hernioplasty. American Journal of Surgery 157: 188–193

5. Fisher R, Hartley J, Winstanley J, Poston GA 1998 Phase II evaluation of the Marlex plug hernia repair. British Journal of Surgery 85 (suppl 1): 36

FEMORAL HERNIA

Appraise

1. It is usually accepted that all femoral hernias are repaired because of the high risk of strangulation, but there are no absolute rules in surgery. Occasionally a patient is seen who is very old and frail, with an incidentally discovered, long-standing femoral hernia that can reasonably be left alone.

2. One of the reasons for offering surgical repair freely is that the operation can be accomplished easily using local anaesthesia.

3. Be aware of the prevascular femoral hernia. Its neck extends laterally in front of the vessels.

4. Try each of the three current open approaches for femoral hernia (Fig. 6.4). They all have merits and they are all safe, provided the operation is skilfully performed. Every surgeon eventually settles upon a favourite approach. We use the low approach for elective operations and McEvedy's for strangulated hernias. Henry's approach, via a Pfannenstiel incision, is of historical interest only.

Low approach (Lockwood)

Access

1. Make an incision 8–10 cm long in the crease of the groin, below the medial half of the inguinal ligament

2. Cut the superficial tissues over the hernia in the line of the skin incision. Look out for the small veins running into the long saphenous vein; ligate and divide them as necessary.

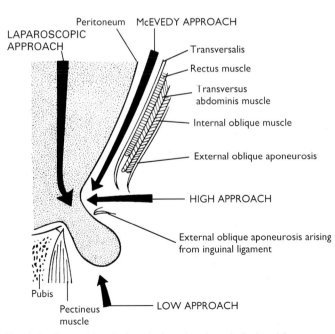

Fig. 6.4 Femoral hernia. A sagittal section through the hernial sac shows the possible approaches.

Action

Hernial sac

1. Expose the fat-covered hernial sac. Often, what appears to be a large swelling is mostly extraperitoneal fat, in which lies a small sac. Clean the sac so that it may be traced proximally beneath the inguinal ligament.

2. Cautiously open the sac by incising it while it is held up between two artery forceps. Remember that the bladder may form the medial wall of the sac. Recognize the inside of the sac by seeing free fluid, a glistening surface and contents that may be reduced into the main peritoneal cavity.

3. Pick up the open edges of the sac with three equally spaced artery forceps, then sweep away the external fat to expose the neck, lying between the inguinal ligament anteriorly and the pectineal ligament posteriorly in the same horizontal plane. Note how deeply the neck of the sac lies.

4. Identify the femoral vein lying just laterally and preserve it from damage.

5. Empty the sac, transfix and ligate the neck with 2/0 (metric 3) absorbable suture.

6. Excise the sac 1 cm distal to the ligature.

Repair

1. The inguinal and pectineal ligaments meet medially through the arched lacunar ligament. The object of the repair is to unite the ligaments for about 1 cm laterally, without producing constriction of the femoral vein (Fig. 6.5).

2. Use 2/0 (metric 3) monofilament nylon or polypropylene, on a small needle. We find a standard 30 mm round-bodied needle can be shaped to fit into the available space – but avoid damaging the tip.

3. Place a small curved retractor over the femoral vein to protect it and draw it laterally. Insert a stitch deeply into the inguinal ligament and use this to draw the ligament upwards, while the needle is insinuated behind it, to take a good bite of the pectineal ligament. Avoid taking too deep a bite or the needle point will break as it strikes the pubic crest. One, two or three stitches or a recrossing 'X' or 'N' stitch may be used but, for ease of access, insert all the stitches before tying any. As the stitches are tightened, keep a retractor over the femoral vein to ensure that it is not constricted.

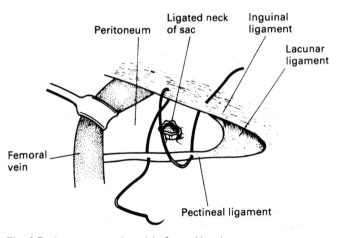

Fig. 6.5 Lower approach to right femoral hernia.

4. Alternatively, the femoral canal may be occluded with a 'plug' of rolled mesh, secured with three sutures.[1]

❓ Difficulty?

1. *Can you not identify the sac in the fatty lump?* Remember that most of the lump may be preperitoneal fat. Gently and carefully incise it and separate it. When the peritoneum is incised you can usually see glistening visceral peritoneum or lobulated omental fat. If the sac contains free fluid it appears bluish and may be confused with the appearance of congested bowel. When the sac is carefully incised the fluid escapes, revealing the contents.

2. If you inadvertently tear the neck of the sac, gently free peritoneum from the peritoneal cavity so that it can be drawn down to form a new neck.

3. If the femoral vein is torn, control the bleeding with pressure from gauze packs for 5 minutes. Meanwhile, order replacement blood for the patient, arterial sutures, tapes, bulldog clamps and heparin solution, and summon assistance. Expose the vein; do not hesitate to approach it from above and below the inguinal ligament. Apply bulldog clamps and tapes above and below the damaged segment. Insert fine 4/0 or 5/0 sutures set 1 mm apart, 1 mm from the torn edges to evert them and close the hole. Flush with heparin at intervals. Release, then remove the clamps and tapes.

4. It is not possible to suture the whole of a prevascular defect. Insert a piece of mesh and suture the opening medial to the vein.

Closure

1. Unite the subcutaneous tissues with fine absorbable stitches.
2. Close the skin, preferably with an absorbable subcuticular suture.

High approach (Lothiesen)

Appraise
1. The advantage of this approach is that it can be used for repairing coexisting inguinal and femoral hernias.
2. For femoral hernia alone it has the disadvantage that it damages the inguinal canal and could lead to a subsequent inguinal hernia.

Access
1. Expose the inguinal canal and dislocate the cord, as for operation for inguinal hernia.
2. Incise the transversalis fascia, as in the Shouldice operation.

Action
Hernial sac
1. Identify the neck of the sac and the external iliac vein.
2. Isolate the neck of the sac and gently withdraw the fundus. If there is difficulty, have the lower skin flap retracted downwards, incise the cribriform fascia and isolate, open and empty the sac from below.
3. Ensure that the sac is empty and that the bladder is not adherent, then transfix, ligate and divide the neck of the sac.

Repair
1. With the index finger, feel the margins of the femoral canal. In front is the inguinal ligament, medially the lacunar ligament, posteriorly the pectineal ligament and laterally the femoral vein.
2. Narrow the triangular gap by inserting non-absorbable sutures of 2/0 (metric 3) monofilament nylon or polypropylene between the pectineal ligament and the inguinal ligament.
3. If the upper approach was selected because there is also an inguinal hernia, deal with an oblique sac now.
4. *Either* close the posterior wall as a Shouldice repair *or* close the incision in transversalis fascia with a non-absorbable suture and carry out a Lichtenstein repair.

Closure
1. Close the inguinal canal, subcutaneous tissue and skin as for an inguinal hernia.

McEvedy's approach

Appraise
We prefer this approach for strangulated hernias as it provides excellent access for assessment of bowel and if necessary for resection. The skin incision, as originally described, left an ugly scar but this can be avoided by placing it more horizontally.

Access
1. Make an incision from 3 cm above the pubic tubercle running obliquely upwards and laterally for 7–8 cm, so as to cross the lateral border of the rectus muscle, which lies more vertically. Reflect the skin flaps so as to display the lateral part of the rectus sheath.
2. Incise the lower rectus sheath about 1–2 cm from, and parallel to, its lateral border. The lateral edge may tend to separate into its two anatomical layers.
3. Lift the lateral edge of the sheath and incise the thin transversalis fascia from about 2.5 cm above the pubic tubercle to mobilize the lower lateral edge of the rectus medially. Ligate and divide the inferior epigastric vessels which cross this line low down. The neck of the hernia is now in view as it enters the femoral canal!

Action
1. Retract the lower skin flap and isolate the sac.
2. Reduce the sac, manipulating it from above and below. Isolate, open and empty it, then transfix, ligate and divide the neck of the sac.
3. For a strangulated hernia (which is the reason for using this approach) the peritoneum may be opened above the neck to facilitate assessment of the bowel.
4. Repair the canal from above.
5. Close the incision in the rectus sheath with 0 (metric 3.5) nylon or polypropylene.
6. Appose the subcutaneous layers and close the skin.

REFERENCE
1. Allan SM, Heddle RM 1989 Prolene plug repair for femoral hernia. Annals of the Royal College of Surgeons of England 71: 220–221

STRANGULATED HERNIA

Appraise

1. Most operations listed as strangulated hernia are carried out for painful, irreducible or obstructed hernias. Some hernias reduce spontaneously when the patient is sedated prior to operation, or when anaesthesia is induced.

2. Strangulation results from venous obstruction, a rise in capillary hydrostatic pressure, transudation of fluid, exudation of protein and cells, and eventual arterial obstruction. Alternatively, the pressure of a sharp constriction ring at the neck of the sac may cause local necrosis of the bowel wall.

3. When the diagnosis is made it is worth trying the effect of reassuring the patient, who is laid supine and told to relax. The head-down position encourages spontaneous reduction. If you are experienced you may try the effect of gentle manipulation to see if the hernia can be reduced, but make sure you do not hurt the patient. There is a slight but real risk that you may reduce the hernia en masse – that is, the hernia remains within the peritoneal sac, the neck of which remains as a constriction, so the strangulation is not relieved.

4. If you can easily reduce the hernia, emergency surgery is unnecessary. Plan for early elective operation.

Prepare

1. Do not rush patients with strangulated hernias to the operating theatre. Make sure you know why the patient has developed strangulation now. Ensure that the patient does not have coincidental disease that makes general anaesthesia and operation hazardous.

2. If strangulation has been present for some time the patient will require fluid and electrolyte replacement. Some patients, especially with strangulated femoral hernias, do not reach hospital for a few days and by then have a severe biochemical disturbance. They may require up to 24 hours of resuscitation to correct the fluid deficit. This takes priority over the operation. It is likely, in such cases, that bowel in the hernia will already be irreversibly ischaemic, so nothing is lost by the delay.

Access

The approach for inguinal and most other hernias is similar to that for an elective operation. For strangulated femoral hernias McEvedy's incision is preferred, as it provides better access to assess, and if necessary resect, bowel. If the low approach is used and bowel resection proves difficult, have no hesitation in opening the abdomen formally.

Assess

1. If the history was short, the sac will frequently be empty by the time you expose it. The relaxation produced by the anaesthetic often succeeds when other conservative methods have failed to reduce a hernia. There is then no merit in exploring the abdomen. Repair the hernia as though this were an elective operation.

2. If bowel is present in the sac, do not let it slip back into the abdomen but gently draw it down into the sac. The bowel is likely to have suffered the greatest damage where it was trapped at the neck of the sac.

3. Feel the margins of the neck of the sac with a fingertip.

4. In Richter's hernia, most frequently associated with femoral hernia, a knuckle of the bowel wall is trapped. The bowel lumen is thus not obstructed but the knuckle may become gangrenous and perforate.

5. Maydl's strangulation is very rare. Two loops lie in the sac but the blood supply to an intermediate loop within the abdomen may be prejudiced so that it is gangrenous.

🔑 Key points

Is the bowel viable?

- If there is a sheen to the bowel wall, if it is pink or becomes pink after release, if the arteries pulsate, if peristalsis is seen, replace the bowel with confidence.

- If the wall is black, green or purple, with no sheen, if there is no pulsation in the mesenteric vessels or it is malodorous, resect it.

- If the bowel is congested, bluish or plum-coloured and still has a sheen, but vascular pulsations cannot be felt, then its viability is doubtful. Remember, however, that extravasated blood in the subperitoneal layer cannot be reabsorbed immediately so the colour may not change. Cover the bowel with warm moist packs for 5 minutes and re-examine it. If it has improved in appearance and mesenteric arterial pulsations are palpable it is probably viable.

- The critical areas are the constriction rings at the point of entrapment. These are white when the bowel is first drawn down but may be greenish or black if they are obviously necrotic. Re-examine doubtful rings after an interval to see if the blood supply returns. If it does not, the bowel must be resected. Occasionally it is possible to invaginate and oversew a doubtful ring.

- Experienced surgeons probably resect bowel less frequently than those who are inexperienced. The mucosa is more vulnerable than the seromuscularis to the effects of ischaemia and if the outer layers survive the mucosa may slough to leave an annular ulcer. When this heals a constriction may develop. This is the intestinal stenosis of Garre. The patient presents after an interval of weeks or months with incipient small bowel obstruction. Provided this is recognized a simple elective abdominal resection can be carried out.

Action

1. If the neck of the hernial sac is constricted, first draw down healthy bowel, then place an index fingertip on each side of the contents, nails facing outwards. Gently dilate the neck of the sac (Fig. 6.6). Make sure the bowel does not slip back. Draw it out to ensure that there is no peritoneal constriction and to expose healthy bowel.

2. If the bowel is viable, return it to the abdomen.

3. If necessary, resect a gangrenous segment of bowel, performing an end-to-end anastomosis.

Repair

After opening the sac and dealing with the contents, repair the hernia as though this were an elective operation, but if possible avoid the use of mesh, for fear of infection.

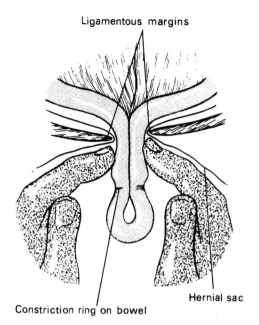

Ligamentous margins

Constriction ring on bowel

Hernial sac

Fig. 6.6 Reducing a strangulated hernia. Healthy bowel is drawn down. The index fingers form a wedge to dilate the ligamentous margins.

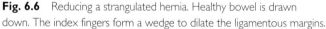

Difficulty?

1. Sometimes the bulk of tissues contained in the hernial sac makes reduction seem impossible. Provided the margins of the neck are defined, gentleness, patience and persuasion will succeed. If only a little at a time is reduced, do not despair because the reduction must get progressively easier.

2. The McEvedy approach avoids most of the difficulties in dealing with the bowel in a strangulated femoral hernia. When reducing a strangulated femoral hernia from below, it is often advised that a grooved director should be passed medial to the neck of the sac, followed by a bistoury to cut the lacunar ligament. We have not found it necessary to use this method and, indeed, find it illogical. Failure to reduce the hernia results from a tight sac neck, not from tight ligamentous margins, which are absent laterally. The femoral vein can be emptied and displaced, producing ample room to reduce the contents.

3. A large mass of fibrotic greater omentum may be adherent within the sac. Do not hesitate to excise the mass, provided the neck of the sac can be isolated, the bowel is not damaged and every blood vessel is safely ligated.

4. If gangrenous bowel slips back into the abdomen and cannot be recovered, repair the hernia, then open the abdomen through a lower midline incision. Find the gangrenous segment and resect it.

UMBILICAL HERNIA

Adult umbilical hernia

Appraise

1. Most hernias in adults are para-umbilical, protruding usually above or below the cicatrix. The contents are most frequently omentum, which is often adherent to the interior of the sac.

2. Some adults, especially of African origin, have true umbilical hernias that have been present throughout life.

3. Umbilical hernia is conventionally treated by early operation for fear of strangulation. However, many patients are grossly obese and elderly, with cardiovascular or respiratory disability and a long-standing hernia that has not been troublesome. Adjure such patients to lose weight and hesitate about offering operation. Ascites may provoke umbilical hernia: find the cause and treat it. In some cases there is extensive malignant disease; surgery is rarely indicated.

4. Operate on strangulated, painful irreducible – but not necessarily painless irreducible – hernias and painful reducible hernias, especially those with small, hard margins.

5. The Mayo repair is widely used. Alternatively a small (less than 2 cm) defect may simply be sutured or a larger defect repaired with a patch as for an incisional hernia.

Access

1. Make a curved incision in the groove above or below the hernia. Extend the cut transversely outwards on each side, for 2–4 cm.

2. Deepen the incision, identify the aponeurosis and expose it around the adjacent half of the circumference of the hernia.

3. If the hernia is small, preserve the umbilical skin by dissecting it off the hernia as a flap. If the hernia is large, make a semicircular incision to include the umbilicus so that the hernia is encircled and excise the stretched skin.

4. Expose the aponeurosis around the remainder of the margin of the hernia.

Action

1. Cut through the thinned-out edge of aponeurosis to expose the peritoneum and gradually work round to display the whole circumference of the neck of the sac.

2. Clear the sac of fatty tissue and cut it right round, at least 2 cm distal to the neck if possible. The contents of the sac are less likely to be adherent here than in the fundus, but free them if necessary. Mark the peritoneal edges with artery forceps.

3. If the contents of the sac are free, reduce them. If they are adherent to the fundus of the sac, free them and return them to the peritoneal cavity. If there is a mass of fibrous omentum, excise it with the fundus of the sac but take care to ligate all the bleeding omental vessels and avoid damaging the transverse colon.

4. Separate the peritoneum from the under surface of the rectus sheath all round, without tearing it.

5. Close the peritoneal neck of the sac with a continuous 2/0 synthetic absorbable suture, producing a transverse linear suture line.

Mayo's repair (Fig. 6.7)

1. Cut the rectus sheath laterally for 2–3 cm on each side. This allows the upper and lower edges to be overlapped.

2. Place a series of horizontal mattress sutures of 0 (metric 3.5) polypropylene or nylon, without tying them. Each stitch picks up the lower edge of the aponeurosis about 1 cm from its edge, penetrates the upper leaf 3–4 cm from its edge and returns through the upper leaf to

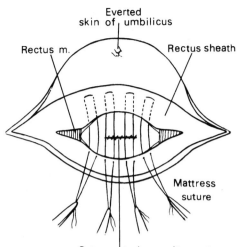

Fig. 6.7 Mayo's repair of umbilical hernia.

catch the lower edge close to the original entry. When the stitches are tied, the lower leaf is drawn up underneath the upper leaf.

3. Sew the overlapping upper edge on to the anterior surface of the lower rectus sheath, using a continuous suture.

Closure

1. If the skin over the fundus was preserved, pick up the under-surface of the navel with a synthetic absorbable stitch and sew it to the rectus sheath to produce a dimple. Suture the skin as a curved line above or below the newly fashioned umbilicus.

2. If the umbilicus was excised, close the skin wound as a transverse suture line.

Infantile umbilical hernia

Appraise

1. Most infantile umbilical hernias protrude through the incompletely closed cicatrix. They appear to be more frequent in infants of African origin. Most of them close spontaneously without surgical repair, so wait for 1–2 years. Repair them only if they increase in size.

2. Infants infrequently develop a supra-umbilical hernia. It will not close spontaneously, so repair it locally through a transverse incision sited directly over the defect.

Access for a true umbilical hernia

1. Approach the hernia through a transverse incision curved beneath the everted umbilicus.

2. Preserve the umbilical skin by turning it upwards as a flap.

Action

1. Expose the aponeurosis and the neck of the sac. The separation is much easier than in acquired hernias.

2. Open the sac, empty it, then close it by suture or transfixion ligature.

Repair

Edge-to-edge repair of the aponeurosis is effective. Make sure the peritoneum is separated sufficiently to allow good bites of sheath to be taken, without piercing the peritoneum. Create a transverse suture line using polypropylene or nylon.

Closure

1. Suture the deep surface of the umbilical skin to the aponeurosis with fine absorbable synthetic material.

2. Close the skin to leave a curved transverse wound, using an absorbable subcuticular stitch.

ABDOMINAL WALL SEPSIS

Wound infection

Appraise

Wound contamination and haematoma are the major factors responsible for wound infection. A reaction to catgut may also contribute while synthetic absorbable sutures seem less liable to do so. Multifilament stitches may perpetuate a wound infection, so monofilament materials are preferred for non-absorbable sutures.

Action

1. The mainstay of treatment is drainage. Often it is possible to achieve this on the ward by removal of a suture from the softest part of the wound, followed by probing with a sinus forceps. If the wound has discharged spontaneously, the opening may need to be enlarged to provide adequate drainage. Always send a specimen for bacteriology.

2. Normally, do not administer antibiotics for wound infection unless there is cellulitis or the patient is at risk from immune deficiency, cardiac disease or prosthetic heart valves, or is already septic.

3. Sometimes when the wound is opened, severe tissue necrosis is discovered. Do not make the error of leaving a small hole and inserting a drain. Re-open the incision, assiduously excise necrotic tissue and leave the wound open.

4. Following drainage of a wound abscess a chronic sinus may persist. Explore the sinus with a pair of fine, sterile mosquito forceps, or a sterile crochet hook, to extract the stitch if possible. If the stitch sinus persists, explore it under local or general anaesthesia to remove the suture material.

Synergistic spreading gangrene

1. This is usually given the name of Meleney, the New York surgeon who described it in 1933. When it affects the scrotum it is called Fournier's gangrene. It may result from the synergistic effects of a number of microorganisms, or from a single organism.

2. Exclude diabetes, immunosuppression, uraemia and hepatic disease.

3. It develops as a slowly extending area affecting the whole thickness of the skin. The advancing edge is typically serpiginous and leaves dead, sloughing skin that separates to expose unhealthy granulation tissue.

4. Start the patient immediately on broad-spectrum antibiotics, such as a cephalosporin and metronidazole, pending the result of bacteriology.

5. The essential action in controlling the infection is to excise all the necrotic tissue, exposing healthy, clean tissue. Leave the wound open and dress it frequently, repeating the excision of any developing necrotic tissue.

6. When the infection has been completely controlled, plan to resurface the denuded area with partial thickness skin grafts.

Necrotizing fasciitis

1. This spreading gangrene primarily affects the abdominal fascia. It may follow surgical operations or injury.

2. Management is with versatile antibiotics and immediate radical excision of all the necrotic tissue to leave healthy living tissue.

Gas gangrene

1. Clostridial infection of abdominal wounds is rare.

2. The patient rapidly develops pyrexia, toxicity and hypotension.

3. The discoloured wound edges are crepitant and may already discharge thin pus, described as smelling 'mousy'.

4. Administer 1 million units of benzyl penicillin and give regular high doses thereafter.

5. As far as possible, and as rapidly as possible, correct the patient's general condition.

6. Under general anaesthesia radically excise the whole area, back to clean, living tissue. Thoroughly wash the raw area with 20 volume hydrogen peroxide.

7. Hyperbaric oxygen at 3 atmospheres has been recommended.

INCISIONAL HERNIA

Appraise

1. Incisional hernia is a deep disruption of the abdominal wound while the superficial layers remain intact. (If the superficial layers also separate then a burst abdomen results.)

2. Herniation may occur early, while the patient is still in hospital. More usually it develops during the following months or years.

3. Incisional hernias are associated with careless suturing, the use of catgut instead of non-absorbable material, haematomas and infection, the insertion of drains through the main incision and damage to abdominal nerves. Jaundice, malnutrition, obesity, postoperative distension and re-exploration through the same incision after a short interval are other contributory factors, as are steroids and immuno-suppression.

4. Incisional hernias rarely strangulate; therefore do not rush to reoperate. We encourage the patient with a wide-necked hernia to try a surgical corset. Some are satisfied with this and avoid an operation.

5. If the patient is overweight advise reduction before surgery. Ensure that infection has completely resolved before proceeding.

6. If mesh is to be used give perioperative antibiotic cover.

Action

1. Excise the old skin scar.

2. If the skin and peritoneum are fused, excise an ellipse of skin wide enough to expose subcutaneous tissue.

3. Dissect back the skin on each side until unscarred subcutaneous tissue is reached, beyond the margins of the defect.

4. Deepen the incision until aponeurosis or muscle is reached, then work towards the margins of the defect.

5. Dissect the edges cleanly and separate the peritoneum from the deep surface all around (unless placing mesh intraperitoneally).

6. Is there anything to be gained by opening and excising some of the stretched peritoneum? If possible, invaginate the sac with a continuous suture. However, adherent contents and a narrow neck may require that the sac be opened to achieve reduction.

7. Multiple defects in the abdominal wall ('buttonhole tears') are most conveniently managed by uniting them and repairing the resulting larger defect.

8. Meticulously stop all bleeding.

Repair

1. There is no advantage in attempting to define the layers of the abdominal wall.

2. Small defects, less than 4 cm, may be sutured, using non-absorbable material (0 or 1G) but this does introduce tension adjacent to the repair so it is suitable only if the edge is strong.

3. Large defects, or poor tissue, are best repaired with a synthetic patch, to avoid a recurrence rate of 40–50%. The mesh may be applied at three levels in the abdominal wall as described below (Fig. 6.8). We prefer the second or third methods on the basis that it is better to patch a bucket on the inside!

4. There are also methods that attach a piece of mesh to each side of the defect and then suture the two together or sandwich the abdominal wall between two layers of mesh. Alternatively, ePTFE mesh may be stapled laparoscopically on the peritoneal surface; polypropylene is stiffer and easier to handle but the bowel must be protected by attaching omentum over the patch.

Onlay patch repair

1. This is the simplest method, placing a patch anterior to the aponeurosis and the defect, which may or may not have been sutured. Polypropylene mesh is most suitable as it is rapidly incorporated in scar tissue. It should extend 4 cm beyond the edge of the defect.

2. Secure the edge of the mesh with interrupted 2/0 polypropylene sutures at 2 cm intervals, reinforced with a continuous over-and-over stitch.

3. Place another continuous suture to fix the mesh where it lies over the edge of the defect.

Extraperitoneal mesh repair

1. This is suitable for midline hernias.

2. The peritoneum, plus the posterior rectus sheath if above the arcuate line, is dissected off the posterior aspect of the rectus muscle laterally and from the aponeurosis in the midline, for about 3 cm.

3. Polypropylene mesh will incorporate more rapidly but polyester is easier to position as it can deform on the bias.

4. Cut a piece of mesh 2 cm larger than the defect at each margin.

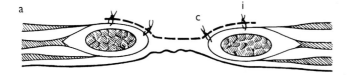

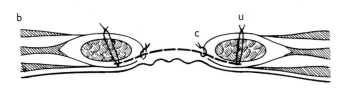

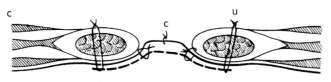

Fig. 6.8 Three alternative levels for placement of mesh in incisional hernia repair: (a) onlay; (b) extraperitoneal; (c) intraperitoneal. Transverse section through abdominal wall. Key: i, interrupted sutures; c, continuous suture; u, 'U' sutures.

5. The mesh is drawn into the space deep to the abdominal wall by interrupted 'U' sutures of 2/0 polypropylene at 2 cm intervals Each passes in through the anterior rectus sheath and rectus, picks up the edge of the mesh and returns to be tied externally.

6. The margin of the defect is then sutured to the surface of the mesh with a continuous over-and-over suture.

Mesh repair at peritoneal level
1. The sac is opened and any adhesions for 4 cm around the rim are freed.

2. Cut a piece of polyester mesh 2 cm larger than the defect in each direction (polypropylene is liable to cause dense intestinal adhesions).

3. Draw the margin of the mesh under the rim of the defect with a series of 'U' sutures of 2/0 polypropylene. These penetrate the peritoneum 2–3 cm from the rim. First place four cardinal sutures and hold them with forceps, adjusting the size of the mesh so that it fits the opening. Then insert more 'U' sutures at 2 cm intervals between one pair of cardinal sutures and tie these. Repeat this for the other three sections.

4. Pick up the mesh and the underlying rim with a continuous over-and-over suture, taking care avoid the bowel.

Closure
1. Drain the large subcutaneous space with one or two suction drains. The tubing tends to curl up in one corner; prevent this by tunnelling the tube under the fascia at one or two points.

2. Appose the subcutaneous fat.

3. Close the skin with an absorbable subcuticular suture.

Aftercare
1. Leave the drains until the daily loss is less than 30 ml.

2. Any subsequent collection should be aspirated, with sterile precautions.

3. In the event of a wound infection, do not rush to remove the mesh; it may survive.

FURTHER READING

Devlin HB, Kingsnorth A 1997 Management of abdominal hernias, 2nd edn. Chapman & Hall, London

Kurzer M, Kark AE, Wantz GE 1999 Surgical management of abdominal wall hernias. Martin Dunitz, London

Nyhus LM, Condon RE (eds) 1994 Hernia, 4th edn. JB Lippincott, Philadelphia, PA

Appendix and abdominal abscess

R. C. N. Williamson and R. M. Kirk

Contents

APPENDICECTOMY

Appraise

1. The diagnosis of acute appendicitis is essentially clinical. It is always better to repeat the taking of a history and re-examine the patient rather than embark on investigations, although investigations may help to rule out other clinically suspected diagnoses.

2. Although appendicectomy is still the commonest reason for laparotomy, remember:

a. Appendicitis is overdiagnosed in children.[1]
b. Girls aged from the menarche to 25 may have other causes than appendicitis for pain and tenderness in the right iliac fossa. Consider re-examining the patient at intervals, ordering a pelvic ultrasound scan or performing laparoscopy in case of doubt.
c. Although elderly patients can develop appendicitis, they may have other causes such as perforating carcinoma of the caecum and diverticulitis. In case of doubt recognize that they may require wide exposure through an enlarged incision at operation.

3. If there is a mass in the right iliac fossa at the time of admission, and the patient shows no clinical features of sepsis, defer appendicectomy unless there is a practical reason to carry it out now. This is safe, *provided* you monitor the patient carefully and operate if:

a. the mass, judged by its initially marked margins, increases or becomes tender
b. the patient's abdomen develops features of obstruction, paralytic ileus or peritonitis
c. the patient becomes toxic, with swinging temperature, rising pulse rate and white blood cell count
d. an ultrasound scan demonstrates an abscess cavity.

As a rule, order a barium enema X-ray when the mass has settled, in patients over the age of 40–50, to exclude caecal carcinoma. It is conventional practice to re-admit patients for interval appendicectomy 1–2 months later. Because many patients who are not operated upon remain symptom-free, it may be justifiable to defer operation indefinitely, after warning patients to seek medical attention if symptoms recur.

4. Diagnostic laparoscopy is carried out by some surgeons whenever they suspect appendicitis, proceeding to laparoscopic appendicectomy if the diagnosis is confirmed. Anxiety that carbon dioxide pneumoperitoneum may increase bacteraemia in the presence of sepsis seems to be unjustified.

5. Avoid removing a normal appendix incidentally during other operations. It is a possible cause of complications such as wound infection – especially following right inguinal hernia repair.

Prepare

The incidence of wound infection is high following operation for acute appendicitis, so routinely insert a 1g metronidazole anal suppository as soon as the decision is made to operate. The earlier it is given beforehand the greater the safety. If the appendix proves to be very inflamed, plan to continue the metronidazole suppositories 8-hourly for 2–5 days. In patients with clinically severe acute appendicitis who are elderly, at high risk, have cardiac disease, an implant such as a hip joint replacement, or diabetes also give cefuroxime prophylactically (1.5g intravenously).

🔑 Key point

- Intend to re-examine the abdomen when the patient is anaesthetized. You may feel a mass in the relaxed abdomen that was impalpable beforehand. Indeed, it is a valuable general rule before any abdominal operation, and may help you determine the best site for the incision.

Access

1. As a routine employ a Lanz incision in a skin crease. This modification of the gridiron incision crosses McBurney's point – the junction of the middle and outer thirds of a line joining the anterior superior iliac spine and the umbilicus. The incision starts 2 cm below and medial to the right anterior superior iliac spine and extends medially for 5–7cm. It may be possible to site it lower down in a young girl so that the scar lies below the waistline of a bikini swimming costume.

2. Use the traditional gridiron incision, 5–8cm long, in line with the external oblique fibres if you anticipate the need to extend the exposure (Fig. 7.1).

The incision crosses McBurney's point at right angles to the spino-umbilical line, one third above, two thirds below. If necessary, the external oblique muscle and aponeurosis can be split in either direction and the internal oblique and transversus muscles can be cut to convert the incision into a right-sided Rutherford Morison incision (see Ch. 4).

3. If appendicitis is but one of a number of likely diagnoses, prefer a lower right paramedian incision.

Opening the abdomen

1. Incise the skin cleanly with the belly of the knife. Divide the subcutaneous fat, Scarpa's fascia and subjacent areolar tissue to expose the glistening fibres of the external oblique aponeurosis. In the gridiron approach these fibres run parallel to the skin incision.

2. Stop the bleeding. Incise the external oblique aponeurosis in the line of its fibres. Start with a scalpel, then use the partly closed blades of Mayo's scissors (Fig. 7.2) while your assistant retracts the skin edges.

3. Retract the external oblique aponeurosis to display the fibres of internal oblique muscle, which run at right angles. Split internal oblique and transversus abdominis muscles, using Mayo's straight scissors (Fig. 7.3).

Open the blades in the line of the fibres and use both index fingers to widen the split. Provided the scissors are not thrust in violently the transversalis fascia and peritoneum are pushed away unopened.

4. Stop the bleeding. Have the muscles retracted firmly to display the fused transversalis fascia and peritoneum.

5. Pick up a fold of peritoneum with toothed dissecting forceps and grasp the tented portion with artery forceps. Release the dissecting forceps and take a fresh grasp to ensure that only the peritoneum is held. Make a small incision through the peritoneum with a knife. Allow air to enter the peritoneal cavity, so that viscera fall away. Use scissors to enlarge the hole in the line of the skin incision. Now protect the wound edges with swabs or skin towels.

Assess

1. Look. Is there any free fluid or pus? If so, take a specimen for microscopy and culture for organisms.

2. Find the caecum, identify a taenia and follow it distally to the base of the appendix. Insert a finger and lift out the appendix by pushing from within, not by pulling from without.

🔑 Key point

- Never pull on the appendix if the distal end is stuck. If it is gangrenous it will tear and release infected material into the peritoneal cavity. Always improve your view, if necessary by extending the incision.

---

3. If the appendix is not evident, move your index finger under the right side of the wound to the right limit of the iliac fossa, left on to the iliacus muscle until you reach the caecum, then gently push it out on to the surface. In some cases you may need to mobilize the caecum by incising the parietal peritoneum in the paracolic gutter, in order to raise the caecum on its mesentery, especially if the appendix is adherently retrocaecal. If the caecum is not evident, remember that it sometimes lies quite high, under the right lobe of the liver.

❓ Difficulty?

- *There is no appendix?* In a small number of patients there is no appendix, either because it did not develop or because it has been digested or has atrophied as a result of previous inflammatory disease. In this case, what is the cause of the patient's clinical features? Carry out a search for disease of nearby organs (see below).

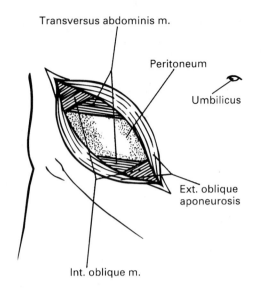

Fig. 7.1 Gridiron incision for appendicectomy. In the Lanz modification the skin incision is transverse but the abdominal muscles are similarly split in the line of their fibres.

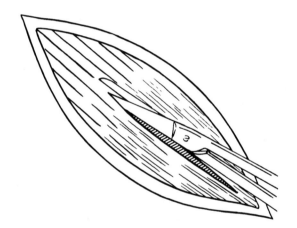

Fig. 7.2 Appendicectomy. The external oblique aponeurosis is split by pushing partly closed scissors in the line of the fibres.

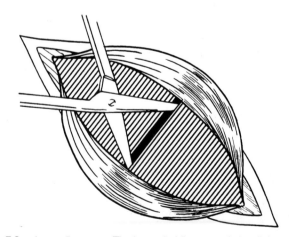

Fig. 7.3 Appendicectomy. The internal oblique muscle is split by opening Mayo's straight scissors in the line of the fibres.

4. Confirm the diagnosis: the appendix, or more usually its tip, is swollen, congested, inflamed, even gangrenous, often with fibrin deposition, turbid fluid or frank pus.

Difficulty?

1. *Is the appendix not inflamed?* Examine its tip to exclude carcinoid tumour (usually a yellowish swelling at the tip), since appendicectomy is usually curative. Adenocarcinoma of the appendix demands right hemicolectomy. Examine the caecum, since an ulcer, inflammation or cancer may present as appendicitis. Pass the distal 1.5 m of the ileum and its mesentery through your fingers to exclude mesenteric adenitis, Crohn's disease or Meckel's diverticulum. Palpate the posterior abdominal wall, ascending colon, liver edge and gallbladder fundus and the lower pole of the right kidney. Now feel below into the right rim of the pelvis, the bladder fundus, right iliac vessels and right inguinal region. In females examine the right ovary and fallopian tube, and attempt to feel the uterus and left ovary and tube.

2. Look for features of a distant cause such as bile-stained fluid tracking down from a perforated peptic ulcer, an inflamed gallbladder or a gynaecological cause. Be prepared to close a standard Lanz incision and make a fresh, well-placed incision, rather than struggle to deal with the problem by extending or stretching the incision in the right iliac fossa. The presence of free fluid, especially if it is turbid, is a guide to embark on wider examination of the abdominal contents.

5. If the appendix is inflamed but not critically fragile, you may confidently exclude Crohn's disease of the terminal ileum and Meckel's diverticulum. If the appendix is very inflamed, and particularly if there is any free fluid that may contain microorganisms, avoid spreading them around the abdomen.

Action
1. Mobilize the appendix from base to tip by gently moving or peeling away adherent structures. Remember that the artery enters from the medial aspect. If the tip is adherent, improve the view. Do not dissect blindly. If necessary, extend the incision. Apply Babcock's tissue forceps to enclose, but not grasp, an uninflamed portion of the appendix, to hold it so you can view the mesentery against the light and identify the artery.

2. Pass one blade of the artery forceps through the mesoappendix and clamp the vessels (Fig. 7.4).

If it is thickened, take the mesoappendix in two bites. Divide the mesoappendix distal to the clamp and ligate the vessel gently but firmly with 2/0 polyglactin 910 or similar material, ignoring the slight backbleeding from the distal cut end.

3. Crush the base of the appendix with a haemostat then replace the clamp 0.5 cm distal to the crushed segment. Ligate the crushed segment. Apply a haemostat on the ligature ends after trimming them.

4. Cut off the appendix just distal to the haemostat. Stop! You have entered the bowel. Place the appendix, held by the Babcock's forceps, together with the knife, into a kidney dish for contaminated articles.

5. Insert a seromuscular purse-string suture of 2/0 polyglactin 910 or similar material, mounted on an eyeless round-bodied needle, in the

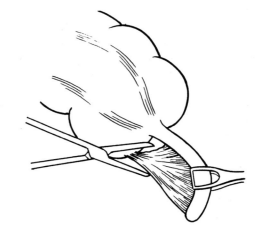

Fig. 7.4 Appendicectomy. Clamping the mesoappendix. The appendix is held up with tissue forceps.

caecum encircling the base of the appendix, at a distance of 10–15 mm from the base. Use the clamp on the appendix stump ligature to push it in while tying the first half-hitch of the purse-string suture (Fig. 7.5). Gently remove the haemostat before tightening the first half-hitch and then completing the reef knot.

Checklist
1. If the appendix is not inflamed, is there another cause for the clinical picture?

2. Examine all the structures you can reach. If there is any enlargement of the mesenteric lymph nodes, remove one for culture, another for histology. Soft, oedematous glands accompanied by a normal-looking terminal ileum often represents mesenteric adenitis.

3. Inspect for free fluid that may represent perforation of a viscus.

4. Check the appendix stump to ensure that it is intact and safely closed.

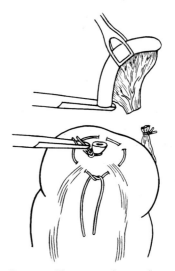

Fig. 7.5 Appendicectomy. The resected appendix, together with the haemostat at its base and the tissue forceps, is placed in a separate dish. The ligated stump of the appendix is invaginated while tying the purse-string suture.

1. If you cannot carry out the steps of the operation safely you must improve the exposure by extending the wound in the line of the skin incision laterally. Extension of the wound medially may encroach on the inferior epigastric vessels but once the rectus sheath is entered, the rectus muscle can be retracted medially.

2. If you cannot free the tip of the appendix, it is sometimes helpful to carry out retrograde appendicectomy. Crush, clamp and ligate the base of the appendix before dividing it. Now the base is free you will be better able to follow it to the tip.

3. If the appendix bursts in spite of gentle manipulations, remove it and look to see if a faecolith has escaped. Wash out any freed material using saline lavage and suction. If there has been any contamination, insert a drain to the superficial tissues, since the peritoneal cavity usually copes well with contamination provided the cause is removed.

4. If the base of the appendix is oedematous and fragile, do not attempt to crush it. If possible, carefully ligate it and cut it off 5 mm distally. If it appears unsafe to insert a purse-string, look for a piece of omentum or other peritoneum to draw over the stump and stitch it to a healthy piece of caecal wall.

5. If gangrene extends on to the caecal wall, first apply a non-crushing clamp gently across the bowel to limit contamination. Resect the gangrenous part to reveal healthy wall that can be closed with a suture line. If the hole cannot be closed, insert a large tube drain into the caecum and suture the edges of the bowel to the skin as a caecostomy. The stoma will close spontaneously in most cases, when the tube is removed after a few days.

6. If there is Crohn's disease and the appendix is not inflamed, do not carry out any procedure.

7. If you find an abscess, drain it but do not explore further or pursue a search for a buried appendix within the cavity. It will most probably be destroyed by the inflammatory reaction.

8. In the presence of purulent peritonitis, carry out appendicectomy. Now gently remove pus and debris and drain the wound. Consider copious saline lavage to cleanse the abdomen (see Ch. 4).

Closure

1. Suture the peritoneum with 2/0 polyglactin 910 or similar material.

2. Insert loose interrupted stitches of the same material in the muscle and aponeurotic layers to appose but not constrict them.

3. Insert a drain to the extraperitoneal tissues if there has been marked contamination, especially if preoperative metronidazole was not given.

4. Appose the subcuticular tissues with fine sutures in an obese patient and close the skin with sutures or clips

Postoperative

1. In the absence of general peritonitis, allow oral fluids after 24 hours.

2. If the appendix was gangrenous, continue metronidazole anal suppositories one each day for 1–2 days. If the appendix was per-

forated, and particularly in a high-risk patient, continue parenteral antibiotics such as cefuroxime 1.5 g 6–8 hourly for 3–4 days.

3. Remove any drain after 2–3 days unless there is still profuse discharge.

4. Monitor the wound if pyrexia develops, and exclude chest and urinary infection.

Key point

● If you decided not to remove the appendix, ensure that you explain this to the patient. A future clinician, seeing a scar in the right iliac fossa may wrongly assume that the appendix has been removed and attribute clinical features to other organs.

Complications

1. Wound infection develops occasionally in patients with mild appendicitis but has a higher incidence in those who have had a gangrenous or perforated appendix removed. Aerobic coliform and anaerobic *Bacteroides* organisms are usually responsible. Examine the wound regularly and remove one or two superficial sutures if there is evidence of infection, to allow any pus to drain.

2. If pyrexia develops, always carry out a rectal examination. Pelvic infection produces localized heat, 'bogginess' and tenderness. Repeat the examination at intervals to detect if an abscess develops and 'points'. Ultrasound or radiological imaging may help if you are uncertain. Finger pressure may release pus but if not, be willing to aspirate it using a needle inserted through the vagina or rectum. Otherwise gently thrust closed, long-handled forceps into the abscess and allow it to drain through the rectum.

3. Reactive haemorrhage is infrequent but occasionally the ligature falls off the appendicular artery. Return the patient to the operating theatre and reopen the wound to catch and religate the artery.

4. Faecal fistula develops in two circumstances. Either the patient has unsuspected Crohn's disease or in florid appendicitis the appendicular stump or adjacent caecum has undergone necrosis. In the presence of necrosis do not over-optimistically rely on suturing the defect. Prefer to insert a large tube in the hole and suture the margins of the hole to the anterior abdominal wall where the tube emerges. The tube can be removed after one week and the fistula usually heals spontaneously.

5. There is a possible late increased incidence of right inguinal hernia.

REFERENCES

1. Simpson ET, Smith A 1996 The management of acute abdominal pain in children. Journal of Paediatrics and Child Health 32(2): 110–112

APPENDIX MASS

Appraise

1. As a rule this is a late presentation of acute appendicectomy.

2. It may result from the adherence of omentum and other viscera

to the inflamed appendix. More usually the appendix has ruptured and an abscess has formed, its walls comprised of the fibrin-lined omentum and adherent viscera.

3. Antibiotics are commonly given even when there are no clinical features of sepsis and the white cell count is not raised. This is usually unnecessary except as prophylaxis in high-risk patients.

4. Provided the patient is well, not tender locally or rectally, and with no features of sepsis or toxicity, treat the patient expectantly. Mark out the margins of the mass and regularly monitor progress. Provided the marked margins of the mass do not extend, features of sepsis do not develop and the white cell count does not increase, wait for the mass to resolve. An opposing view is early operation.[1]

5. Ultrasound scanning or computerized tomography are valuable to exclude an abscess and if necessary allow it to be drained percutaneously. If it extends into the pelvis it can be drained transrectally under ultrasonic guidance.[2]

6. If septic signs develop, or if percutaneous drainage of an abscess is not feasible or fails, then carry out open drainage without delay.

7. The subsequent management of patients with a resolved abscess remains controversial. Conventionally, the patient is re-admitted for interval appendicectomy after about 3 months. At such operations one frequently finds no evidence of the appendix. If no further action is taken it is only rarely that recurrent appendicitis will develop.[3]

Access

1. Define the mass when the patient is relaxed under anaesthesia.

2. Employ a standard Lanz incision. You may encounter oedema as you reach the deeper layers of the abdominal wall. This warns you that you are about to enter an abscess cavity.

3. Alternatively you may enter the abdomen and find the mass on the posterior wall.

Action

1. If you find on entering the abdomen that you are within the abscess cavity, do not rush to explore the wound. Take a specimen of the contents of the cavity for bacterial culture and to determine the antibiotic sensitivity of the contained organisms. Gently and thoroughly aspirate all pus and debris. Explore the cavity with your finger to decide whether it is safe to enlarge the opening without damaging viscera or disrupting the cavity wall.

2. If you gain an improved view you may see the appendix and be able to remove it safely. Sometimes the terminal part has separated and you will need to remove it piecemeal.

Key point

● Do not misinterpret the presence of a short, apparently normal appendix. This is the stump left after the distal part has dropped off and is lying in the abscess cavity. Look carefully for it. If you do not find it, it will need to be digested by a long process of macrophage and microphage activity.

3. Sweep your finger round the cavity to identify any loose contents and remove them. Thoroughly aspirate any pus.

4. If you cannot find the appendix or if it is unsafe to open up the

abscess cavity, insert a tube or corrugated drain, closing the wound layers loosely around it.

5. If, when you open the abdomen, you enter the peritoneal cavity and find a mass lying on the posterior wall, pack it off from the remainder of the abdomen and gently explore the mass to determine if there is a plane of cleavage into the interior. Remember, inflamed tissues are friable; respond to the findings and be willing to stop if you encounter difficulty.

6. The mass or abscess may lie retrocaecally, retroileally, or within the pelvis. Be prepared to pack off the rest of the abdomen and mobilize the caecum by incising the peritoneum in the paracaecal gutter, so you can gently lift it off the mass. Now explore the mass to decide whether to enter it or leave it.

7. Whether you open the mass or leave it, insert a drain into the peritoneal cavity to provide a track for any pus.

REFERENCES

1. Handa N, Muramori K, Taguchi S 1997 Early appendectomy versus an interval appendectomy for appendiceal abscess in children. Fukuoka Acta Medica 88(12): 389–394
2. Kuligowska E, Keller E, Ferrucci JT 1995 Treatment of pelvic abscesses: value of one-step sonographically guided transrectal needle aspiration and lavage. American Journal of Roentgenology 164(1): 201–206
3. Price MR, Haase GM, Sartorelli KH, Meagher DP Jr 1996 Recurrent appendicitis after initial conservative management of appendiceal abscess. Journal of Pediatric Surgery 31(2): 291–294

SUBPHRENIC AND SUBHEPATIC ABSCESS

Appraise

1. Following major surgical procedures, operations performed in the presence of infection or sometimes spontaneously following, for example, perforation of a viscus, an abscess may form. It could result from retained foreign bodies, necrotic tissue, inadequate drainage of blood or contaminated fluid, or subclinical anastomotic or spontaneous leakage. The abscess may develop above the liver (subphrenic), below the liver (subhepatic), along either paracolic gutter, between loops of bowel in the mid-abdomen, or in the true pelvis.

2. 'Subphrenic' should be reserved for an abscess lying immediately below the diaphragm. On the right it lies above the right lobe of the liver, on the left it lies above the left lobe of liver, gastric fundus and spleen (Fig. 7.6). Right subhepatic collections may be anterior (paraduodenal) or posterior (above the right kidney – Fig. 7.7). Left subhepatic collections may lie anterior to the stomach and transverse colon, or posteriorly in the lesser sac.

3. Make the diagnosis from the development of rigors, swinging pyrexia, toxicity and leucocytosis. In the presence of subphrenic abscess the hemidiaphragm may be paralysed, as demonstrated on screening, and a 'sympathetic' pleural effusion often collects above the diaphragm. If leakage from a viscus or anastomosis has developed, or in the presence of gas-forming organisms, a fluid-level is often visible on plain X-ray, with gas above it. Aspirate a specimen of pus for culture and determination of antibiotic sensitivity. Ultrasound scan

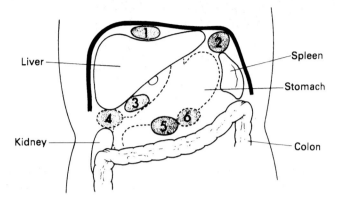

Liver

Spleen

Stomach

Kidney

Colon

Fig. 7.6 Common sites of abscess above and below the liver: 1, right subphrenic; 2, left subphrenic; 3, right anterior subhepatic; 4, right posterior subhepatic (hepatorenal); 5, left anterior subhepatic; 6, left posterior subhepatic (lesser sac).

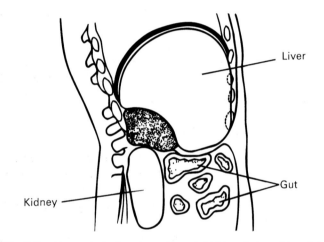

Liver

Gut

Kidney

Fig. 7.7 Abscess in the hepatorenal pouch (right posterior subhepatic). This type of posterior collection may be drained by an extraperitoneal approach from behind, through the bed of the 12th rib, or from an anterolateral direction.

is a valuable means of identifying an abscess. Computerized tomography and radiolabelled white blood cell scans may reveal abscesses not revealed by simpler methods.[1]

4. Once an abscess is identified and localized by clinical signs or imaging methods, a percutaneous needle can be inserted to confirm the presence of pus and aspirated material can be cultured and tested for antibiotic sensitivity.

5. At the same time percutaneous catheter drainage can be instituted and often succeeds.[2] An ultrasound- or CT-guided needle is inserted while avoiding damage to adjacent structures. A flexible guide wire is passed through the needle, which is then withdrawn. A bevel-tipped catheter is passed over the guide wire into the cavity and the guide wire is withdrawn. This is the Seldinger technique. Multilocular abscesses are often unsuccessfully treated in this way but may be successfully drained laparoscopically.[3]

6. Open operation is necessary for very large or recurrent abscesses, loculated abscesses, those containing blood, necrotic or inspissated material and those in which the cause continues, such as leakage from the gut or an anastomosis.

7. The choice of approach depends on the site of the abscess. Ideally, an extrapleural, extraperitoneal approach avoids the possibility of contaminating the peritoneal or pleural cavities. As a rule this is possible only for posterior collections, although a right anterior subphrenic abscess can sometimes be approached extraperitoneally. Multiple or loculated abscess cavities usually demand a transperitoneal approach.

REFERENCES

1. Goldman M, Ambrose NS, Drole Z et al 1987 Indium[111]-labelled leucocytes in the diagnosis of abdominal abscess. British Journal of Surgery 74: 184–186
2. Fulcher AS, Turner MA 1996 Percutaneous drainage of enteric-related abscesses. Gastroenterologist 4(4): 276–285
3. Lam SC, Kwok SP, Leong HT 1998 Laparoscopic intracavitary drainage of subphrenic abscess. Journal of Laparoendoscopic and Advanced Surgical Techniques (Part A) 8(1): 57–60

Oesophagus

John Bancewicz and R. M. Kirk

Contents

ENDOSCOPY

Appraise

1. Endoscope every patient with dysphagia except when this is fully explained by the presence of neurological or neuromuscular disease.

2. Endoscope patients with suspected disease in the oesophagus producing pain on swallowing (odynophagia), heartburn, bleeding, or if accidental and iatrogenic damage are suspected.

Prepare

1. Ensure that the endoscope, the ancillary equipment and necessary spares are available, function correctly and are appropriately sterile. The endoscope must be thoroughly prepared between procedures according to the maker's instructions. Fibreoptic instruments, biopsy forceps and similar instruments are scrupulously cleaned using neutral detergent and usually disinfected with 2% alkaline glutaraldehyde. This is capable of eliminating all infective organisms, including HIV. Keep abreast of the literature on methods of sterilization. Initial cleaning is done by hand. Washing and sterilization is performed mechanically in an automatic machine to avoid exposure of endoscopy room staff to glutaraldehyde fumes.

2. Modern gastrointestinal endoscopes are versatile, have remarkably flexible tips and can be passed with minimal sedation and pharyngeal anaesthesia in most patients. They are safe, relatively comfortable for the patient and allow examination of the stomach and duodenum beyond. Use the end-viewing instrument routinely since it gives the best general view. Through it can be passed biopsy forceps, cytology brushes, snares, guide-wires for dilators and needles for injection. Argon plasma coagulation or Nd–YAG laser may be applied through it for the palliation of inoperable neoplasms or for the treatment of Barrett's oesophagus. The technology of endoscopes is steadily improving and the rigid oesophagoscope is, to all intents and purposes, obsolete.

3. Obtain signed informed consent from the patient.

4. Remove dentures from the patient.

5. Except in an emergency have the patient starved of food and fluids for at least 5 hours. In an emergency, pass a naso-oesophageal or nasogastric tube to empty the oesophagus and stomach to prevent reflux and aspiration, before giving a general anaesthetic or passing a flexible endoscope under local anaesthesia.

6. Obtain a preliminary barium swallow X-ray if there is a suspected pharyngeal pouch.

7. Attach a pulse oximeter probe to the patient's finger and ensure that there are sufficient staff in the endoscopy room for safe care of a sedated patient.

8. Spray the pharynx with lignocaine solution just before passing the endoscope.

9. Insert a small plastic cannula into a peripheral vein and through it inject slowly 2–5 mg of midazolam until the patient's eyelids just begin to droop. Remember that it takes 2 minutes for the full effect of midazolam to develop.

Fibreoptic endoscopy

1. Lay the patient on the left side with hips and knees flexed. Place a plastic hollow gag between the teeth. Ensure that the patient's head is in the midline and that the chin is lowered on to the chest.

2. Lubricate the previously checked end-viewing instrument with water-soluble jelly.

3. Pass the endoscope tip through the plastic gag, over the tongue to the posterior pharyngeal wall. Depress the tip control slightly so that the instrument tip passes down towards the cricopharyngeal sphincter. Do not overflex the tip or it will be directed anteriorly and enter the larynx. Visualize the larynx and pass the endoscope just behind it.

4. Ask the patient to swallow. Do not resist the slight extrusion of the endoscope as the larynx rises but maintain gentle pressure so that it will advance as the larynx descends and the cricopharyngeal sphincter relaxes. Advance the endoscope under vision, insufflating air gently to open up the passage. Aspirate any fluid. Spray water across the lens if it becomes obscured. If no hold-up is encountered, pass the tip through the stomach into the duodenum then withdraw it slowly, noting the features. Remove biopsy specimens and take cytology brushings from any ulcers, tumours or other lesions.

5. If a stricture is encountered note its distance from the incisor teeth. Sometimes the instrument will pass through, allowing the length of the stricture to be determined. Always remove biopsy specimens and cytology brushings from within the stricture. Decide if the stricture should be dilated now because it is benign and requires no further treatment, or because it is malignant and the patient will benefit from improved oral feeding prior to surgical treatment, or because it is unsuitable for surgical treatment and palliative dilatation is indicated, possibly with intubation.

Assess

1. Note the level of each feature. The cricopharyngeal sphincter is approximately 16 cm from the incisor teeth. The deviation around the aortic arch is 28–30 cm, the cardia lies at 40 cm and here the lining changes abruptly from the pale, bluish, stratified oesophageal to the florid, pinker, gastric columnar-cell epithelium.

2. Oesophagitis is usually from gastro-oesophageal reflux, but is not necessarily associated with hiatal hernia. Consult a colour chart that illustrates the grades of oesophagitis. Most commonly there are red streaking erosions just above the cardia. Oesophagitis may be seen above a benign stricture. Occasionally, in advanced achalasia one may see a mild diffuse oesophagitis from contact with fermenting food residues. Thick white plaques indicate monilial infection, usually in association with oral involvement. Confirm the diagnosis by taking mucosal scrapings.

3. Sliding hiatal hernia produces a loculus of stomach above the constriction of the crura with a raised gastro-oesophageal mucosal junction. To determine the level of the hiatus, ask the patient to sniff, and note the level at which the crura momentarily narrow the lumen. Reflux and oesophagitis may be visible. A rolling hernia is visible only from within the stomach by inverting the tip of a flexible instrument to view the apparent fundic diverticulum.

4. Frank ulceration in the oesophagus is unusual, but may be due to severe reflux disease. In Barrett's oesophagus the lower gullet is lined with modified gastric mucosa and an ulcer may develop in the columnar-lined segment. In all cases of Barrett's take biopsies of the columnar segment from all four quadrants at 2 cm intervals. In patients with dysplasia even more biopsies are required for accurate assessment. Use 'jumbo' forceps. Ulcerating carcinomas may develop at any level. In most western countries the majority of cancers are adenocarcinomas and arise in the lower oesophagus in association with Barrett's oesophagus. Take multiple biopsies and cytological brushings from a number of areas of all ulcers.

5. Strictures from peptic oesophagitis or, rarely, ulceration in a Barrett's oesophagus develop at any time from birth onwards, but more frequently occur in middle or old age. Almost always there is a coincidental hiatal hernia. If there is no hernia below the stricture suspect cancer. Also suspect cancer if there is food residue above a stricture. Food residue may also be seen in achalasia and may be the only diagnostic clue. Take multiple biopsies and brushings for cytology. The cause of Schatzki's ring is unknown. It is usually asymptomatic, seen radiologically at the junction between gastric and oesophageal mucosa. Caustic strictures develop at the sites of hold-up of swallowed liquids at the cricopharyngeus, at the aortic arch crossing and at the cardia. Webs or strictures in the upper oesophagus are uncommon. However, it is not unusual to see a patch or ring of ectopic gastric mucosa in the upper oesophagus 1–2 cm below cricopharyngeus, the so-called 'inlet patch'. Stricture may arise from external pressure, of which by far the most common cause is bronchogenic carcinoma.

6. Mega-oesophagus may be seen in achalasia of the cardia, but is now uncommon as most cases are diagnosed long before dilatation takes place. Mega-oesophagus may also be seen in the South American Chagas' disease and in some cases of advanced scleroderma.

7. Pulsion diverticula are seen above the cricopharyngeus muscle (Zenker's diverticulum or pharyngeal pouch) and above segments of presumed spasm. Traction diverticula in the mid-oesophagus develop as a result of chronic inflammation of mediastinal glands, especially from tuberculosis.

8. Oesophageal varices are usually recognized just above the cardia as convoluted varicose veins, which may extend into the upper stomach.

OESOPHAGEAL EXPOSURE

Neck (Fig. 8.1)

1. The cervical oesophagus may be approached from either side. Operations for the removal of pharyngeal pouch or cricopharyngeal myotomy are usually carried out from the left side. Approach to the lower cervical oesophagus on the left endangers the thoracic duct; therefore whenever possible approach it from the right side.

2. The anaesthetized intubated patient lies supine on the operating table with the head turned to the opposite side from which the exploration will be made, resting on a ring with the neck extended. After preparing the skin, wrap the head, endotracheal tube and hair within a sterile towel.

3. Incise along the anterior border of sternomastoid muscle, through platysma muscle, cervical fascia, omohyoid muscle, ligating and dividing the middle thyroid vein to enter the space between the oesophagus, trachea and thyroid gland medially and the sternomastoid muscle and carotid sheath laterally. The inferior thyroid artery crosses the space: ligate and divide it only if it interferes with the dissection, preferring to retain it if the oesophagus is to be mobilized for subsequent anastomosis.

4. Rotate the whole oesophageal–tracheal–thyroid column towards the opposite side, bringing into view the tracheo-oesophageal groove, and display the posterior surface of the oesophagus and lower pharynx. Beware of inserting a Langenbeck's retractor into the tracheo-oesophageal groove since it may well crush the recurrent laryngeal nerve.

5. If the oesophagus is to be separated from the trachea, carefully identify the recurrent laryngeal nerve to preserve it. Gently insinuate blunt forceps between the trachea and oesophagus, taking care not to damage either the oesophagus or the membranous posterior wall of

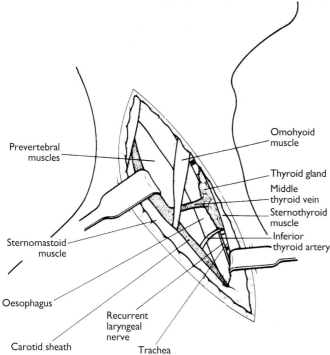

Fig. 8.1 Exposure of the cervical oesophagus on the right side. Sternomastoid muscle and the carotid sheath are drawn laterally. The space between these structures and the midline column of the pharynx and oesophagus, larynx, trachea and thyroid gland is crossed by the omohyoid muscle, middle thyroid vein and the inferior thyroid artery.

the trachea. The recurrent laryngeal nerve on the opposite side cannot be seen and is endangered. Insert a curved Moynihan's or Lahey's forceps between the tubes, turn the point posteriorly to make contact with the anterior vertebral muscles on the opposite side. Insert a finger behind the oesophagus to reach the forceps point and guide it through so that a tape can be fed into its jaws. Now withdraw the forceps, leaving the tape encircling the oesophagus. This can be the starting point for further dissection.

Thoracic

Right thoracotomy (Fig. 8.2)

1. The anaesthetized patient, intubated with a double-lumen tube to allow exclusion of the right lung, lies on the left side. Carry out right thoracotomy at the level of the fifth or sixth rib (see Ch. 26).

2. Ask the anaesthetist to collapse the right lung. Draw it downwards and forwards to reveal the mediastinal pleura. The oesophagus cannot be seen but the azygos vein can be seen arching over the lung root. Incise the mediastinal pleura, mobilize, doubly ligate and divide the azygos vein. This reveals the oesophagus running posterior to the trachea and lung root. The lower oesophagus is not visible between the left atrium and the vertebral column as it veers to the left. Expose it by diving the pulmonary ligament until the inferior pulmonary vein is exposed. Then divide the mediastinal pleura anterior to the descending aorta. The upper stomach can be approached after dilating or incising the diaphragmatic crus to enlarge the hiatus.

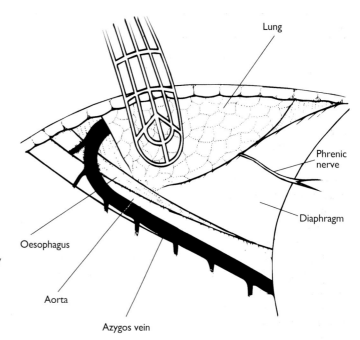

Fig. 8.2 Diagram of approach to the oesophagus through the right pleural space. The right lung is retracted anteriorly.

Left thoracoabdominal approach

1. The lower thoracic oesophagus and upper stomach are best approached using a combined thoracoabdominal approach (see Fig. 8.3).

2. Lay the anaesthetized intubated patient on the right side, left leg extended, right leg flexed at hip and knee, both arms flexed with forearms before the face as though performing the hornpipe dance. Allow the patient to lie back with the shoulders at 30° from the vertical. Fix the patient's hips with an encircling band; support the left upper scapula against a padded post.

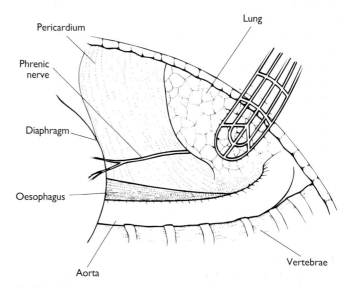

Fig. 8.3 Diagram of approach to the lower oesophagus through the left pleural space. The left lung is retracted anteriorly.

3. Prepare the skin and drape the area with sterile towels.

4. Start the incision just above the umbilicus, carry it obliquely upwards and to the left to cross the costal margin along the line of the seventh or eighth rib, extending to the posterior angle of the chosen rib. Deepen the incision to enter the thorax along the line of the rib, cutting and removing 1 cm of the costal margin. Incise the diaphragm radially towards the oesophageal hiatus or peripherally parallel to the chest wall. The latter method spares the phrenic nerve.

5. In case of doubt make the abdominal or thoracic part of the incision first: assess the condition and now, if indicated, extend it fully.

6. After completing the procedure, close the diaphragm with strong absorbable material. Suture the abdomen in the usual manner. Close the chest after inserting an underwater-sealed drain.

Abdominal (Fig. 8.4)

1. The lower oesophagus is approachable through the abdomen and oesophageal hiatus.

2. Make an upper midline incision extending to the costal margin, opening the peritoneum just to the left of the falciform ligament. Ligate the ligamentum teres. Divide it and the falciform ligament.

3. Draw down the stomach while an assistant elevates the left lobe of the liver with a flat-bladed retractor. The lower oesophagus can be felt at the hiatus.

4. If necessary, cut the left triangular ligament and fold the left lobe of the liver to the right. To improve the view of the oesophagus remove the xiphoid process and if necessary split the lower sternum subcutaneously.

5. To display the lower thoracic oesophagus, transversely incise the peritoneum and fascia over the abdominal oesophagus for 5 cm, preserving the anterior vagal trunk. If greater exposure is necessary insert a finger into the posterior mediastinum. Turn it forwards to separate the pericardium from the upper surface and incise the crus and diaphragm anteriorly for 5–7 cm.

6. In patients of suitable build, the oesophagus can be viewed almost up to the carina of the trachea if the heart is gently elevated with a flat retractor. It is usually unnecessary to close the incision in the crus and diaphragm.

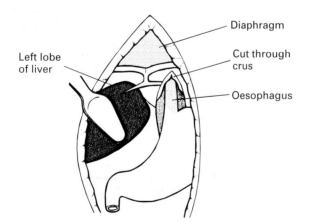

Fig. 8.4 Transabdominal approach to the lower oesophagus. The left lobe of the liver is folded to the right. If necessary, the diaphragmatic crus can be incised anteriorly.

OPERATIVE CONSIDERATIONS

Appraise

1. Most other parts of the bowel are covered with serosa that rapidly forms fibrinous adhesions, sealing small defects and preventing leaks. The oesophagus has no serous coat except on the anterior wall of the abdominal segment.

2. A considerable part of the oesophageal wall is composed of longitudinal muscle. Longitudinally placed sutures thus have a tendency to cut out. The powerful longitudinal muscle produces shortening of the transected oesophagus when it contracts. Unless this is allowed for, the most carefully placed sutures may be torn out.

3. When the oesophagus is completely relaxed it has a remarkably large lumen. Commonly, the action of the circular muscle makes the diameter appear to be small. However it can be stretched quite easily to facilitate the placement of sutures. If this is not done closely spaced sutures may become widely separated on stretching, and leakage can easily occur between them.

4. The blood supply to the oesophagus is tenuous when it is mobilized.

5. The healthy oesophagus is easily damaged but disease may make it exceptionally fragile.

6. A diseased or partially obstructed oesophagus is contaminated. Prophylactic antibiotics must be given to cover the operation.

7. Although oral feeding may be stopped temporarily following oesophageal surgery, swallowed saliva must still pass through.

8. Intrathoracic oesophageal leakage produces posterior mediastinitis and if the pleura is damaged a pleural collection develops. The best hope for the patient's survival if major leakage occurs is rapid clinical recognition with early reoperative repair and drainage. Minor leaks may be treated conservatively.

Anastomosis

1. The tenuous blood supply of the oesophagus makes it rarely possible to excise a segment, mobilize the cut ends and carry out an end-to-end union, except in neonates. Anastomosis is therefore usually to stomach, jejunum or colon.

2. Sutured anastomoses have been described using many different methods and materials, with up to three layers of interrupted sutures. This only demonstrates again that it is the meticulous care with which an anastomosis is performed rather than the technique used that determines the outcome.

3. Mechanical circular stapling devices are often useful. Do not assume that perfection automatically follows their use. As with sutures, staplers give results commensurate with the care with which they are used. Which to choose? The stapling device saves a little time. It may allow an anastomosis to be accomplished where suturing is difficult high in the abdomen, under the aortic arch, or high in the thorax – but if it fails, suturing is usually impossible and a higher resection is necessary. The stapling gun has an inevitable crushing effect on the tissues. If a dilated and thickened oesophagus is to be joined to the cut end of bowel, the resulting tissue bulk cannot be accommodated in the staple gun. It is safer to use a sutured anastomosis. Hand suturing is usually preferable in the neck since there may be insufficient bowel accessible below the anastomosis for insertion of the gun.

Sutured anastomosis

1. Have you made sure that the oesophagus and conduit, which may be stomach, jejunum or colon, can be joined without tension and are not twisted? When the oesophagus contracts, the powerful longitudinal muscle causes remarkable shortening. However, longitudinal muscle is of little value in retaining sutures, which easily cut out between the muscle fibres, so the strength of the anastomosis must depend upon the submucous coat and to some extent on the mucosa. Now make sure that the conduit has a good blood supply by noting the colour and by feeling good pulsations in the supplying arteries, and ensuring that the draining veins are not overdistended. It is difficult to judge the blood supply to the oesophagus – the best means of ensuring that it is adequate is to mobilize it as little as possible above the point of section. If you are not certain, do not proceed. The anastomosis is the most critical part of the operation.

2. Make sure the hole in the conduit matches the oesophageal lumen when it is slightly stretched. Place the oesophagus and conduit together as they will lie when joined. Insert traction stitches through all coats of both viscera, not quite at each end but a little posteriorly (Fig. 8.5).

When these are drawn apart they will slightly stretch the posterior walls and keep them in apposition, while leaving the anterior edges slack. Place a traction suture in the middle of each of the anterior edges, by which they can be drawn apart to display the posterior edges as they are united.

3. Suture material may be absorbable such as polyglycolic acid, monofilament polyglyconate, polydioxanone or braided polyglactin 910 or braided lactomer 9-1. It may be non-absorbable such as polyamide or polyester. Use very fine material such as 4/0 or 5/0. Although many surgeons still use silk, catgut and even stainless-steel wire with great success, the strength and reliability of synthetic materials make them attractive. They cause little reaction and the absorbable materials tend to retain their strength for longer than catgut.

4. The argument about continuous versus interrupted stitches continues. To achieve edge-to-edge contact, the ends must lie as they will when united, not be brought 'back to back' (Fig. 8.6).

Suturing may start at one end and continue round but it is wise to ensure that the last few stitches are placed in the middle of the anterior walls rather than at the ends, where the amount of tissue grasped and

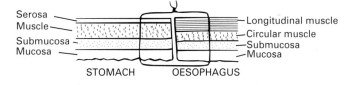

Fig. 8.6 Diagram of edge-to-edge oesophagogastric anastomosis using an all-coats stitch.

the distance between stitches is difficult to judge. Place stitches 2–3 mm apart, with 2–3 mm bites that penetrate all layers accurately. Make sure that every stitch catches the mucosa on each side. When the anastomosis is nearly complete, insert the last few but do not tighten or tie them until they have all been inserted. In this way you can ensure that every stitch is truly an all-coats stitch.

5. As you draw stitches taut and tie them, remember that there will be some swelling of the tissues within the next few hours. If you have pulled the sutures too tight, they will cut through. Concentrate on placing each suture perfectly. Prefer to cut out and replace any that you are not satisfied with, rather than inserting extra 'bodging' stitches that may merely damage the blood supply. At the end, gently rotate the anastomosis to examine it – but remember that even more important is the integrity of the mucosal apposition.

Stapled anastomosis
1. Make sure that the oesophagus and bowel can be joined together without tension, are not twisted and that both ends have a good blood supply.

2. Transect the oesophagus. Insert a purse-string suture into the cut end of the oesophagus, using a running all-coats over-and-over stitch around the cut edge (Fig. 8.7).

3. Assess the size of the oesophageal lumen by gently opening the jaws of an empty swab-holding forceps within it to allow the insertion of a test sizing head or use a measuring device that simultaneously stretches and measures the lumen. Select a suitable-sized stapling head.

4. Open the circular stapling device to its maximum extent, separate the anvil from the spindle and then retract the stem by 'closing' the gun without the anvil. Introduce the anvil into the lower oesophagus. Tipping the anvil sidewise may make introduction easier if it is a snug fit. Tighten and tie the previously inserted purse-string suture. Check that the purse string has drawn the oesophagus close to the stem. If there is a gap insert a second purse string.

5. If the stomach is to be used, create a temporary anterior

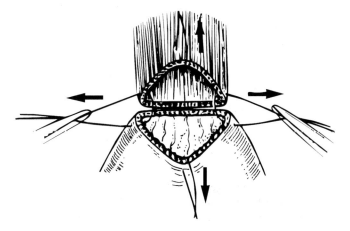

Fig. 8.5 Oesophageal anastomosis. The traction stitches are used to stretch the anastomosis.

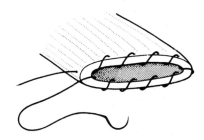

Fig. 8.7 Running purse-string suture inserted into the cut end of the oesophagus.

gastrotomy and insert the spindle of the stapler into the fundus at least 2 cm from any suture or staple line. 'Open' the instrument so that its sharp point comes through the stomach (Fig. 8.8). If the jejunum or colon are joined end-to-side, insert the stapler without the anvil head through the cut end, which will be closed later. Protrude the stem through the antimesenteric wall at a suitable point.

6. Attach the anvil on its spindle to the instrument and bring together the conduit and the oesophagus by closing the anvil down on to the cartridge. Check that there is no twisting and that nothing is interposed, nothing is protruding.

7. Release the safety catch.

8. Compress the handles fully and firmly until a definite crunch is felt. The gun has now been 'fired'.

9. Separate the jaws slightly. Gently rotate the device and draw it clear of the stapled anastomosis. Completely withdraw the instrument.

10. Remove the anvil head and check the toroidal ('doughnut-shaped') oesophageal and viscus cuffs trimmed from the inside of the anastomosis. Make sure they are complete and then place them in fixative solution prior to histological examination.

11. Insert a finger through the anastomosis to check it. If an aspiration tube is to be passed, ask the anaesthetist to pass it now and guide it through the anastomosis with a finger.

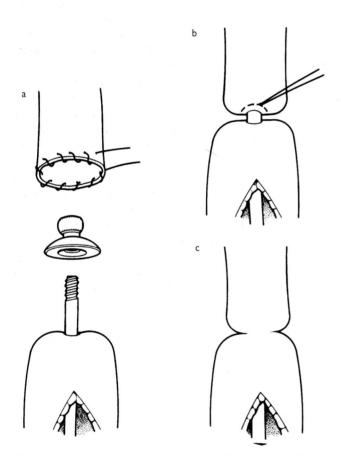

Fig. 8.8 A stapled oesophageal anastomosis; (a) the stapler shaft has been pushed through a hole in the stomach – the anvil is attached so that it can be introduced into the oesophagus; (b) the purse-string suture is tightened; (c) the device is actuated, producing an anastomosis.

12. Close the opening through which the instrument and finger were passed.

13. Carefully check that the anastomosis is complete all the way round and lies without tension.

GASTRO-OESOPHAGEAL REFLUX DISEASE

Appraise

1. The continence of the gastro-oesophageal junction is maintained by a combination of anatomical and physiological factors.

2. Gastro-oesophageal reflux disease (GORD) occurs when the function of the lower oesophageal sphincter is impaired.

3. Careful clinical assessment remains paramount in making the diagnosis and determining its effects on the life of the patient. Endoscopy is valuable to monitor the state of the mucosa and to detect the complication of Barrett's oesophagus, which is a premalignant condition. If symptoms of reflux cannot be confirmed by endoscopy, 24-hour lower oesophageal pH recording is useful. Assessment of GORD and its complications by radiology is inaccurate and therefore plays little part.

4. Uncomplicated reflux can frequently be managed without surgical treatment. Many patients are overweight.

5. Consider surgery if severe symptoms continue in spite of compliance with medical advice.

6. The best indication for surgery is persistent regurgitation. This responds poorly to medication and can be remarkably disabling.

7. Barrett's oesophagus is the result of reflux and seems to be increasing in incidence.

8. The most popular antireflux operation is the Nissen circumferential fundoplication. This can be performed by conventional open surgery through the chest or abdomen, but the laparoscopic method is now standard.

Transabdominal floppy Nissen fundoplication

Access (Fig. 8.9)

1. Elevate the head end of the operating table.

2. Use an upper midline abdominal incision, opening the peritoneum to the left of the ligamentum teres and falciform ligament.

3. Mobilize the left lobe of the liver and fold it to the right.

Action (Fig. 8.10)

1. Resist the temptation to approach the oesophagus as the first manoeuvre. In open surgery it is much easier to perform a Nissen fundoplication if the fundus of the stomach is mobilized first.

2. Divide most of the short gastric vessels that tether the stomach to the spleen. Use metal clips for haemostasis, but be careful not to pull them off with a swab. There is often a second layer of vessels entering the posterior aspect of the fundus directly from the splenic artery. Divide these also.

3. When the fundus has been mobilized continue sharp dissection around the hiatus to expose the lower oesophagus and the crural margins. Identify the anterior and posterior vagal trunks and preserve them.

4. Do not use blunt dissection. This causes bleeding and may damage a friable oesophagus. Do everything under vision.

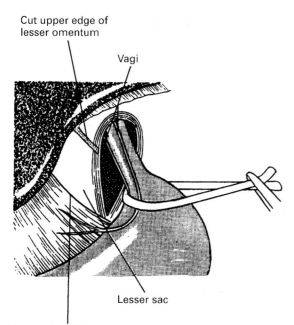

Fig. 8.9 Abdominal approach to the repair of hiatal hernia. The hernial sac has been excised to define the margins of the hiatus, and the upper edge of the lesser omentum has been detached from the diaphragm. Either an anterior or posterior repair may now be performed.

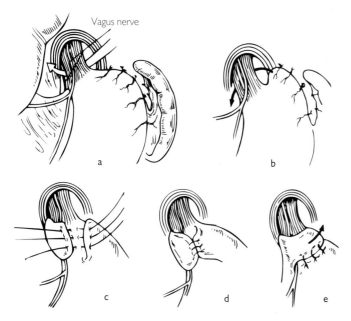

Fig. 8.10 Transabdominal Nissen fundoplication; (a) free the oesophagus in the hiatus, while preserving the vagi and branches; isolate, doubly ligate and divide the upper short gastric vessels; (b) gently fold the freed fundus behind the lower oesophagus to emerge on its right side; (c) insert three or four non-absorbable sutures to pick up the fold, the lower oesophagus and the anterior wall of the stomach to the left of the oesophagus; include the submucosa but not the mucosa; avoid piercing or damaging the vagi; (d) gently tie the sutures – you should be able to insert a finger beneath the cuff so formed; (e) rotate the cuff to the left in order to insert two or three sutures fixing the lower edge of the oesophagogastric junction.

5. On the right side, divide the upper portion of the gastrohepatic omentum, to display the right margin of the hiatus. Leave the hepatic branches of the vagus nerve intact, together with an accessory hepatic artery.

6. Trim the sac, consisting of stretched peritoneum and phreno-oesophageal ligament, from the lower oesophagus.

Posterior repair

1. Ask the anaesthetist to pass a 50F Maloney tapered mercury dilator into the stomach. This has a soft flexible tip and can be passed with safety.

2. Displace the gullet forwards and stitch the margins of the hiatus together behind it using two to four non-absorbable sutures. Leave a space between the hiatus and the stented oesophagus that will admit a finger or a 36F Hegar dilator. With practice the dilator may be omitted, but take care not to overtighten the hiatus to avoid postoperative dysphagia.

3. Excise the fat pad that lies in front of the cardia. Take care not to damage the anterior vagus when doing this. There are some surprisingly large blood vessels in the pad that must be ligated.

4. Now gently fold the gastric fundus behind the lower oesophagus so that the greater curvature emerges above the lesser curvature. The posterior vagus nerve may be included in the wrap or the wrap may be placed between the posterior vagus and the oesophagus. Both methods have their advocates and are equally acceptable.

5. The fundus of the stomach should fold around the oesophagus with ease and should lie in place when released. If it tends to retract the fundus has not been adequately mobilized.

6. Insert a non-absorbable suture, such as braided polyamide or expanded PTFE, to pick up the upper anterior wall of the stomach on the left of the oesophagus, the lower oesophagus immediately above the cardia and the part of the stomach that has been folded behind and to the right of the oesophagus. Each stitch is deep enough to incorporate the submucosa but not to pierce the mucosa. Tighten the stitch, so that the two folds of stomach are brought together in front of the oesophagus. Check that a finger or 36F Hegar dilator can be passed easily between the wrap and the oesophagus, which contains the 56F dilator. The wrap must be really floppy to avoid postoperative dysphagia and gas bloat. Insert a second stitch 1 cm above the first one. The completed fundoplication must not be more than 1 cm long anteriorly. If it is too longer there will be an increased risk of dysphagia and gas bloat. Insert a second row of two sutures over the first two to give added security, but do not lengthen or tighten the fundoplication with these sutures.

7. Resist the temptation to insert extra stitches and hitches. They do more harm than good.

8. Ask the anaesthetist to withdraw the mercury dilator and the nasogastric tube.

FURTHER READING

Agwunobi AO, Bancewicz J 1998 Simple laparoscopic gastropexy as the initial treatment of paraoesophageal hiatal hernia. British Journal of Surgery 85: 604–606

Anderson JR 1990 Oesophageal injury: part I. The changing face of the management of instrumental perforations. Gullet 1: 10–15

Bate CM, Keeling PWN, O'Morain C et al 1990 A comparison of omeprazole and cimetidine in reflux oesophagitis: symptomatic, endoscopic and histological evaluations. Gut 31: 968–970

De Meester TR, Wang CI, Wernly JA et al 1980 Technique, indications and clinical use of 24-hour oesophageal pH monitoring. Journal of Thoracic and Cardiovascular Surgery 79: 656–670

Donahue PE, Bombeck CT 1977 The modified Nissen fundoplication – reflux prevention without gas-bloat. Chirurgie et Gastroenterologie 11: 15–21

Hallissey MT, Ratliff DA, Temple JG 1992 Paraoesophageal hiatus hernia: surgery for all ages. Annals of the Royal College of Surgeons of England 76: 25

Oesophageal cancer

H. Akiyama, H. Udagawa and R. M. Kirk

Contents

INTRODUCTION

1. The epidemiology of squamous oesophageal carcinoma is the most varied of any tumour. A number of benign diseases predispose to its development including corrosive alkali burns, achalasia, the Paterson–Kelly–Plummer–Vinson syndrome and a history of irradiation. In addition, Barrett's oesophagus may lead to the development of adenocarcinoma.

2. The tumour spreads circumferentially and longitudinally within the mucosa (intra-epithelial spread), and spreads also in the submucosa and the muscle layer continuously or sometimes apart from the main tumour (intramural metastasis). It invades the trachea, bronchi, lungs, thoracic duct, recurrent laryngeal nerves, pericardium and aorta. This tumour notoriously spreads to the lymph nodes, not just locally but also at a considerable distance.

Appraise

1. Because oesophageal carcinoma is so often advanced at the time of diagnosis, some surgeons feel that treatment should be palliative.

2. There is general agreement that radical resection is indicated in otherwise fit patients with early lesions that have invaded the submucosa, the muscle layer and even the adventitia, provided they have no detectable nodal involvement (T1/213 N0).

3. Adequate resection of oesophageal carcinoma requires a tumour-free margin to completely avoid the development of recurrent malignant dysphagia.

RESECTION OF CARCINOMA OF THE LOWER OESOPHAGUS

Appraise

Our routine operation for carcinoma of the abdominal oesophagus and the cardia is resection of the lower thoracic oesophagus together with a cuff of the gastric cardia or entire stomach followed by jejunal interposition or Roux-en-Y reconstruction. This is done through a left thoracoabdominal approach (Fig. 8.a.1). Primary oesophageal carcinoma of the lower thoracic oesophagus needs right thoracotomy for lymph node dissection.

Access

1. Place the anaesthetized, intubated patient on the right side, with the left shoulder rotated back against a support attached to the operating table, or use a self-retaining mat.

2. Open the left upper abdomen obliquely along the line of the sixth or seventh intercostal space, starting in the midline halfway between the umbilicus and the tip of the xiphisternum and extending to the left costal margin.

3. Palpate the liver and the pelvis to detect distant spread. Determine the fixity of the cardia and feel for extensive lymph node involvement that would make resection useless.

4. If resection seems feasible, cut across the costal margin and along the seventh or eighth left rib to its neck. Open the chest close to the upper border of the rib. In elderly patients with fixed ribs be prepared to excise a few centimetres near the neck of the ribs above or below to allow adequate access.

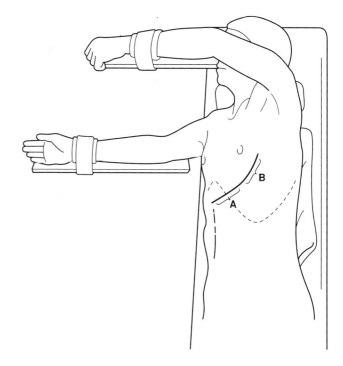

Fig. 8a.1 Left thoracoabdominal approach to the lower oesophagus. Line A is for initial abdominal exploration. When the tumour is resectable, the incision is extended (B). (Modified with permission from Akiyama H 1990 Surgery for cancer of the esophagus. Williams & Wilkins, Baltimore, MD.)

5. Cut the diaphragm radially 10–25 cm towards the right crus. You can cut through the diaphragm later and resect the crural muscle with the oesophagus if necessary. Insert a self-retaining rib retractor and gently open it in stages.

6. Stop all bleeding meticulously.

7. Anchor the incised edge of the incised diaphragm to the edge of the skin incision so that the left lung will not prolapse and interfere with the operative field during the intra-abdominal procedure.

Assess

1. Determine the extent of spread to the gastric cardia and glands along the left gastric vessels and around the celiac axis.

2. Even if the stomach and associated glands appear to be uninvolved, the left gastric area should be removed, including the root of the left gastric artery. If the cardia or upper stomach is widely involved, total gastrectomy is preferable. If the tumour is fixed, or if there are multiple hepatic or intraperitoneal metastases, resection is inappropriate.

Resect

Abdominal procedure

1. Open the lesser sac, dissecting the greater omentum from the transverse colon and severing the avascular portion of the gastric lesser omentum.

2. Ligate and cut each artery and vein of the stomach at the root according to the planned resection procedure.

3. Cut the stomach (for proximal gastrectomy) or the duodenal bulb (for total gastrectomy) with a linear stapling device.

4. Remove the anchoring stitch from the diaphragm and pass a tape through the hiatus. Pull the tape down to get good exposure of the left thoracic cavity.

Thoracic procedure

1. Gently free the lower lobe of the left lung, dividing the pulmonary ligament, taking care not to injure the pulmonary vein.

2. Locate the lower thoracic aorta and incise the mediastinal pleura just anterior to it. Dissect the anterior surface of the aorta. Ligate and cut the proper oesophageal arteries, which are rather rarely found in the lower mediastinum. Elevate and pull forward the lower lobe of the lung to display the posterior mediastinum.

3. Incise the mediastinal pleura just posterior to the pericardium. Gently mobilize the lower oesophagus, leaving the mediastinal adipose tissue on the oesophageal side and taking care not to accidentally injure the azygos vein and the thoracic duct on the left side.

4. Transect the oesophagus, ensuring there is at least 2 cm normal gullet above the tumour, in the specimen.

Unite

1. Jejunal interposition

Isolate a jejunal loop usually based on the second ot third jejunal artery. Take the cranial cut end retrocolically through the hiatus to be joined with a stapling device to the oesophageal stump. Join the caudal end to the gastric remnant.

2. Roux-en-Y

If total gastrectomy has been carried out, employ a Roux loop (see p. 108).

3. Oesophagogastrostomy

If the gastric remnant is long enough, intrathoracic oesophago-gastrostomy is possible.

OPERATIONS FOR THORACIC OESOPHAGEAL CARCINOMA

Ivor Lewis resection for mid-oesophageal carcinoma

This two-step operation is the classic method for dealing with mid-oesophageal carcinoma. The first step is the abdominal operation in which the whole stomach is mobilized for reconstruction leaving the right gastric and gastroepiploic vessels as feeding and draining vessels. The second step is the thoracic operation involving oesophageal resection and reconstruction using the pulled-up stomach as an oesophageal substitute. By careful positioning it is possible for two surgical teams to work simultaneously.

Radical curative surgery – extensive lymph node dissection (Akiyama)

Japanese surgeons have been performing extensive lymph node dissection for about 15 years. They include the extensive (three-field) lymph node dissection promoted by Akiyama and other Japanese surgeons. The operative mortality is satisfactory and the 5-year survival rate exceeds 50% for those who undergo a curative resection.

Reliable preoperative assessment of the tumour is mandatory by endoscopy, conventional ultrasound of the neck and abdomen, endoscopic ultrasound, and computerized tomography. The basis of the operation is the Ivor Lewis procedure but the lymph nodes are cleared in the lower neck, the mediastinum and the upper abdomen.

FURTHER READING

Akiyama H 1980 Surgery for carcinoma of the esophagus. In: Current problems in surgery. Year Book Publishers, Chicago

Akiyama H 1990 Surgery for cancer of the esophagus. Williams & Wilkins, Baltimore

Akiyama H, Tsurumaru M 1988 Basic principles of resectional therapy for cancer of the esophagus. In: Jamieson GG (ed) Surgery of the oesophagus. Churchill Livingstone, Edinburgh, pp 605–610

Akiyama H, Udagawa H 1999 Surgical management of esophageal cancer: The Japanese experience. In: Daly et al (ed) Management of upper GI cancer. WB Saunders, London (in press)

Stomach and duodenum

D. Johnston and R. M. Kirk

Contents

ENDOSCOPY

Appraise

1. Diagnostic endoscopy using flexible fibreoptic endoscopes has become so easy that even inexperienced clinicians can safely pass the instrument and interpret most abnormalities.

2. Endoscopy does not compete with radiology but is complementary to it. Consider endoscopy whenever there is any possibility of a lesion lying within its scope. It often provides authoritative diagnosis because of the facility to remove guided biopsy specimens or cytological brushings.

3. It is no longer ethical practice to operate on a patient for suspected oesophago-gastro-duodenal disease without carrying out endoscopy when this is available, even when the diagnosis seems certain.

4. Endoscopy is mandatory before operations for gastrointestinal bleeding.

5. Following previous gastric surgery, radiology may be difficult to interpret and endoscopy allows the mucosa to be studied visually and by histology of biopsy specimens.

6. During an operation when an unexpected diagnostic difficulty is encountered, an endoscope can be passed down to allow examination of the interior of the upper gastrointestinal tract by the surgeon or a colleague.

7. When strictures are encountered they may be dilated using bougies or balloons. Malignant strictures may be enlarged using the Nd–YAG (neodymium–yttrium–aluminium–garnet) laser before passing the endoscope through them to view the viscus beyond. The endoscope tip can be reversed to view the stricture from below to ensure that no damage has been sustained. If necessary a splinting tube may be impacted in the stricture to prevent it from recurring.

8. Polyps may be snared and the base can be coagulated with diathermy current. With some double-channelled instruments, the polyp can be steadied with forceps while the snare is accurately placed.

9. With specially designed instruments it is possible to cannulate the ampulla of Vater for biliary and pancreatic duct radiology after injecting radio-opaque medium, or aspirate fluid for cytology. A diathermy wire can be used to perform sphincterotomy at the ampulla. Stones can be removed using a modified Dormier basket or a Fogarty-type balloon. They can be fragmented with shock waves. A stricture of the bile duct can be dilated using bougies or angioplasty-type balloons. It can then be cannulated with an indwelling drainage tube leading through the obstruction into the duodenum.

10. Percutaneous endoscopic gastrostomy has replaced operative gastrostomy for most purposes.

Prepare

1. The easiest endoscope to pass is a slim end-viewing instrument originally designed for paediatric use, but other types offer wider suction and biopsy channels through which larger forceps can be passed for biopsy, grasping foreign bodies or snaring polyps. The very flexible ends of end-viewing endoscopes make them very versatile, but side-viewing instruments are of value in special circumstances, notably when cannulating the ampulla of Vater (Fig. 9.1).

2. Make sure that the instrument, light source, suction apparatus, biopsy forceps, and air insufflation pump all work satisfactorily and that the instrument has been sterilized according to the manufacturer's recommendations. Sterilization of instruments during an endoscopy list demands careful organization to guard against transmission of microorganisms such as *Salmonella* spp, *Pseudomonas aeruginosa*, *Mycobacterium* and also hepatitis B virus (HBV) and immunodeficiency virus (HIV). Thorough cleaning is followed by immersion in 2% alkaline, activated glutaraldehyde or 10% succine dialdehyde for a minimum of 4 minutes. Since these substances are toxic, irritant and may cause allergic reactions, the endoscopes must be thoroughly washed afterwards.

3. Obtain written, informed consent from the patient.

4. The patient takes no food or fluids overnight before a morning endoscopy but may be allowed a light breakfast if the endoscopy is scheduled for the afternoon or evening. When there is no evidence of gastric delay, endoscopy is often worthwhile even when the patient has taken food or fluids within 4 hours. In an emergency, attempt endoscopy even if the patient has had a recent meal, determining to remove the

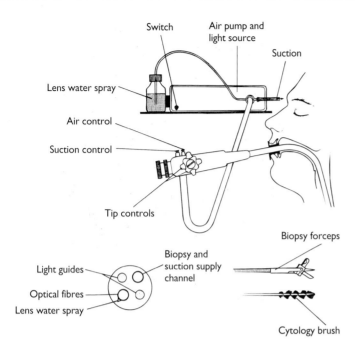

Fig. 9.1 Flexible fibreoptic endoscopy.

endoscope, pass a large gastric tube and wash out the stomach with water if necessary, using an electric sucker or Senoran's evacuator.

5. Apply protective gloves and spectacles before starting the procedure.

6. Ensure that the patient has no dentures. Anaesthetize the pharynx with an aerosol spray of 4% lignocaine or by giving amethocaine lozenges to be sucked 60 minutes and 30 minutes before the examination. The patient may be premedicated using papaveretum 20 mg with hyoscine hydrobromide 0.4 mg by intramuscular injection 1 hour before the procedure or a slow intravenous injection of up to 50 mg of pethidine (meperidine). For simple diagnostic endoscopy diazepam 10–40 mg given over a period of 3–4 minutes intravenously through an indwelling butterfly-type needle, just before the instrument is passed, is generally sufficient sedation. Other short-acting benzodiazepines, such as lorazepam, or midazolam titrated in 2.5 mg increments, until the patient's speech becomes slurred, may be used as alternatives. Further increments of sedative can be given and if the procedure becomes painful, small doses of pethidine can be given. Elderly or infirm patients given analgesics and sedatives are at risk of hypoxia, especially during prolonged procedures. If peristaltic activity is excessive, give hyoscine butylbromide 20–40 mg through the indwelling butterfly needle.

7. Insert a plastic mouthpiece between the patient's teeth or gums through which the instrument will slide easily. Smear the endoscope shaft with water-soluble lubricant. Secretion and mucus are less likely to adhere to the lens if it is smeared with silicone liquid and lightly polished to leave a thin film.

8. The patient may be laid on the left side, with no pillow but with the head steadied by an assistant who maintains neck flexion, discouraging the patient from extending his/her neck, which tends to make the instrument pass into the larynx. The patient's pronated left hand lies on the right chest, the right hand grasps the edge of the bed. Both knees and hips are flexed. Alternatively, the patient may lie supine but with the head of the bed raised. Stoical patients can be examined while they sit on a chair provided they are given minimal or no sedation and provided the instrument is passed with great skill and gentleness.

9. Before passing the instrument, carefully inspect any barium meal radiographs to assess potential difficulties and pinpoint areas requiring special attention.

10. It is less tiring and restricting if the view is transmitted to a television screen.

Access

1. Slightly flex the tip of the instrument. Pass it through the mouthpiece, over the tongue, keeping the flexed tip strictly in the midline pointing towards the cricopharyngeal sphincter. As the tip reaches the sphincter there is a hold-up. Ask the patient to swallow. The tip will be slightly extruded, and do not resist this, but suddenly the obstruction disappears as the sphincter relaxes and the instrument can be smoothly passed into the stomach after unflexing the tip.

2. If there is any difficulty, insert the index and middle fingers of the left hand alongside the mouthpiece to guide and control the tip of the endoscope to the correct place.

   DO NOT USE FORCE.

3. Look down the instrument and concentrate on safely passing the instrument through the oesophagus and stomach and into the duodenum, noting incidentally if there is any abnormality. Insufflate the minimum of air to open up the passage. Hold the eyepiece with the left hand, adjusting the tip controls with the left thumb. Hold the shaft of the endoscope with the right hand close to the patient's mouth, advancing, withdrawing and rotating it as necessary. When the gastric angulus is passed, flex the tip to identify the pylorus. Advance the tip, keeping the pylorus in the centre of the field until the tip slips through.

4. The side-viewing endoscope has a rounded tip that makes it easier to negotiate the pharynx. If there is any doubt about the free passage, always examine the patient first with an end-viewing endoscope. Become familiar with the tip control and angle of view before passing it. When it has passed into the stomach, rotate it to bring into view the relatively smooth, straight lesser curve which ends at the arch of the angulus, below which can be seen the pylorus in the distance. Angle the instrument up towards the roof of the antrum while advancing the instrument. The view of the pylorus is lost momentarily as the tip slips through into the duodenum. Paradoxically, if the shaft is slightly withdrawn the instrument is straightened and the tip advances further into the duodenum. Rotate the shaft to bring the medial duodenal wall into view and as the instrument enters the second part of the duodenum the ampulla of Vater is usually seen as a nipple, often with a hooded mucosal fold above it.

Assess

1. Withdraw the end-viewing instrument in a spiral fashion to bring into view the whole circumference of the duodenum and stomach. Withdraw the side-viewing endoscope while rotating it 180° either side to view the whole circumference. Do not overinflate the stomach and duodenum with air. In the duodenum and distal stomach, keep the endoscope still and watch the peristaltic waves form and pass distally, to estimate the suppleness of the walls and exclude rigidity from infiltration or disease. With the tip of the end-viewing instrument lying in the body of the stomach, flex it fully while gently advancing the shaft to bring the fundus

and cardia into view. Flex the side-viewing instrument to produce the same view. From just above the cardia the end-viewing instrument displays the pinchcock action of the diaphragmatic crura at each in-spiration. If gastric mucosa is seen above this, there is a sliding hiatal hernia. The gastric mucosa is pink and shiny: at the crenated transition to the thinner and more opaque oesophageal squamous mucosa, the colour becomes paler and sometimes slightly bluish. Islands of pink gastric mucosa may be seen above the line of transition.

2. If the view disappears, withdraw the instrument and insufflate a little air. If the lens is obscured, clean it with the water jet or wipe it against the mucosa to free it of adherent mucus.

3. Remove biopsy specimens under vision from any suspicious sites, including tumours, the edges of ulcers, irregularities of the mucosa and suspected inflammation. Take specimens from different places, preferably from each quadrant of an ulcer.

4. Cytological diagnosis is extremely helpful: pass the brush through the biopsy channel and rotate it against the suspicious area. Withdraw it and wipe it against clean glass slides, which are sprayed with fixative or placed in special jars containing fixative. The brush may be agitated in a separate jar of fixative – this will be subsequently centrifuged and the cells stained and examined.

Postoperative

1. Lay a heavily sedated patient on the left side, slightly face-down, under the care of a trained nurse who will watch him until he recovers fully. If he has any respiratory obstruction this must be overcome: chest physiotherapy will help him to cough up his retained secretions. Do not allow any fluids or foods to be given until the patient is fully recovered and until the effect of pharyngeal anaesthesia has worn off – usually 4 hours.

2. Carefully clean and check the instrument.

ACCESS IN THE UPPER ABDOMEN

1. *Gastric cardia*: Tilt the whole patient slightly head-up.

2. *Kocher's duodenal mobilization*: This manoeuvre (Fig. 9.2) raises the head of the pancreas contained within the duodenal loop into its embryological midline position, restrained by the structures in the free edge of the lesser omentum above, the superior mesenteric vessels below, and the body and tail of the pancreas to the left. Incise the peritoneum and underlying fascia of Toldt for 5 cm, placing the incision 1 cm from and parallel to the convex border of the second part of the duodenum. Insinuate your fingers beneath the descending duo-denum and pancreatic head. A natural plane of cleavage opens up between the embryological layers that were present when the duodenum was freely suspended in the peritoneal cavity.

> ### Key point
>
> • Did you make a firm diagnosis before operation? Mucosal lesions within hollow organs are best assessed from within the lumen by radiology and endoscopy, not by examination of the exterior at operation.

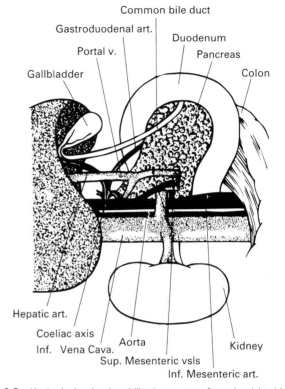

Fig. 9.2 Kocher's duodenal mobilization, as seen from the right side of the patient.

SUTURING AND STAPLING THE STOMACH AND DUODENUM

Suturing

1. The traditional absorbable material, 2/0 chromic catgut, has served well. Stronger, more reliably absorbed synthetic materials that elicit less inflammatory reaction have been created by the manufacturers. Finer thread can be safely used, thus introducing less foreign material. All sutures are severely weakened by crushing, abrasion and rough hand-ling, especially when drawing them through the tissues and tying knots.

Many surgeons still insert an outer non-absorbable layer. As an alternative to silk or linen thread, non-absorbable 3/0 or 4/0 braided polyamide may be used, but slowly absorbing synthetics are probably better.

2. Innumerable papers have been written about the best ways of suturing stomach and intestine. There is but a single common factor and that is the care with which sutures are inserted and tied. If you bring together edges of stomach or bowel that have a good blood supply, are not under tension and are apposed carefully with sutures that do not strangulate the included tissue, they will heal. The one layer that must always be included in the stitches, as shown by Halsted, is the submucosa.

Ligatures

As with sutures, ligatures are applied using the finest possible materials, although silk and linen are still popular because of their excellent handling properties. Metal clips are reliable to clamp blood vessels but they easily catch in swabs and can be dragged off.

Staples

The development of reliable instruments for joining bowel has potentially great value in gastroduodenal surgery. However, they are not as versatile as sutures. If you are a trainee, by all means learn to use stapling instruments but more importantly take every opportunity to master the accurate placement of sutures.

There are two over-riding indications for using stapling instruments. The first is when the difficulties of suturing, perhaps because of inadequate access that cannot be improved, make stapling safer. The second is when speed is essential, perhaps during a major operation.

GASTROTOMY AND GASTRODUODENOTOMY

Appraise

1. Gastric, gastroduodenal and duodenal incision allows the interior of the bowel to be examined to confirm, biopsy or treat a suspected lesion such as an ulcer, tumour or source of bleeding.

2. Gastrotomy allows access from below to the lower oesophagus. Strictures are often dilated more safely from below than from above. If a prosthetic tube such as Mousseau–Barbin or Celestin is to be pulled through an oesophageal stricture, it is necessary to carry out gastrotomy.

Access

1. As a rule, open the stomach on the anterior wall midway between the greater and lesser curves.

2. To recover a tube or dilate the gullet, open the proximal stomach only sufficiently to pass a finger or bougie or for the prosthetic tube to emerge.

3. For the purpose of diagnosis, start with a small incision, 3–4 cm long, the proximal end of which is 5–6 cm from the pylorus. This incision ensures that the intact pylorus or mucosal diaphragm can be examined and it may be unnecessary to destroy the pyloric muscular ring. The incision can be extended proximally or, if it becomes necessary, distally through the pyloric ring on to the anterior wall of the duodenal bulb.

4. To view the interior, first aspirate all the contents. Retractors may be placed to hold open the stomach so that it can be examined by adjusting the theatre light to shine through the opening. The stomach can be manoeuvred manually to bring different parts of the interior into view. Frequently the gastric wall can be evaginated through the incision so that it can be examined and any lesion excised or biopsied. If the pylorus is not too narrow, small retractors may be placed in it to allow the duodenal bulb to be viewed, and if it is wide, an unscarred duodenal bulbar wall may be evaginated through it on a finger. If there is difficulty in viewing the duodenum to exclude or confirm disease, a peroral endoscope may be introduced through it. Sometimes when fibreoptic endoscopy is ineffective before operation, perhaps resulting from inability to evacuate the gastric contents, the stomach may be emptied and endoscopy can then be performed. The gastrotomy can be temporarily occluded with a clamp to allow the stomach to be inflated but as a rule the stomach can be held open to allow endoscopy to be accomplished without the need for inflation.

Closure

1. Close a gastrotomy in one or two layers, leaving a longitudinal suture line.

2. It is conventional practice to close a gastroduodenotomy as a Heineke–Mikulicz pyloroplasty. This may be accomplished using a single edge-to-edge row of sutures, a two-layer invaginating suture or a row of staples. However, this destroys the pyloric metering function and if truncal vagotomy is not carried out, it may be preferable to carefully close the incision to create a longitudinal scar, bringing the edges together without invagination in a single layer, taking care to appose the pyloric edges perfectly. If highly selective vagotomy is performed, close the gastroduodenotomy longitudinally, to preserve the sphincter. Cover the suture line with a layer of omentum as an extra precaution.

3. Use ingenuity to incorporate the gastrotomy in plans for other procedures. A distal gastrotomy may be incorporated in a gastroenterostomy. The proximal part of a long gastroduodenotomy may be closed longitudinally and the distal part converted into a pyloroplasty if necessary. If gastrectomy is intended, temporarily close the gastrotomy with stitches or staples to limit soiling to a minimum.

OPERATIVE GASTROSTOMY

Appraise

Gastrostomy offers a valuable method of feeding patients who are unable to swallow because of oesophageal obstruction, bulbar palsy and other causes. Patients with mechanical obstruction who will have reconstructive surgery utilizing the stomach as a conduit should not normally have a temporary gastrostomy since this will interfere with subsequent reconstructive surgery. They are better served by a jejunostomy.

Stamm's gastrostomy is almost universally used now (Fig. 9.3).

PERFORATED PEPTIC ULCER

Appraise

1. Record the patient's age, blood pressure and the presence or absence of serious associated disease such as cardiac, respiratory or renal failure. If the patient is over 60 years old, with systolic blood pressure below 100 mmHg and serious comorbidity, he is likely to die if operated on, so conservative management may be preferable.

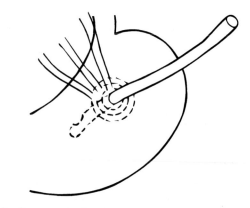

Fig. 9.3 Stamm gastrostomy.

2. Not all patients who have a perforated peptic ulcer should have an operation. Patients seen within 8 hours, in whom a confident diagnosis is made and who are haemodynamically stable, may be treated conservatively. Ensure that the tip of an 18F nasogastric tube is accurately placed in the most dependent part of the stomach. A disadvantage is that peritoneal toilet cannot be performed. Proceed to operation at once if the patient develops pyrexia, tachycardia, pain, distension or increasing intraperitoneal gas on X-rays.

3. Perforated gastric ulcer carries a higher mortality than perforated duodenal ulcer, because the patients are, on average, older and less 'fit' generally. Most gastric ulcer perforations are successfully managed by simple suture after excising a specimen from the edge for histology.

4. Perforated gastric carcinoma may be amenable to the same operation as would be carried out electively.

5. The diagnosis has been confirmed through the laparoscope and followed by repair using sutures or staples, and this may become an accepted method of diagnosis and treatment.

Access
Use a midline or right paramedian incision from the xiphisternum to the umbilicus, 10–12 cm long.

Assess
1. Remove all instruments from the field with the exception of a retractor for your assistant and the sucker tube for yourself.

2. Aspirate any free fluid after collecting a specimen for laboratory examination. Gastric juice is usually bile-stained.

3. Examine the duodenal bulb and the stomach, especially along the lesser curve. If necessary, open the lesser sac of omentum through the lesser or gastrocolic omenta to view the posterior gastric wall.

4. Remember that multiple perforations can occur.

5. Always remove a biopsy specimen from the edge of a gastric ulcer.

6. If you cannot find the perforation after a diligent search, explore the whole abdomen, if necessary extending the incision downwards. Examine in particular the gallbladder and sigmoid colon. If you are still puzzled, consider the possibility of Boerhaave's syndrome (spontaneous rupture of distal oesophagus).

7. If you are a surgeon in training and find yourself in difficulty because of either failure to discover the cause or indecision about the best course of action, or because the required procedure is beyond your capabilities, do not hesitate to contact your chief for advice and assistance.

🔑 Key point

- Your function at this emergency operation is to perform the simplest procedure that will correct the catastrophe. If you do more than this, will you be able to justify it to yourself and others if the patient succumbs?

Simple closure
1. Place two or three parallel sutures of 2/0 chromic catgut or 3/0 synthetic absorbable material on eyeless needles through all coats, passing in 1 cm proximal to the ulcer edge and emerging 1 cm distal

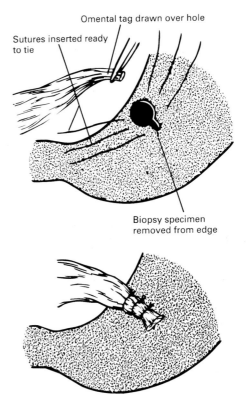

Fig. 9.4 Suture of a perforated peptic ulcer.

to the ulcer (Fig. 9.4). Do not pick up the opposite wall as this will obstruct the lumen. When all the sutures are in place tie them just tightly enough to appose the edges.

2. If a stitch starts to cut through as you tighten it, do not continue. Pick up a convenient fold of omentum and place it over the perforation between the suture ends, and tie the suture over it to occlude the hole. Insert further stitches to reinforce the obturating action of the omentum, to make sure the hole is adequately sealed.

3. Even when closure seems secure, do not hesitate to suture omentum over it.

4. Aspirate any free fluid from above and below the liver, from within the lesser sac, from the right paracolic gutter and from the pelvis.

Checklist
1. Re-examine the closure of the perforation.
2. Aspirate in the collection areas once more.

Drain?
If the perforation was sutured without delay, if the closure is secure and peritoneal toilet was adequate, drainage is unnecessary. Make sure the insertion of a drain does not replace careful technique.

HEINEKE–MIKULICZ PYLOROPLASTY

Appraise
1. Reformation of the pylorus has the effect of increasing the size of the lumen and also destroys the pyloric sphincteric metering function. It can be used to overcome stricture of the pylorus and also to improve

gastric emptying following truncal vagotomy. Following proximal gastric vagotomy, the distal stomach or 'antral mill' remains innervated so that gastric emptying is not usually prejudiced and pyloroplasty is not required.

2. Pyloroplasty is simple to perform in most circumstances and has enjoyed great popularity as an adjunctive operation with truncal vagotomy for duodenal ulcer.

Action

1. Gently mobilize the pyloroduodenal region by Kocher's manoeuvre and place a large pack behind the upper duodenal loop to bring it forwards in the wound.

2. Make a longitudinal incision through all coats starting on the anterior wall of the duodenal bulb, carried through the pylorus and on to the anterior gastric antral wall (Fig. 9.5).

The incision, 4–5 cm long, should be centred on the narrowest part of the pyloroduodenal canal.

3. Aspirate the contents and inspect the interior of the distal stomach and proximal duodenum. Sometimes there is a mucosal diaphragm with no evidence of ulcer in patients with typical features of pyloric stenosis in whom an endoscope would not pass.

4. Gently apply tissue forceps to the middle of the upper and lower cut edges, and draw them apart, allowing the proximal and distal limits of the incision to come together, transforming the longitudinal cut into a transverse slit.

5. Close the incision, starting from the upper tissue forceps and ending at the lower forceps. The traditional technique is to insert an invaginating continuous all-coats layer reinforced with a second seromuscular layer of sutures. The invaginated edges temporarily produce some hold-up and many surgeons insert a single layer of all-coats sutures placed closely together, uniting the walls edge to edge without invagination.

GASTROENTEROSTOMY

Appraise

1. Gastroenterostomy was originally applied to the relief of pyloric obstruction from distal gastric carcinoma. It offers an important method of relief when gastrectomy cannot be carried out because the growth is locally too extensive or has already metastasized.

2. Gastroenterostomy was used for the relief of benign pyloric stenosis from duodenal ulceration, but in the absence of stenosis it diverts some of the acid away from the ulcer, which usually heals. A proportion of patients eventually develop an ulcer at the stoma, although this may be delayed for many years.

3. As a general rule surgeons now use only anterior juxtapyloric gastroenterostomy for benign disease (Fig. 9.6).

Access

Use a right upper paramedian or midline incision 15 cm long.

Assess

Explore the abdomen. If the patient proves to have extensive and inoperable carcinoma with no evidence of impending distal obstruction, carry out limited exploration only, but remove a biopsy specimen.

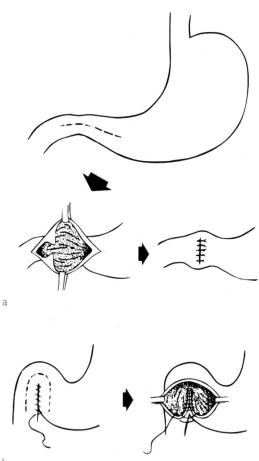

Fig. 9.5 Pyloroplasty; (a) Heineke–Mikulicz pyloroplasty; (b) Finney pyloroplasty.

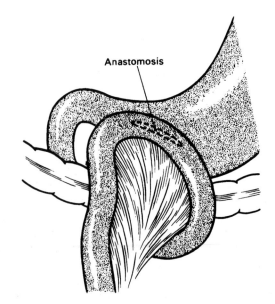

Fig. 9.6 Juxtapyloric anterior gastroenterostomy.

Action

1. Pick up a longitudinal fold of anterior gastric wall and grasp it with one of Lane's twin clamps. Choose a fold as close to the pylorus as possible if this is for benign pyloric obstruction or accompanies vagotomy for ulcer. Choose a fold as high as possible if this is to bypass an unresectable distal gastric carcinoma.

2. Lift up the greater omentum and transverse colon to identify the duodenojejunal junction. Draw the first loop of jejunum up over the colon and greater omentum to the stomach, with the short but not taut afferent loop against the proximal part of the clamped gastric fold and the efferent loop against the distal end of the fold. Place the second twin clamp along the apposed bowel, avoiding the mesentery, to occlude the lumen but not the blood supply. Lock the clamps together.

3. Unite the adjacent gastric and jejunal walls with a running seromuscular stitch on an eyeless needle. Leave the ends long so that the stitch can be continued to encircle the anastomosis.

4. Open the stomach and jejunum parallel to the seromuscular stitch and 0.5 cm from it on each side, for 4–6 cm if this is for benign disease and for as long as possible if it is to bypass malignant obstruction.

5. Apply specially coloured towels to isolate the area and keep separate instruments during the next part of the operation when the potentially infected interior of the bowel will be exposed.

6. Unite the adjacent gastric and jejunal walls with a running all-coats stitch. Carry the stitch round the corner on to the anterior wall to complete the anastomosis. As the anterior gastric and jejunal walls are brought together, invert the edges. A Connell mattress stitch may be used as an alternative to the simple over-and-over stitch but take care that the blood vessels are picked up and tied along the edges, since the Connell stitch is not haemostatic.

7. Remove the twin clamps, discard and take sterile replacements for the soiled towels, instruments and gloves.

8. Carry the seromuscular stitch round the end on to the anterior wall and complete it to encircle the anastomosis, burying the all-coats stitch.

Checklist

1. Examine the anastomosis and make sure it is patent.

2. Make sure there is no tension on the loop of jejunum. Draw the transverse colon and greater omentum to the right so there is no weight of bowel to drag on the anastomosis.

Technical points

1. The anastomosis can be fashioned using a linear cutter stapling device.

2. Suture material and stitches vary from surgeon to surgeon. We have described a sutured anastomosis using two layers of continuous absorbable stitches. A single all-coats stitch is also quite adequate. Many surgeons insert interrupted non-absorbable stitches such as silk on the outer, seromuscular layer. It is not the material or type of stitch but the care with which they are inserted that determines whether the patient will recover without complications.

3. The use of non-crushing clamps is argued about by surgeons. Certainly many successful surgeons use them routinely when they can be conveniently applied to prevent the leakage of bowel content into

the wound, and to hold the stomach and bowel perfectly apposed while the anastomosis is fashioned. If you use clamps, apply them to the bowel only and not across the mesentery. Apply them sufficiently firmly to occlude the arteries as well as the veins, otherwise the bowel becomes congested and oedematous.

BILLROTH I PARTIAL GASTRECTOMY

Appraise

1. Billroth I gastrectomy was originally used to resect distal gastric carcinoma. It is now rarely used. The distal stomach is resected and the proximal remnant is united to the duodenum (Figs 9.7, 9.8).

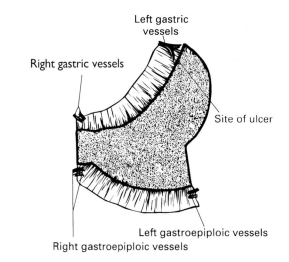

Fig. 9.7 Billroth I partial gastrectomy. The removed specimen.

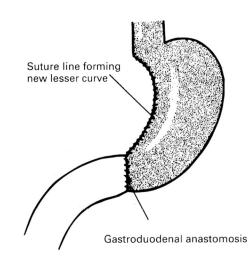

Fig. 9.8 Billroth I partial gastrectomy. The gastroduodenal anastomosis is complete, after re-forming the lesser curve of the stomach.

POLYA PARTIAL GASTRECTOMY

Appraise

The most frequent indication for gastrectomy is distal carcinoma. Polya gastrectomy is now preferred to Billroth I gastrectomy because it allows a full-width stoma to be constructed, which is unlikely therefore to become obstructed if the tumour recurs. Since the duodenum is closed and not used for anastomosis, distal spread of growth is less serious than when gastroduodenal anastomosis is used. The preferred method of resecting distal carcinoma is by radical subtotal gastrectomy with Polya or Roux-en-Y reconstruction (see later).

Access

Make a right upper paramedian or midline incision that skirts the umbilicus, extending downwards from the xiphoid process for 20 cm. Ligate and divide the ligamentum teres and divide the falciform ligament.

Assess

1. Explore the whole abdomen. If the operation is for carcinoma, start in the pelvis and lower abdomen, para-aortic region and root of the mesentery, proceeding to the liver before touching the stomach in order to avoid carrying malignant cells around the peritoneal cavity.

2. Carefully examine the stomach and duodenum to confirm the diagnosis and assess the strategy of the operation. If necessary, open the lesser omentum or gastrocolic omentum to examine the posterior wall of the stomach and contents of the lesser sac, including the glands around the coeliac axis and along the superior border of the pancreas.

Resect

1. Make a hole in an avascular area of the gastrocolic omentum to the left of the gastroepiploic vascular arch. Identify the posterior gastric wall and separate it from the pancreas and transverse mesocolon.

2. Clamp in sections, divide and ligate the gastrocolic omentum, extending on the left up to and including the main left gastroepiploic vessels and the first one or two short gastric vessels. Avoid damaging the spleen directly or by exerting heavy traction on the stomach. To the right, divide and ligate the main right gastroepiploic vessels as they lie near the inferior border of the pylorus. The separation of this vascular tissue can be accomplished rapidly using a stapling device that places two clips across the tissue and cuts between them in a single action. Avoid damaging the middle colic vessels, which lie within 1 cm.

3. Clamp, divide and ligate the right gastric vessels after identifying and isolating them as they run to the left in the lesser omentum just above the duodenal bulb and pylorus. Divide the lesser omentum proximally, if possible preserving an accessory hepatic artery if one is present.

4. Free the first 1–2 cm of duodenum after applying fine artery forceps on the small vessels posteriorly, dividing and ligating them with fine ligatures. Now apply a Payr's clamp across the duodenum just beyond the pylorus. Place a second clamp just proximal to this to occlude the stomach. If there is insufficient room for this, apply a non-crushing clamp across the distal stomach. Transect the duodenum just above the distal Payr clamp, ensuring that no gastric mucosa remains attached to the duodenum. Cover the cut distal stomach with a swab.

5. Dissect the duodenum free for 2–3 cm so that it can be safely closed applying fine forceps and ligatures to the vessels, keeping close to the duodenal wall. The common bile duct lies near the posterior and superior parts of the proximal duodenum and may be drawn out of its normal relationship by scar tissue. The gastroduodenal artery runs close to the medial wall of the duodenum.

6. Close the duodenal stump. First use a running over-and-over spiral stitch that encircles the clamp and the enclosed crushed duodenum. Gently ease out the clamp, tightening the stitches *seriatim* as it is withdrawn. Tie the stitch. Insert a second invaginating sero-muscular suture to cover the first stitch line or insert a purse-string suture and invaginate the first suture line as it is tightened and tied. If possible, insert a third stitch that picks up and draws together the ligated right gastric and right gastroepiploic vessel stumps, the anterior duodenal wall and the peritoneum over the head of the pancreas.

The duodenal stump may be closed using a linear stapling device. This places a double row of staples across the duodenum. If it is to be used it is applied just beyond the pylorus in place of the Payr crushing clamp, and a proximal clamp is placed across the distal stomach. Activate the stapling device to staple and seal the duodenum, which is transected using a scalpel applied closely to the upper edge of the stapler. Alternatively, close the distal stomach and duodenal stump with GIA® staplers. It is wise to invaginate or reinforce the everted staple line with a layer of sutures.

7. Radical subtotal gastrectomy is described later, but non-radical partial gastrectomy is appropriate in frail patients and in those who have a resectable carcinoma but already have metastatic deposits in the liver or elsewhere that make radical resection impossible.

8. Exert a little tension on the left gastric vessels by elevating the pyloric end of the stomach. Identify the artery by feeling for the pulsations. Isolate the vessels from the lesser curve of the stomach, doubly clamp, divide and ligate them.

9. Select the line for the transection of the stomach (Fig. 9.9).

10. Ask the anaesthetist to withdraw the nasogastric tube until the tip lies above the line of transection.

11. Plan to provide a full width gastroenterostomy to guard against recurrent tumour causing obstruction.

Unite (Fig. 9.10)

1. Place one of the twin gastroenterostomy clamps across the stomach 2 cm above the proposed line of transection, from greater to lesser

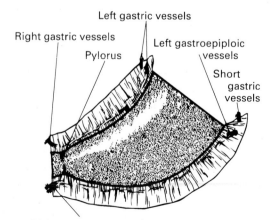

Right gastric vessels

Pylorus

Left gastric vessels

Left gastroepiploic vessels

Short gastric vessels

Right gastroepiploic vessels

Fig. 9.9 Polya partial gastrectomy. The removed specimen.

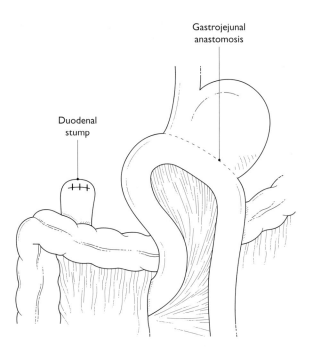

Fig. 9.10 Polya partial gastrectomy. The antecolic gastrojejunal anastomosis, with afferent loop joined to lesser curve, is complete. The duodenal stump is closed.

curve. Place a long non-crushing clamp across the stomach 3 cm distal to the twin clamp and parallel to it. The stomach will be transected just above this clamp. Fold the distal part of the stomach upwards. Reach down and identify the duodenojejunal junction. Draw up to the stomach the first loop of jejunum, with afferent loop to lesser curve with no slack but not tight. The efferent loop is placed at the greater curve. Place the second of the twin clamps across this loop of bowel, occluding only the lumen and not the mesentery. Marry and lock the clamps together.

2. Run a continuous seromuscular stitch to unite the adjacent gastric and jejunal walls.

3. Incise the full width of the posterior gastric wall 0.5 cm above the clamp, taking care at this time to leave the anterior wall intact. Make a parallel incision in the jejunum, 0.5 cm from the seromuscular suture line. Join the adjacent gastric and jejunal edges with an all-coats stitch on an eyeless needle. Now cut through the anterior wall of the stomach 1 cm distal to the clamp and remove the specimen of distal stomach. Continue the all-coats stitch round on to the anterior wall and along it to completely encircle the anastomosis. Remove the clamps, discard and take sterile replacements of the towels, gloves and instruments. Complete the seromuscular suture line on to the anterior wall to encircle the anastomosis.

4. Alternatively, the gastroenterostomy can be accomplished using stapling devices. Place and actuate a long, straight stapling device across the stomach at the proposed line of section and cut off the distal gastric specimen with a scalpel run along the distal edge of the stapler. Remove the stapler. Bring up a proximal loop of jejunum and suture it to the posterior wall of the stomach 5 cm above the staple line, placing a seromuscular stitch at each end, with the afferent loop to the lesser curve, the efferent loop to the greater curve. Make a stab wound in the greater curve aspect of the posterior wall of the stomach 2 cm proximal to the staple line and make a matching stab wound in the jejunum at the origin of the efferent loop. Insert the two limbs of the stapler separately into the holes, with the tips pointing to the lesser curve. Ensure that there is no interposed tissue, lock the two limbs together and actuate the instrument. Four lines of staples will have united stomach to jejunum and the knife will have cut a stoma between the centre rows of staples. Unlock and withdraw the stapler. Carefully check that the staple lines are perfect. Place tissue forceps at the ends of the inner and outer staple lines and separate the forceps to create an everted linear defect in the anastomosis. Place a short, straight stapler across the everted lips of the defect, tighten and actuate it. Cut off the excess tissue, remove the stapler and check the line of closure carefully, if necessary reinforcing the whole anastomosis all round with sutures.

> ### 🔑 Key point
>
> - The inside of the stomach and bowel are infected with micro-organisms. While fashioning anastomoses, isolate the interior of the bowel from the peritoneal cavity and wound edges by using separate towels, instruments and gloves. When the bowel is repaired, discard and replace them with sterile gloves, towels and instruments.

Checklist

1. Examine the anastomosis. See that it is perfectly fashioned and intact. If necessary insert extra sutures. Ensure that you can invaginate the gastric and jejunal walls through the stoma.

2. Check each of the main vascular ligatures. Retie them if they are insecure.

3. Check the spleen. Aspirate all the blood from under the left cupola of the diaphragm and recheck it just before closing the abdomen to ensure that there has been no further collection of blood.

4. Make sure the duodenal stump is safely closed. Should you leave a drain down to it? If so, does this replace careful technique and should you therefore reclose the duodenum or reinforce the closure?

5. Examine the colon to ensure there is no damage to it, or the mesocolon or middle colic vessels. Draw the greater omentum, transverse colon and mesocolon through to the right so there is no weight of colon resting on the anastomosis.

6. Aspirate any blood from under the right cupola of the diaphragm, from under the liver and in the right prerenal pouch. Finally, aspirate any blood that has collected in the pelvis.

GASTRODUODENAL BLEEDING

Appraise

1. Bleeding is the most life-threatening complication of peptic ulcer. Its management is best carried out by experienced clinicians, endoscopists and surgeons acting as a team. Dedicated units achieve much better survival than those undertaking it as part of a general service.

2. Erosive bleeding sometimes complicates bleeding elsewhere, sepsis, burns, head injury and major trauma. Drugs such as steroids and non-steroidal anti-inflammatory drugs (NSAIDs) can cause erosive bleeding or be associated with ulcer bleeding. Alcohol causes acute gastritis with bleeding from this or, following retching, Mallory–Weiss tears around the cardia.

3. Carry out endoscopy as soon as possible to determine the cause, site, state and number of lesions. Look for continuing bleeding and the presence of visible vessels, which indicate that the bleeding is likely to continue or recur. Even if you cannot identify the source you can usually exonerate particular areas, for example excluding oesophageal varices.

4. Relative indications for operation when other methods of control have failed remain:

a. continuing bleeding that fails to respond to other measures
b. bleeding that recurs
c. patient more than 60 years old
d. gastric ulcer bleeding
e. cardiovascular disease patients, who do not withstand hypotension well. This makes it dangerous to defer operation if bleeding is serious and not controllable.

Action

1. Bleeding duodenal ulcer is preferably treated at present by pyloroplasty or duodenotomy, and suture of the bleeding vessels (Fig. 9.11).

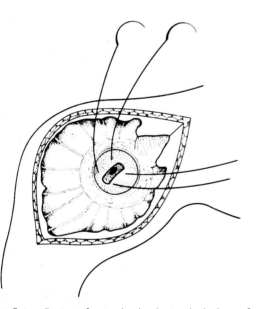

Fig. 9.11   Suture-ligature of gastroduodenal artery in the base of posterior duodenal ulcer, using 2/0 silk.

GASTRIC CARCINOMA

Appraise

1. At present the best hope of cure is radical resection. Gastric carcinoma is usually resistant to radiation therapy, but responses to chemotherapy are improving.

2. Unfortunately, most tumours present late. In Japan a high proportion of early cancers are detected by screening or open access endoscopy and are successfully treated by surgery.

3. Endoscopy with cytology and biopsy is the best method of screening and diagnosis. It is valuable in detecting early gastric cancer.

4. The ability to determine the extent of the tumour before operation saves many patients from fruitless exploration.

5. Careful studies, carried out mainly in Japan, have demonstrated the sequential spread of cancer from various sites in the stomach to the lymph nodes. Local nodes within 3 cm of the primary tumour are designated N1, the next nodes to be affected are N2, the third tier is N3 and distant spread is N4.

6. En bloc resection of the tumour with the N1 nodes is designated a D1 resection, with the N1 and N2 nodes a D2 resection. D2 resection is the standard procedure. On occasion a D3 resection may be performed, incorporating the N3 nodes.

7. Removal of the primary tumour is valuable even when the growth has spread beyond the limits of radical resection.

8. When resection is impracticable, try to relieve existing or impending obstruction. Distal obstruction can usually be bypassed using a proximal gastrojejunostomy.

D2 RADICAL ABDOMINAL TOTAL GASTRECTOMY

Appraise

1. Radical resection is carried out on patients who have no evident involvement of the peritoneum distant from the tumour or of N3 and N4 nodes. Any local invasion of contiguous structures must be resectable with the stomach, such as proximal duodenum, a segment of small bowel, transverse colon, pancreas, liver lobe or parietal wall.

2. If radical resection cannot encompass all the detectable growth, carry out a more modest palliative resection if possible. Ensure that the resection margin is well clear of growth, because a resection that does not protect the patient against stomal recurrence and obstruction is not worth carrying out. If there are extensive metastases, even palliative resection is probably inappropriate. Bypass existing or impending pyloric obstruction with proximal gastroenterostomy.

Access

1. Make a long vertical midline incision skirting the umbilicus, or a paramedian incision.

2. If necessary excise the xiphoid process. Be prepared to mobilize the left lobe of liver and fold it to the right.

Assess

1. Do not immediately palpate the stomach. Note any ascites and peritoneal deposits. Start your complete exploration from the pelvis and work towards the stomach in order not to disperse malignant cells.

Exclude pelvic deposits and, in the female, ovarian seedlings. Examine the greater omentum for deposits and then raise it to feel the para-aortic nodes and those around the root of the mesentèry, and the right colic and middle colic arteries. Examine the full length of the small and then large intestine, seeking peritoneal deposits on the bowel wall, the mesentery and the parietal peritoneum. Look for incidental disease. Throughout the examination confirm the pulsations in the arteries, noting atheromatous rigidity, aneurysms and venous or lymphatic obstruction.

2. Now draw the omentum caudally to examine the upper compartment. Feel both lobes of the liver and adjacent diaphragm, gallbladder and free edge of the lesser omentum, the spleen, kidneys and adrenal glands. Starting at the oesophageal hiatus and working distally, look and feel for tumour involvement, fixity, glands and also incidental disease. Systematically move distally, avoiding handling or squeezing the tumour if possible.

3. Palpate the duodenum and initially split the floor of the aditus to the lesser sac to feel the head of the pancreas between finger and thumb. Now palpate the body and tail of the pancreas through the lesser omentum and transverse mesocolon, then the region of the coeliac axis just above the neck of the pancreas. This part of the examination cannot be exact and must be repeated as the dissection allows. If you are seriously in doubt whether to proceed, incise the lesser omentum in an avascular area near the liver and examine the coeliac axis and emerging arteries and assess the spread across the lesser sac. To assess the left part of the lesser sac and body and tail of the pancreas, carefully make a hole in the base of the transverse mesocolon to the left of the middle colic vessels. If you are doubtful about involvement of the head of the pancreas, perform Kocher's manoeuvre in order to palpate it adequately. None of these manoeuvres commits you to proceed with radical resection if you discover unsuspected spread.

🔑 Key point

- If you are still in doubt, plan to mobilize the stomach without dividing any vital structures until you have ensured that resection is appropriate and achievable. This may entail a change in the order of the procedure, approaching the suspect area from different aspects.

Resect

1. Lift the great omentum and dissect it from the transverse colon. There is a bloodless plane of fusion between the folded omentum, which was part of the dorsal mesogastrium, and the anterior leaf of mesocolon. Gently peel off the omentum, taking care not to damage the anterior leaf of mesocolon or the middle colic and marginal vessels. Continue on to the pancreas until you reach its upper border. Take care to avoid damaging the pancreas or its blood vessels.

2. At the left extremity of the greater omentum the left gastro-epiploic vessels pass forwards in the gastrosplenic omentum from the hilum of the spleen. Carefully dissect out the lymph nodes at the origin of the left gastroepiploic artery, then doubly ligate and divide the artery and vein.

3. At the right extremity of the greater omentum the right gastroepiploic vessels pass forwards from the gastroduodenal vessels.

Carefully isolate them and the subpyloric lymph nodes before doubly ligating and dividing them at their origins.

4. Now draw the distal stomach caudally to put on stretch the free edge of the lesser omentum. Carefully make a transverse incision in the anterior leaf above the pylorus to reveal the right gastric vessels and the suprapyloric lymph nodes. Dissect the nodes and doubly ligate and divide the right gastric blood vessels.

5. Gently burst through an avascular area of the lesser omentum close to the liver and extend this towards the cardia, keeping close to the liver. Look for and divide between ligatures the accessory hepatic artery crossing from the left gastric artery.

6. Perform Kocher's mobilization of the duodenum so that the first part can be dissected from the head of the pancreas. The blood vessels are short and fragile. In order to avoid damaging the pancreas, apply fine haemostatic forceps on the vessels a few millimetres from the duodenal wall, divide the vessels between the tips of the forceps and the duodenal wall, then pick up the short duodenal cut ends to ligate them. Do not allow the dissection to wander away from the duodenal wall while mobilizing 5–6 cm beyond the pylorus, or you risk damaging the bile duct and pancreas.

7. Apply two pairs of thin crushing clamps across the duodenum, the distal clamp being placed so as to leave 1 cm of freed duodenum to close and invert. Alternatively use a GIA® or similar mechanical stapler. Isolate the area with distinctive coloured towels. Transect the duodenum between the two pairs of clamps, cover the proximal cut end with a swab and fold it upwards. Close the distal cut end of duodenum as described in the section on gastrectomy for benign disease.

8. From the site of ligature of the right gastric artery, strip the peritoneum, connective tissue and lymph nodes from the hepatic artery, proximally along the upper border of the pancreas, to the coeliac artery.

9. Have the distal stomach elevated by an assistant, to tauten the left gastric vessels in their peritoneal fold. In the free edge of the fold lies the left gastric vein; identify, doubly ligate and divide this first. Now extend the dissection of the hepatic artery to the coeliac artery, in order to dissect all the glands from this area, including those around the origin of the splenic artery. Elevate the gland mass into the column of tissue around the now cleaned origin of the left gastric artery. Doubly ligate and divide the left gastric artery. We always place two ties on the proximal cut stump or transfix it with an arterial suture.

10. Have the stomach drawn caudally and to the patient's left, to place the cardia on stretch. Complete the division of the lesser omentum until the right side of the cardia is reached; now gently clean the upper lesser omentum, connective tissue and right cardiac lymph nodes from the gastric lesser curve down to the selected site of transection. The nerves of Latarjet will be transected during this manoeuvre.

11. Turn the distal stomach cranially again, to examine the upper posterior wall, ensuring that it is free of adhesions – there is often a vein, arching backwards in a peritoneal fold from the posterior gastric fundus, which bleeds annoyingly if it is torn.

12. Complete the gastric mobilization by dividing the lesser omentum right up to the diaphragm and dividing the gastrophrenic ligament close to the diaphragm. Posteriorly, there is a vein arching

backwards from the upper stomach that must be ligated or occluded with haemostatic clips and divided. Removal of the spleen ± distal pancreas is not always necessary.

13. The stomach is now attached only to the oesophagus. Gently free this in the hiatus. Transect the anterior and posterior vagal trunks and decide on the level of transection. Do not divide the oesophagus until either the posterior oesophagojejunal outer Lembert suture line is in place after turning the specimen upwards over the patient's chest to prevent the oesophagus from retracting out of sight, or until most of the purse-string suture has been inserted for use with a circular stapling device. Prevent retraction of the oesophagus into the chest by:

a. application of a Crafoord or Satinsky clamp, and
b. slow intravenous injection of up to 20 mg hyoscine butylbromide.

14. If a nasojejunal tube is to be used, have it drawn up into the lower oesophagus. It can be pulled down when making a sutured anastomosis when the posterior all-coats suture is in place and pushed on into the jejunum. If a stapled anastomosis is made, have the anaesthetist push it on with a twisting motion when the stapler is withdrawn.

Unite

1. Oesophagojejunostomy is preferably performed using a Roux-en-Y jejunal loop (see Ch. 10). Transect the jejunum close to the ligament of Treitz and divide sufficient primary vascular arcades to allow the distal portion to be taken up to the oesophagus. Transect the bowel beyond the duodenojejunal junction and join the cut proximal end into the side of the Roux loop 50 cm downstream. If a sutured oesophagojejunal anastomosis is used, close the end of the jejunum in two layers, or staple it. The loop should be led up to the oesophagus posterior to the transverse mesocolon. Make sure it lies without tension or twisting. Insert a posterior running suture line of Lembert stitches joining the posterior wall of the oesophagus to the posterior wall of the Roux loop about 5 cm from the closed end. Now transect the oesophagus below the suture line and remove the specimen. Create a hole in the antimesenteric border of the jejunum exactly matching the oesophageal lumen. Insert a stitch through all coats of the oesophagus and jejunum at each end so they can be slightly stretched. Carefully insert a circular all coats stitch to produce perfect union. Now carry the posterior Lembert stitch on to the anterior wall to encircle the anastomosis, trying to draw up the jejunal wall to cover the inner, all coats stitch. Discard and replace the soiled towels, instruments and gloves.

2. The oesophagojejunal anastomosis may be accomplished using one of the circular stapling devices. Before the oesophagus is completely transected, most of an encircling all coats purse-string suture is inserted and the specimen is then resected below it and removed. Introduce a size-testing head so that the correct size of stapler can be used. An end-to-side Roux anastomosis does not require a separate stab since the instrument, without the anvil, can be passed in through the cut end of bowel, which will be closed in two layers or stapled after it is withdrawn.

Now feed the anvil head into the cut end of oesophagus, tighten and tie the purse-string suture and close the anvil head on to the cartridge after ensuring there is no extraneous tissue trapped and that the oesophagus and jejunum lie without tension or twist. Release the safety catch and actuate the gun. Open it, remove it, check the intactness of the anastomosis and of the doughnut-shaped rings on the spindle. Close the portal of entry of the device in two layers. If the oesophageal wall is very thick, dissect back a cuff of muscularis so that it is not included in the stapler. After uniting the oesophagus to jejunum, insert a layer of stitches drawing the muscle coat on to the jejunum around the stapled anastomosis.

Anastomosis has been made easier by the development of improved circular stapling devices in which the anvil head and the spindle can be detached together. A temporary pointed trocar can be fitted to the main instrument and pushed through the wall of the bowel, then removed. Introduce the anvil on its spindle into the lower oesophagus and tighten and tie the previously inserted purse-string suture. Attach the anvil on its spindle to the instrument and bring together the jejunum and oesophagus by closing the anvil down on to the cartridge. Actuate the stapler. Always, before loosening the stapler, feel again around the anastomosis to ensure that nothing is interposed, nothing is protruding. In case of doubt about the integrity of the anastomosis, retain the closed stapler and use it to rotate the anastomosis while inserting reinforcing sutures around the circumference of the stoma. Only now release and remove the stapler. We must admit to the temptation to perform this manoeuvre routinely.

Check

1. Stop all bleeding.

2. Ensure that the anastomoses are perfect, the bowel is a good colour, untwisted and not stretched and the mesentery lies free.

3. Check all the other structures that have been disturbed. The hiatus does not need to be repaired if total gastrectomy has been carried out. The liver must be replaced if the left lobe was folded to the right. Repair the transverse mesocolon if there is a hole through which small bowel may prolapse.

Closure

1. Drain the cut end of the pancreas if splenopancreatectomy has been performed and leave the drain in situ for 6–10 days to form a track. Pancreatic fistula is common and very dangerous if the corrosive juices cannot freely drain externally.

2. Close the abdomen in routine fashion.

RADICAL THORACOABDOMINAL TOTAL GASTRECTOMY

1. Never embark upon this operation without first obtaining a tissue diagnosis with endoscopic biopsy or cytology or frozen-section histology at operation. Never embark upon it without making every effort by preoperative and operative assessment to exclude metastatic tumour.

2. As a rule, this is a radical operation undertaken for carcinoma of the proximal stomach or cardia which can apparently be totally encompassed by this major resection of the stomach, lower

oesophagus, omenta, spleen, body and tail of the pancreas, with all the primary lymph nodes and the next tier, completing a D2 resection.

3. It is accomplished through a left thoracoabdominal incision (Figs 9.12, 9.13) or via separate abdominal and right thoracic incisions. It can be carried out through a single midline abdominal incision only if the upper stomach is free of growth and in that case it is merely an extension of radical partial gastrectomy to include the upper fringe of stomach in the resection. Transabdominal total gastrectomy is usually contraindicated, except in very thin patients, if the growth extends proximally to within 2–3 cm of the gastro-oesophageal junction, since at least a 3 cm segment of apparently uninvolved lower oesophagus should be resected.

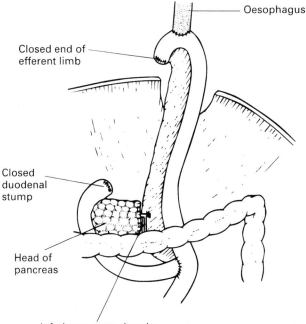

Fig. 9.13 Radical total gastrectomy. The oesophagojejunal anastomosis is complete, using a Roux loop of jejunum taken behind the mesocolon. The duodenal bulb is closed, and the duodenal loop is joined end-to-side to the jejunum.

FURTHER READING

Akiyama H 1979 Thoracoabdominal approach for carcinoma of the cardia of the stomach. American Journal of Surgery 137: 345–349

Cuschieri A, Fayers P, Fielding J et al 1996 Post-operative morbidity and mortality after D1 and D2 resections for gastric cancer. Lancet 347: 995–999

Japanese Research Society for Gastric Cancer 1981 The general rules for the gastric cancer study in surgery and pathology. Part I: Clinical classification. Part II: Histological classification of gastric cancer. Japanese Journal of Surgery 11: 127–145

Johnston D 1977 Division and repair of the sphincteric mechanism at the gastric outlet in emergency operations for bleeding peptic ulcer. Annals of Surgery 186; 723–726

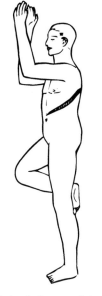

Fig. 9.12 Left thoracoabdominal approach to total gastrectomy, as seen from above the patient. The shaded section shows the extent of the incision.

Small bowel

R. C. N. Williamson and T. R. Worthington

Contents

EXAMINATION OF THE SMALL BOWEL

1. *Diverticula*. These are quite common. Meckel's diverticulum arises from the distal ileum. Acquired diverticula may affect the duodenum, jejunum and to a lesser extent the ileum, and are frequently multiple. Do not remove incidental diverticula, but excise localized groups if they are causing symptoms, such as pain or bleeding.

2. *Inflammation*. Crohn's disease may affect any part of the alimentary canal but especially the terminal ileum. Affected segments of bowel are inflamed, thickened, narrowed and often covered with fibrinous exudate. The mesentery is thickened and encroaches on a greater proportion of the circumference of the bowel; adjacent lymph nodes are enlarged. Look for evidence of disease elsewhere in the small and large bowel. Segmental resection is usually indicated for chronic Crohn's enteritis (see below). Tuberculous and yersinial infection can produce similar changes of ileitis; if in doubt remove a gland for bacteriological and histological examination. Coeliac disease particularly affects the jejunum. The diagnosis is indicated by dilatation of subserous and mesenteric lymphatics, thinning and pigmentation of the bowel wall and splenic atrophy, and it is confirmed by full-thickness biopsy (see below). Small-bowel ulcers and strictures may occur spontaneously or follow either radiotherapy, transient strangulation in an external hernia or the ingestion of potassium tablets.

3. *Infarction*. The viability of the small bowel must be carefully checked after reduction of a strangulated hernia or untwisting of a volvulus in adhesion obstruction. Any frankly necrotic or perforated loops should be excised. If you are in doubt about the viability of a dusky segment, return it to the abdomen and wait for 5 minutes (timed by the clock). The return of a shiny, pink appearance, pulsation of the mesenteric vessels (or bleeding if pricked) and peristalsis across the affected segment indicate viability. If you are still in doubt, resect. Clinical judgement will usually determine intestinal viability, but

possible adjuncts are the use of a small Doppler ultrasound probe and injection of fluorescein with examination under ultraviolet light. Constriction rings may be carefully invaginated, using interrupted seromuscular sutures.

4. *Tumours*. Serosal deposits occur in carcinomatosis peritonei and may cause kinking and obstruction of the small bowel, requiring side-to-side bypass. Primary neoplasms are less common. Benign tumours include adenoma, leiomyoma, lipoma and Peutz–Jeghers hamartomas; they can cause intussusception. Carcinoid tumours favour the ileum, but may be multiple and metastasizing; they are hard with a yellowish cut surface. Malignant tumours comprise adenocarcinoma, lymphoma and leiomyosarcoma in that order of prevalence. Primary neoplasms should be excised or, if irresectable, bypassed and biopsied.

Biopsy

1. Duodenal lesions can be biopsied endoscopically under direct vision.

2. Small intestine endoscopy (enteroscopy) is now feasible.

3. Operative biopsy of the small intestine is seldom indicated.

4. Mesenteric lymph nodes can be biopsied with relative impunity. Where possible, select a node close to the bowel wall and avoid dissecting deep in the root of the mesentery. Carefully incise the peritoneum and dissect out the entire node, using diathermy to coagulate its small blood vessels.

INTESTINAL ANASTOMOSIS

General principles

1. Several hundred intestinal anastomoses are carried out each week in Britain, and the vast majority heal rapidly by primary intention.

2. Remember that most of the intestinal canal is contaminated with bacteria, disproportionately so towards the distal end.

3. Ensure that the bowel ends are pink and bleeding freely, and leave the mesentery attached to the bowel right up to the point of intestinal transection.

4. Tension puts the mesenteric vessels on stretch and tends to distract the bowel ends. It usually results from inadequate mobilization, especially of the colon. Though readily avoidable, twisting of the mesentery can also render an anastomosis ischaemic. The mesenteric/mesocolic defect should normally be repaired after completing an intestinal anastomosis to prevent postoperative internal herniation, but take care in so doing not to compromise the vessels supplying the bowel ends.

5. Distended loops of bowel are heavy and difficult to handle.

Moreover, healing is impaired, probably because the bowel wall is thinner and somewhat ischaemic. Distended small bowel may be decompressed by milking contents upwards into the reach of the nasogastric tube or by enterotomy and insertion of a sucker. Gaseous distension of the large bowel can be relieved by introducing a needle obliquely through its wall. Try to avoid leaving hard faecal lumps proximal to a colonic anastomosis. If possible, milk them beyond the site of intended colonic transection.

Key point

- The key to a successful anastomosis is the accurate union of two viable bowel ends with complete avoidance of tension.

Hand-suturing techniques

1. Traditionally, bowel is united in two layers, using catgut or another absorbable suture material (e.g. polyglactin 910) for the inner, all-coats layers and an outer stitch (called after its inventor, Lembert) to join the seromuscular layers. In certain sites only a one-layered anastomosis can sometimes be achieved, e.g. colorectal and biliary–enteric anastomoses and oesophagojejunostomy.

2. Surgeons have long disputed the best suture material, the best type of stitch and the best methods of fashioning a suture line. We believe that these technical points are less important than the principle stated above: to achieve accurate and tension-free coaptation of two healthy mucosal surfaces.

3. A continuous (running) stitch is undoubtedly quicker and it achieves good haemostasis. It is therefore appropriate for straightforward gastric, enteric and colonic anastomoses.

4. Interrupted sutures allow slightly greater precision and may be more convenient than a continuous stitch when there is marked disparity in the size of the bowel ends to be united or the anastomosis is technically difficult. In inaccessible situations (e.g. colorectal anastomosis deep in the pelvis or hepaticojejunostomy) it may be wise to insert the entire posterior row of interrupted sutures before trying any individual stitch.

5. Many surgeons routinely use two layers of continuous absorbable sutures for gastric and intestinal anastomoses. If impaired healing is anticipated, e.g. in Crohn's disease, consider whether an inner layer of continuous catgut or polyglactin 910 and an outer layer of interrupted silk would provide added security. Non-absorbable sutures are usually indicated when joining small bowel (or colon) to the oesophagus, pancreas or rectum; suitable materials include silk (2/0 or 3/0), polypropylene, monofilament nylon and stainless-steel wire.

6. Insert each stitch separately and invert the bowel edges as the suture is tightened. Once the bowel edge is inverted, prevent the suture material from slipping by getting your assistant to follow up. Alternatively, follow up yourself, using the taut suture as a means of steadying the bowel against the thrust of the needle. The objective is a snug, water-tight anastomosis. Excessive tension risks strangulating the bowel incorporated in the stitch and perhaps causing subsequent leakage.

7. Do not place the sutures so close to the edge of the bowel that they might tear out nor so deep that they turn in an enormous cuff of tissue and narrow the bowel; usually 3–5 mm is about the correct

depth of 'bite'. Be sure that the all-coats suture does in fact incorporate all coats of the bowel wall. Some surgeons deliberately exclude the mucosa. This is usually termed extramucosal anastomosis. If you use this method take great care that every stitch takes a good 'bite' of the most important layer, the strong submucosa.

8. The seromuscular stitch unites the adjacent bowel walls outside the all-coats stitch. Sometimes the posterior seromuscular layer is inserted before opening the gut, e.g. in side-to-side anastomoses (Fig. 10.1).

After the all-coats stitches have been inserted, the seromuscular sutures are carried round the ends of the anastomosis and across the front wall, ultimately encircling the anastomosis so that the all-coats stitches can no longer be seen. For end-to-end anastomoses in small and large intestine it may be simpler to complete the all-coats layer before placing any Lembert sutures. Thereafter, the seromuscular layer can be inserted all the way round by rotating the bowel.

9. The all-coats stitch is accepted as the paramount stitch for holding bowel edges, since it catches the strong submucosa. There are many ways of inserting these stitches; three popular methods are described below:

a. *Continuous over-and-over suture.* Approximate the two edges of cut bowel. Starting at one end, insert a corner stitch from outside to in, then over the adjacent edges of bowel and out through the other corner. Tie the suture and clip the short end. Pass the stitch back through the nearest bowel wall, over the contiguous cut edges and back through the full thickness of both walls. Continue over-and-over stitches to the opposite corner (Fig. 10.2).

After the last stitch is inserted right into the corner, take it back through the nearest corner leaving a loop on the mucosa so that the stitch emerges from the outer wall of the bowel (Fig. 10.3).

Now sew the front walls together by passing the stitch over and over, from out to in and then from in to out (Fig. 10.4). Continue until the anastomosis has been encircled and the edges inverted, then tie off the ends of suture material. This over-and-over stitch is haemostatic.

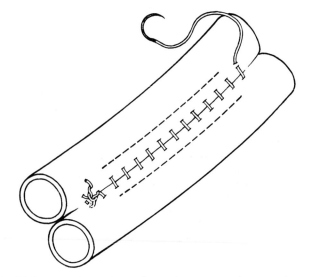

Fig. 10.1 A continuous layer of posterior seromuscular sutures has been inserted before fashioning a side-to-side anastomosis. The dotted lines indicate the lines of incision of the bowel.

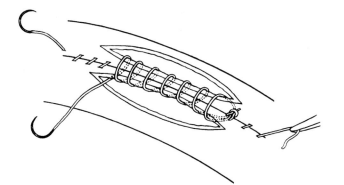

Fig. 10.2 The all-coats stitch is being inserted in a continuous over-and-over fashion. Care is taken to include mucosa and muscularis in each bite.

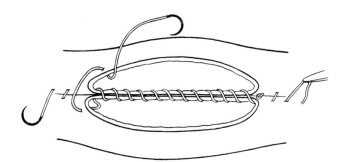

Fig. 10.3 The all-coats stitch is continued round the corner. A single loop-on-the-mucosa stitch starts the return over-and-over stitch.

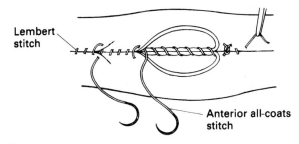

Lembert stitch

Anterior all-coats stitch

Fig. 10.4 The anterior all-coats stitch is continued; then the anterior seromuscular stitch completes the anastomosis.

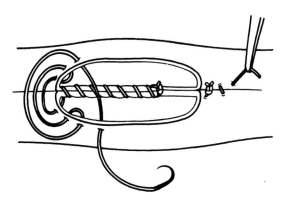

Fig. 10.5 Starting from the middle of the back wall, an over-and-over stitch has been inserted as far as the corner. Two or three Connell stitches are placed to turn the corner, followed by an anterior over-and-over stitch. A separate suture is used to fashion the other half of the anastomosis.

b. *Continuous over-and-over plus Connell suture.* Commence in the middle of the posterior wall by placing a stitch between the adjacent cut edges of bowel and tying it on the luminal surface. Now continue towards one corner with over-and-over stitches. At the corner the needle passes from in to out on the nearside cut surface, then crosses to the far edge and is passed in and out to leave a loop on the mucosa (Fig. 10.5).

The needle returns to the near edge and another loop-on-the-mucosa (Connell) stitch is inserted. These Connell stitches turn the corner neatly. Once you are round the corner, leave this stitch and return to the middle of the posterior wall. Use a new length of suture material, unless there is a needle at each end of the original length. Insert and tie a stitch close to the site of the original ligature, tie the two short ends of suture material and proceed towards the opposite corner, using Connell sutures to negotiate the corner again. Either continue with Connell stitches along the anterior wall from each end or return to over-and-over stitches once you are round the corners. Tie off the ends of suture material in the middle of the anterior wall. The Connell stitch is not fully haemostatic, so all bleeding points must be secured.

c. *Interrupted suture.* Insert a stitch from out to in and in to out at each corner. If the anastomosis is easily accessible, tie each stitch at this stage. Clip the ends of suture material and get your assistant to hold the clips to exert traction on the posterior cut edges of bowel (Fig. 10.6).

Insert a row of posterior sutures 2–3 mm apart, tying the knots on the luminal surface. If the anastomosis is relatively inaccessible, avoid tying any sutures until the entire posterior row has been inserted. Then approximate the bowel ends and tie the sutures snugly and in order, proceeding from one corner to the next. Now place an anterior row of interrupted sutures. It is easier to tie the knots on the outside at this stage, and inversion does not appear to be essential. Indeed, some surgeons practise edge-to-edge or eversion techniques routinely for intestinal anastomosis, preferring not to turn in a ridge of tissue that might obstruct the lumen.

Mechanical stapling techniques
1. Stapling machines are now available to carry out most types of gastrointestinal anastomosis. Disposable and angled instruments are

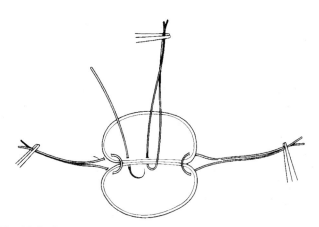

Fig. 10.6 End-to-end anastomosis using interrupted sutures. The two corner stitches are tied with the knots on the outside, but for the remainder of the posterior wall the knots are placed on the inside. If access is restricted, each suture is inserted and held in a clip before any one is tied (as shown).

available for use in particular circumstances, and the metal staples come in different lengths to accommodate the different tissue thicknesses encountered. For end-to-end anastomosis (e.g. colorectal, oesophagojejunal) the stapling gun is introduced into the intestinal lumen downstream, brought out through the distal cut end of bowel and then insinuated into the proximal cut end.

The largest anvil should be chosen that will fit comfortably into the proximal lumen. Proximal and distal gut are snugged tightly around the central rod (Fig. 10.7), using purse-string sutures, and the anvil is then approximated to the cartridge by closing the instrument.

When the gun is fired, a circular double row of stainless-steel staples is inserted and at the same time a complete 5 mm rim of each bowel end (the 'doughnut') is resected. The machine is then withdrawn, the 'doughnuts' are checked and the anastomosis is complete.

2. For side-to-side anastomosis a different instrument is used, resembling a pair of scissors. One 'blade' is inserted into each of the two intestinal segments to be united, and the blades are closed. Firing the gun advances a knife, which divides the adjacent surfaces of bowel between two parallel rows of staples.

3. Yet another set of instruments has been designed to place a double row of staples across the end of a segment of intestine or stomach. The staple line can be 30, 55 or 90 mm long. After firing the staples, the instrument is left attached and used as an anvil on which to transect the gut. Some surgeons prefer to bury the staple line with a continuous Lembert suture.

🔑 **Key point**

- Using a mechanical stapler does not guarantee a perfect result. It is just as important to prepare healthy bowel ends and avoid tension as it is in hand-sewn anastomoses, and a different set of technical details has to be learnt.

---

4. Stapling machines reduce the time involved in fashioning an anastomosis and facilitate certain operations that can be difficult to complete by hand, such as oesophageal transection, oesophago-gastrectomy (Fig. 10.7) or low anterior resection of the rectum. The introduction of disposable stapling guns obviates the need for careful maintenance of the reusable instrument and may reduce the substantial costs involved in mechanical stapling. On the other hand there are many situations where the stapler is inappropriate (e.g. choledocho-jejunostomy) or unnecessary (most small-bowel anastomoses). Aim to be versatile and try to acquire experience in both methods of gastrointestinal anastomosis.

Types of anastomosis

End-to-end anastomosis

This is the simplest way of restoring intestinal continuity after partial enterectomy and/or colectomy. After removal of the resected specimen, clean and approximate the bowel ends. The anastomosis is usually created in two layers, using a continuous absorbable suture (e.g. 2/0 or 3/0 polyglactin 910 or chromic catgut) swaged on to an eyeless needle (Fig. 10.8).

Insert the all-coats stitch, using one of the techniques described above or a variant that you have been shown. Remove the intestinal

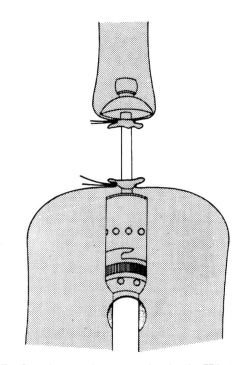

Fig. 10.7 Oesophagogastric anastomosis, using the EEA stapling gun inserted through a small gastrotomy. After tying each purse-string suture around the central rod, the anvil is approximated to the cartridge and the staples are discharged.

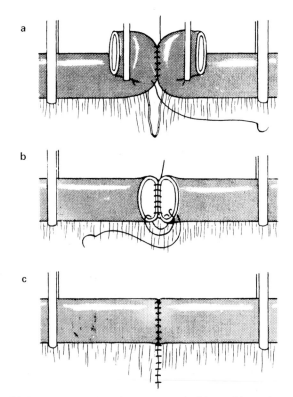

Fig. 10.8 End-to-end intestinal anastomosis: (a) and (b) two layers of stitches being inserted; (c) the completed anastomosis with the mesentery repaired.

clamps and check that the anastomosis is airtight and watertight by gently squeezing intestinal contents across it. Now insert the circumferential seromuscular stitch, taking care not to turn in too thick a cuff of tissue. Make sure the thumb and forefinger can invaginate bowel wall on each side through the anastomosis. Some surgeons prefer to unite the bowel ends with a posterior layer of Lembert sutures before embarking on the all-coats stitch, but we only resort to this manoeuvre with end-to-end anastomosis if we anticipate subsequent difficulty in placing the posterior seromuscular layer. Lastly, unite the cut edges of mesentery and/or mesocolon on each aspect with interrupted catgut sutures, taking care to avoid damaging the vessels.

Oblique anastomosis

When the ends of bowel are disproportionate in size, they may be matched by incising the antimesenteric border of the narrow bowel longitudinally (Fig. 10.9a).

This manoeuvre is useful in joining obstructed to collapsed bowel or ileum to colon. In neonates with congenital intestinal atresia, the lumen of the distal bowel is particularly narrow and this type of 'end-to-back' anastomosis is necessitated. The mesentery of the proximal bowel is also disproportionately big and should be shortened with a few gathering stitches before being united to the distal cut edge of mesentery. When two segments of narrow intestine must be united, they may both be opened along their antimesenteric borders, which are then joined back-to-back (Fig. 10.9b). The mesenteries are now on opposite sides of the anastomosis and cannot always be neatly approximated. Poth has described an elegant variant of this technique, in which the end of the larger segment is sutured to the end-to-lateral aspect of the smaller segment of bowel (Fig. 10.10).

End-to-side anastomosis

This is most commonly used when creating a Roux-en-Y anastomosis. Approximate the cut end to the side of bowel to which it will be joined and insert a posterior seromuscular suture (Fig. 10.11).

Incise the antimesenteric border of the side of bowel to accommodate the cut end. Insert the all-coats stitch as before, remove the clamps and complete the seromuscular stitch. Lastly, join the cut edge of mesentery to the side of the intact mesentery.

Side-to-side anastomosis

This can be used to joint two loops of bowel without resection, or to unite intestine to stomach, bile duct, etc. (Fig. 10.12).

It may also be employed as an alternative to end-to-end anastomosis after intestinal resection, in which case the cut ends of bowel should first be closed and invaginated. The advantages of the side-to-side anastomosis are that the segments of bowel to be united have no interruption to their blood supply at all and that the incisions can be made exactly congruous. The disadvantages are that there are more suture lines involved and that there may be some degree of stasis and bacterial overgrowth.

Lay the segments to be joined side by side in contact for 8–10 cm and insert a posterior seromuscular stitch. Incise the antimesenteric borders for about 5 cm and insert an all-coats stitch. Remove the clamps and complete the anterior seromuscular layer of stitches. When side-to-side anastomosis follows bowel resection, suture the cut edge of mesentery to the adjacent intact mesentery on each side of the anastomosis.

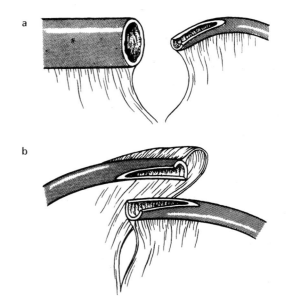

Fig. 10.9 Oblique anastomoses: (a) end-to-back anastomosis – the narrow bowel has been opened along its antimesenteric border so that its lumen matches the end of the wider bowel; (b) back-to-back anastomosis – two narrow segments of bowel have been opened along their antimesenteric borders to create a wide anastomosis.

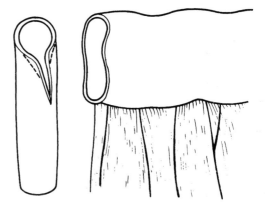

Fig. 10.10 End-to-lateral anastomosis. Poth's variation of the oblique anastomosis may be used to unite ileum to colon. The corners on the ileal segment are trimmed along the dotted lines.

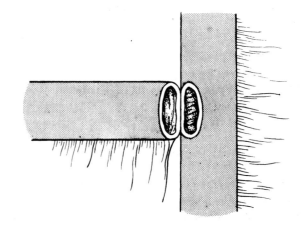

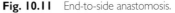

Fig. 10.11 End-to-side anastomosis.

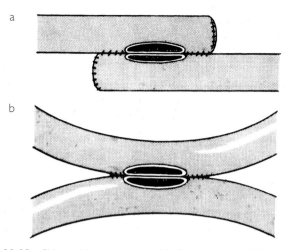

Fig. 10.12 Side-to-side anastomoses: (a) after transection of the bowel, with closure of each end; (b) two segments are joined without dividing the bowel.

ENTERECTOMY (SMALL-BOWEL RESECTION)

Appraise

1. Resection is often indicated for congenital lesions of the small bowel (atresia, duplication), traumatic perforation, critical ischaemia (from mesenteric trauma, strangulation or arteriosclerosis), Crohn's disease or other cause of stricture, and tumours of the bowel or its mesentery. Resection is sometimes indicated for fistula, diverticulitis, intussusception and a symptomatic blind loop. Small portions of the duodenum and ileum are removed during partial gastrectomy and right hemicolectomy respectively.

2. There are several reasons for being conservative in the management of *Crohn's disease*: the indolent nature of the disease, its relapsing course and its strong tendency (> 50%) to recur anywhere in the intestinal tract, but especially at and just proximal to the anastomosis. Despite many advances in the treatment of Crohn's disease, the course of the disease in any given patient remains unpredictable. There is little agreement as to which factors predispose a patient to recurrence. A multivariate analysis has shown that the only independent predictors of earlier postoperative recurrence after initial operation are an initial presentation with peritonitis, secondary to perforation, and a longer preoperative disease duration. Do not resect for Crohn's ileitis discovered incidentally during laparotomy for suspected appendicitis. On the other hand, most patients with chronic Crohn's enteritis eventually require resection of the affected segment because of subacute obstruction, fistula or abscess. Bypass is obsolete: the defunctioned segment is unlikely to heal, bacterial overgrowth of the blind loop may aggravate diarrhoea and there is a long-term risk of carcinoma. For 'burnt-out' stenotic areas of bowel, strictureplasty is an alternative to resection.

3. When operating for *radiation enteropathy* certain principles should be observed. The extent both of the original cancer and the radiation damage should be established. Where possible, bypass or exclusion procedures should be avoided: the leakage rate is probably no lower than after resection and anastomosis, and the defunctioned bowel may still give rise to problems such as bleeding and fistula. Wide resection is the optimal approach, ensuring that at least one side of the subsequent anastomosis employs healthy (non-irradiated) bowel.

Prepare

1. In the presence of an obstructing lesion, ensure that the patient is adequately resuscitated before operation with nasogastric intubation and intravenous rehydration. In non-obstructed patients undergoing small-bowel operations, a nasogastric tube should be passed after induction of anaesthesia.

2. Healthy ileum has a resident bacterial flora, and in the presence of obstruction the entire small bowel may be colonized. It is sensible to cover all operations likely to involve intestinal resection with appropriate prophylactic antibiotics, e.g. a cephalosporin plus metronidazole given preoperatively by a single intravenous shot.

3. Nutritional status may be impaired in some patients requiring small-bowel resection, for example those with Crohn's disease, cancer, radiation enteropathy or enterocutaneous fistula. In the absence of obstruction or fistula, supplemental enteric feeds may reverse the nutritional defect, but some patients will require a period of preoperative parenteral nutrition.

Access

1. Adequate exposure of the entire small bowel can be provided by a number of different incisions. We usually employ a midline incision that skirts the umbilicus and can be extended in either direction as necessary.

2. Remember that the small bowel quite often adheres to the back of a previous laparotomy incision, and take particular care during abdominal re-entry. The chances are that an accidental perforation will not be located in a segment of bowel that you would in any case have intended to remove.

Access

1. Expose and examine the entire small bowel. Continue by examining the stomach, large bowel and remaining abdominal viscera.

2. If a loop of small bowel has been strangulated in an external hernia, for example, release the obstruction and check the viability of the bowel after allowing a minimum period of 5 minutes for possible recovery in doubtful cases.

3. Healthy small intestine possesses both a considerable functional reserve and the capacity to adapt to partial tissue loss by compensatory villous hyperplasia of the portions that remain. Nevertheless, do not gratuitously sacrifice healthy bowel, particularly terminal ileum, which has specialized transport functions. Except when operating for primary malignant tumours it is quite unnecessary to excise a deep wedge of mesentery, which might increase the extent of small bowel requiring removal. In Crohn's disease do not remove more than a few centimetres of gut on either side of the affected segment, but include any fistulas or sinuses. It is more than likely that further resection will be required in future, and microscopic inflammation of the bowel at the resection margin does not appear to increase subsequent anastomotic recurrence. Conventional right hemicolectomy is unnecessary for small-bowel Crohn's disease; conservative ileocaecal resection should be undertaken.

4. Sometimes a partial resection of small bowel can be performed, leaving the mesentery intact. Appropriate conditions include Richter's hernia, Meckel's diverticulum and small tumours arising on the antimesenteric border.

Action

1. Isolate the diseased loop of bowel from the other abdominal contents by means of large, moist packs or a special towel.

2. Hold up the bowel and examine the mesentery against the light. Note the vascular pattern.

Standard resection

1. Determine the proximal and distal sites for dividing the bowel, and select the line of vascular section in between; keep fairly close to the bowel wall (Fig. 10.13), except when resecting a neoplasm (Fig. 10.14).

Incise the peritoneum along this line on each aspect of the mesentery. This manoeuvre is most easily accomplished by inserting one blade of a pair of fine, curved scissors beneath the peritoneum and cutting superficially to expose the mesenteric vessels.

2. Using small artery forceps, create a small mesenteric window right next to the bowel wall at each point chosen for intestinal transection. Starting at one end, insinuate a curved artery forceps through this window and back through the mesentery (denuded of peritoneum) 1–2 cm away, thus isolating a small leash of mesentery with its contained vessels. Either doubly ligate this leash in continuity and divide between ligatures, or divide between artery forceps, ligating the mesentery beneath each pair of forceps. Proceeding in this manner, divide the mesentery right up to the bowel wall at the further end of the line of peritoneal incision. Take care in placing and tying each ligature; if the knot slips, there can be troublesome haemorrhage. We use polyglactin 910 or silk ties (2/0 or 3/0 according to the thickness of the mesentery).

3. Apply four intestinal clamps (Fig. 10.13). The first two clamps are crushing clamps (Payr's, Lang Stevenson's or Pringle's). They should be applied obliquely at the points of intended intestinal transection, so that slightly more of the antimesenteric border is resected than of the mesenteric border; the obliquity reduces the risk of a tight anastomosis. Now apply a non-crushing clamp about 5 cm outside each crushing clamp, having milked the intervening bowel free of contents.

4. Place a clean gauze swab beneath the clamps at each end (to catch spills), and divide the bowel with a knife flush against the outer aspect of each crushing clamp. Place the specimen and the soiled knife in a separate dish, which is then removed.

5. Cleanse each bowel end, using small swabs or pledgets of gauze soaked in cetrimide. Then remove the protective gauze swab and proceed to intestinal anastomosis. In an attempt to limit contamination, some surgeons divide the intestine between two pairs of light crushing clamps (i.e. six clamps in all) and insert the posterior seromuscular layer of sutures before removing the outer clamps and excising the narrow rim of crushed tissue (Fig. 10.14).

6. Perform a two-layer, end-to-end anastomosis, as described in the previous section.

Partial resection

1. A diverticulum on the antimesenteric border may be locally excised. Clamp and cut it off at the neck, then close the defect in two layers as a transverse linear slit. Try to avoid narrowing the intestinal lumen during this procedure.

2. A diamond-shaped area of the antimesenteric border may be included in the resection of a localized tumour or wide-mouthed Meckel's diverticulum. Apply two light crushing clamps (Lang Stevenson's or Pringle's) across the antimesenteric border, meeting in a V (Fig. 10.15). Incise the bowel flush with the outer aspect of each clamp, and close the wall in two layers, leaving a transverse suture line.

3. A similar defect results if the antimesenteric lesion is excised through a longitudinal ellipse. Approximate the ends of the ellipse, pull apart the sides and close transversely as before.

Checklist

1. Take a last look at the anastomosis. Check that the bowel is pink, that haemostasis is secure and that all mesenteric defects are closed.

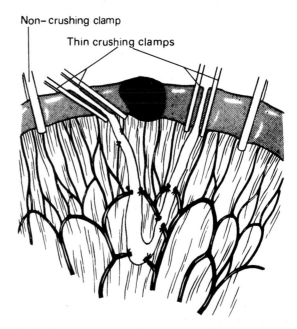

Fig. 10.14 Resection of a small-bowel tumour. A deeper wedge of mesentery is included than in operations for benign disease (see Fig. 10.13). As before, the narrower segment of bowel (on the left) is transected obliquely, removing more of the antimesenteric border with the specimen.

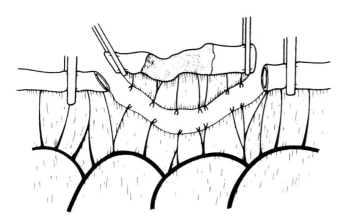

Fig. 10.13 Resection of an ischaemic segment of small bowel including a shallow wedge of mesentery. The narrower bowel end has been cut obliquely to match the wider end.

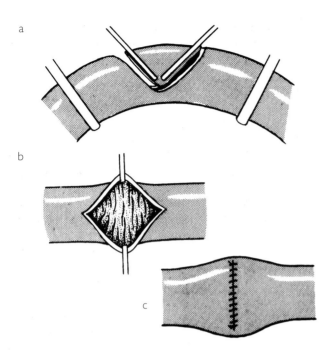

Fig. 10.15 Partial resection of small bowel: (a) a wedge of antimesenteric bowel is removed; (b) the defect is opened out transversely; (c) closure across the long axis of the bowel prevents narrowing.

2. It is easy to lose a swab among the coils of small intestine. Check the entire abdominal cavity and make sure that the swab count is correct. Remove any ends of suture material that might provoke subsequent adhesions. Replace the intestine and the greater omentum in their normal anatomical position.

3. Suck out the peritoneal cavity. Place a fine-bore suction drain to the region of the anastomosis.

Aftercare

1. Anticipate a period of postoperative ileus, during which the patient is maintained on intravenous fluids. The nasogastric tube should be left on open drainage and aspirated regularly for the first 24–48 hours. Allow 30 ml of water per hour by mouth. The tube can usually be removed when bowel sounds return, the volume of aspirate drops below the volume of fluid taken by mouth and there is passage of flatus. Peristalsis returns to the small bowel before the stomach and colon regain their motility.

2. Remove the drain when the fluid loss diminishes, generally at 2–3 days.

3. If restoration of oral feeding is very delayed, consider whether a period of parenteral nutrition would be appropriate.

Complications

1. Wound infection is a potential risk of any procedure involving an intestinal anastomosis. Good surgical technique in limiting contamination from bowel contents will certainly reduce the incidence. If wound sepsis develops, remove sufficient sutures to allow the pus to drain, irrigate the wound, obtain bacteriological cultures and (in severe cases) institute appropriate antibiotic therapy. Once the infection is controlled, the wound will usually heal without the need for secondary suture.

2. As with any abdominal operation there is a risk of chest infection

Difficulty?

1. *Is the bowel obstructed?* Decompress obstructed jejunum by milking its contents upwards until they can be aspirated through the nasogastric tube. Decompress obstructed ileum by inserting a sucker tube, either into the end of the proximal bowel after releasing the clamps or via a separate enterotomy. Do this without allowing bowel contents to spill.

2. In the presence of obstruction there may be marked disparity between the diameters of the bowel ends. In practice moderate incongruities can be overcome by adjusting the size of bite while suturing proximal to distal bowel. The diameter of the distal bowel can be increased by transecting it more obliquely (sparing the mesenteric border) and by opening it along the antimesenteric border. If there is gross disparity, consider oblique or side-to-side anastomosis (see preceding section).

3. Resection and anastomosis can usually be completed outside the abdomen. Sometimes this is not possible, in which case you may not be able to apply all the clamps described above (either four or six). Try and retain the non-crushing clamps placed at a distance from the anastomosis, if possible. In difficult circumstances, concentrate on completing the all-coats suture without defect, if necessary using interrupted sutures. You may subsequently be able to insert seromuscular sutures around all or most of the circumference.

4. *A haematoma develops in the mesentery or in the submucosa at the point of intestinal transection.* Compression of the area with a swab will usually stop the bleeding. Alternatively, gently close swab-holding forceps or non-crushing clamps across the bleeding point and wait for a few minutes. If the bleeding is not fully controlled, incise the peritoneum, find the bleeding point, pick it up with fine artery forceps and ligate it. Check the colour of the bowel to confirm that the blood supply is not prejudiced.

5. *One or other intestinal end becomes dusky during the anastomosis.* Time will usually declare the issue. Non-viable bowel will not heal, so if you are in any doubt it is better to excise a few more centimetres of bowel and make a fresh start. Leave the mesentery attached to the bowel as close as possible to the point of transection, and check for visible pulsations in the edge of the mesentery.

resulting from atelectasis. Vigorous physiotherapy will often avert the need for antibiotics.

3. Occasionally a collection of infected material will develop within the abdominal cavity. Abscess sites may be subphrenic, subhepatic, pelvic or adjacent to the anastomosis. The patient develops fever and leucocytosis. Ultrasound scan will localize the collection and allow percutaneous drainage in many cases.

4. A leaking anastomosis will often present with pain, fever, tachycardia and erythema of the wound or drain site before intestinal contents begin to discharge. The management of an established small-bowel fistula is described at the end of this chapter.

5. It is occasionally necessary to undertake massive resection of the small bowel, e.g. for volvulus complicating an obstruction. Repeated enterectomies in Crohn's disease can similarly remove a substantial percentage of the small intestine. Increased frequency of bowel actions may follow loss of a third to a half of the small bowel,

and more extensive resections produce short bowel syndrome.[1] During the initial phase of recovery and adaptation, anticipate and replace losses of fluid and electrolytes, notably potassium. Give codeine or loperamide to control diarrhoea. The body compensates better for proximal than distal enterectomy. After an extensive ileal resection regular injections of vitamin B_{12} may be needed indefinitely; cholestyramine may diminish the irritative diarrhoea that results from bile-acid malabsorption. Consider nutritional support by the enteral or parenteral routes in severe short bowel syndrome. Cimetidine or, rarely, vagotomy may be needed for gastric acid hypersecretion.

REFERENCES

1. Bristol JB, Williamson RCN 1985 Postoperative adaptation of the small intestine. World Journal of Surgery 9: 825–832

ENTERIC BYPASS

Appraise

1. Small-bowel loops may become obstructed as a result of carcinomatosis peritonei or a particularly dense set of adhesions, sometimes deep in the pelvis. Irradiated small bowel may fistulate into other organs, such as the bladder or vagina. In these unfavourable circumstances it is often better just to bypass the affected segment of intestine (Fig. 10.16) rather than embark on a difficult and hazardous disentanglement. In radiation enteritis choose overtly normal bowel for the anastomosis, since healing is likely to be impaired.

2. Resection is almost always a better option than simple defunction

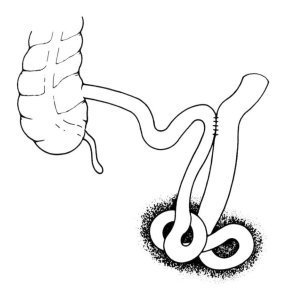

Fig. 10.16 Bypass procedure for small-bowel obstruction resulting from irresectable pelvic cancer. A side-to-side anastomosis is fashioned between a (proximal) distended loop of bowel and a (distal) collapsed loop.

in Crohn's disease of the small bowel. For irresectable carcinoma of the caecum, however, side-to-side bypass is indicated between the terminal ileum and the transverse colon (ileotransversostomy).

Action

Bypass of an irresectable lesion

1. A midline incision is usually appropriate. Aim to anastomose healthy bowel on either side of the diseased segment. Side-to-side anastomosis avoids the risk of closed-loop obstruction developing in a sequestered loop of bowel.

2. Occasionally if there are multiple sites of actual or imminent obstruction, two or more side-to-side anastomoses between adjacent loops may cause less of a short circuit than one enormous bypass.

3. Approximate a distended loop of proximal intestine to a collapsed loop of distal small bowel (Fig. 10.16) or transverse colon. Pack off the remaining viscera. Consider decompression of the obstructed loops.

4. Carry out a two-layer, side-to-side anastomosis, as previously described. Take care with the anastomosis and subsequent wound closure, since healing may be impaired, but do not prolong the operation unnecessarily if the patient has advanced disease.

Aftercare and complications

The principles of management are as for enterectomy (see previous section). Short bowel syndrome is inevitable after subtotal (about 90%) jejunoileal bypass, although adaptation can still be anticipated.

STRICTUREPLASTY

Appraise

This technique is virtually confined to patients with Crohn's disease causing a single (or a few) strictures in the small intestine. It can avoid the need for resection and may therefore be appropriate for patients with disease at several sites or those with recurrent disease and a limited length of residual small bowel. Florid inflammatory change or bowel containing several strictures within a relatively short segment is better treated by local resection. Sometimes one or more strictureplasty can be combined with resection to reduce the total length of bowel excised.

Assess

The tightness of the stricture(s) can be assessed by making a small enterotomy and passing a balloon catheter. Moderate strictures (e.g. 20–25 mm diameter) may be treated by balloon dilatation, but tight strictures (< 20 mm diameter) require either strictureplasty or resection.

Action

1. Carry a longitudinal full-thickness incision across the stenotic area and for 1 cm into the 'normal' bowel on either side.

2. Close the bowel transversely, using either one or two layers of 3/0 polyglactin 910 sutures. Test that the anastomosis is airtight and watertight.

3. This modification of the Heineke–Mikulicz pyloroplasty is suitable for short stenoses.

THE ROUX LOOP

Appraise

1. A defunctioned segment of jejunum provides a convenient conduit for connecting various upper abdominal organs to the remaining small bowel. Originally described by César Roux in 1907 for oesophageal bypass, the technique has proved invaluable in gastric, biliary and pancreatic surgery. Its uses in these circumstances are considered in the relevant chapters. Creation of the fundamental loop is described below.

2. Roux-en-Y anastomosis has two advantages over the use of an intact loop: it can stretch further and it is empty of intestinal contents, thus preventing contamination of the organ to be drained (e.g. bile duct). Active peristalsis down the loop encourages this drainage.

3. Probably the commonest indications for Roux-en-Y anastomosis are biliary drainage in irresectable carcinoma of the pancreatic head and reconstruction after total gastrectomy (Fig. 10.17) or oesophagogastrectomy.

4. Intact loops are used for cholecystoenterostomy, gastro-enterostomy and Polya (Billroth II) reconstruction after partial gastrectomy.

Action

1. Select a loop of proximal small bowel, beginning 10–15 cm distal to the ligament of Treitz. Hold up the jejunum and transilluminate its mesentery to display the precise blood supply, which varies from patient to patient. The number of vessels requiring division depends on the length of conduit required.

2. Starting at the point chosen for intestinal transection, incise the peritoneal leaves of the mesentery in a vertical direction (Fig. 10.18).

Divide at least one vascular arcade and the smaller branches that lie between the arcade vessels and the bowel. Ligate these vessels neatly in continuity and avoid using artery forceps, which can bunch up the tissues and prevent mobilization of the loop. Now divide the bowel between clamps.

3. If a longer loop is required, sacrifice two or three main jejunal vessels, preserving an intact blood supply to the extremity of the bowel via the arcades (Fig. 10.18). The peritoneum may require further incision to facilitate elongation of the loop without tension. Individual ligation of the arteries and veins is recommended, using fine silk sutures. Check the viability of the bowel at the tip of the loop, and sacrifice the end if it is dusky.

4. Straighten out the efferent limb and take it up by the shortest route for anastomosis to the oesophagus, stomach, bile duct, common hepatic duct or pancreatic duct. It is often easier to close the end of the limb and fashion a new subterminal opening of the correct diameter. Make a window in the base of the transverse mesocolon, to the right of the duodenojejunal flexure, for passage of the Roux loop. At the end of the operation suture the margins of this defect to the Roux loop to prevent internal herniation.

5. Restore intestinal continuity by uniting the short afferent limb to the base of the long efferent limb, using an end-to-side anastomosis. Ensure that the efferent limb is at least 30 cm long and that the afferent loop is joined to its left-hand side.

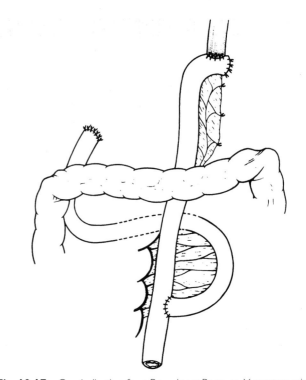

Fig. 10.17   One indication for a Roux loop: Roux-en-Y anastomosis between the oesophagus and jejunum after total gastrectomy.

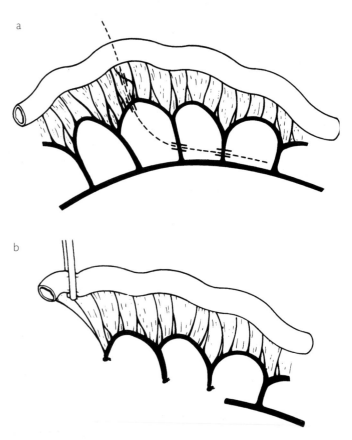

Fig. 10.18   Creation of a long Roux loop: (a) three arcade vessels have been divided; (b) the bowel is transected at a point previously selected and the loop is mobilized.

ENTEROTOMY

Appraise

1. Probably the commonest reason for making an incision into the lumen of the small bowel is to decompress the intestine proximal to the site of an obstruction. The enterotomy should be made halfway between the ligament of Treitz and the site of obstruction, so that the sucker can be inserted both proximally and distally to reach all the distended loops. It is usually possible to avoid enterotomy in a high obstruction by advancing the nasogastric tube through the duodenum and squeezing luminal contents upwards until they can be aspirated. In other circumstances the decompressing sucker can be inserted through the proximal cut end of bowel, if enterectomy is planned, or through the caecum and ileocaecal valve after appendicectomy.

2. Sometimes enterotomy is needed to extract a foreign body, for example in gallstone ileus or bolus obstruction.

3. Traumatic enterotomy can result from blunt or penetrating abdominal injuries. After a closed injury there is typically a rosette of exposed mucosa on the antimesenteric border of the upper jejunum. After knife or gunshot injuries, look for entry and exit wounds; holes in the small bowel nearly always come in multiples of two.

Action

Decompression enterotomy

1. The objective is to empty the small bowel without contaminating the peritoneal cavity. Pack off the area and apply non-crushing clamps on either side of the site chosen for enterotomy. Insert an absorbable purse-string stitch, make a small nick through the wall of the bowel and introduce a Savage decompressor, which consists of a long trocar and cannula connected to the sucker tubing.

2. Pass the sucker up and down the bowel, removing first one clamp and then the other. The assistant feeds the distended loops of gut over the end of the sucker, while the surgeon controls the force of suction by placing a finger over a side-port on the decompressing cannula. Sometimes the bowel appears to be only partly deflated, because of interstitial oedema.

3. After emptying the bowel, remove the sucker, tighten and tie the purse-string and discard the contaminated packs. Place a second purse-string suture or Lembert sutures to bury the wound.

Extraction enterotomy

1. It may be possible to knead a foreign body, especially a bolus of food, onwards into the caecum. If so, it will pass spontaneously per rectum. Do not persist with this manoeuvre if it is difficult.

2. Before opening the bowel, pack off the area carefully. Try and manipulate an impacted foreign body upwards for a few centimetres, away from the inflamed segment in which it was lodged.

3. Apply soft clamps across the intestine on either side of the enterotomy site. Open the bowel longitudinally over the foreign body or tumour and gently extract or resect the lesion. Close the bowel transversely in two layers to prevent stenosis.

4. In gallstone ileus examine the right upper quadrant of the abdomen. Consider whether it is appropriate to proceed to cholecystectomy, choledochotomy and possible closure of the biliary–enteric fistula. Since the patient is often elderly and unfit, relief of the intestinal obstruction must be the dominant consideration. Examine the rest of the small bowel to exclude a second gallstone.

Traumatic enterotomy

1. Excise devitalized tissue and close the intestinal wounds(s) in two layers. An associated haematoma in the mesentery should be explored, with ligation of any bleeding points. Check the viability of the bowel thereafter, and if in doubt resect the damaged segment with end-to-end anastomosis.

2. Examine the other abdominal viscera for concomitant injuries.

ENTEROSTOMY

Appraise

1. A feeding jejunostomy permits enteral nutrition in patients who are unable to take sufficient food by mouth. It should always be placed as high as possible in the jejunum.

2. A terminal ileostomy replaces the anus after total colectomy for multiple neoplasia, ulcerative proctocolitis or Crohn's colitis.

Increasingly, defunctioning loop ileostomies are being used as forms of faecal diversion. In comparison with transverse colostomy, it produces predictable volumes of relatively inoffensive faecal effluent and it is a truly defunctioning stoma to which an appliance can easily be attached. Split ileostomy (separated stomas) will completely defunction the distal bowel and has been advocated in selected cases of colitis.

Action

Feeding jejunostomy

1. Expose the upper jejunum through a small left upper paramedian or transverse incision. Trace the bowel proximally to the duodeno-jejunal flexure. Select a loop a few centimetres distal to this point, so that it will easily reach the anterior abdominal wall.

2. Insert a catgut purse-string suture on the antimesenteric border of the bowel. Make a tiny enterotomy in the centre of the purse-string and introduce a T-tube (14 F) into the lumen of the bowel (Fig. 10.19). Tighten the purse-string snugly around the tube.

4. Whichever tube is used, it should be introduced first through a stab incision in the abdominal wall and then into the jejunum. Traction on the tube will approximate the bowel to the underside of the abdominal wall, where the intestine should be sutured to the peritoneum.

Terminal ileostomy (Fig. 10.20)

1. Excise a circular disc of skin and subcutaneous fat, 3 cm in diameter, at the site marked preoperatively. Make a cruciate incision in the exposed anterior rectus sheath, split the fibres of the rectus muscle and open the posterior sheath and peritoneum. The defect should comfortably accommodate two fingers.

2. The terminal ileum will previously have been clamped and transected. Now exteriorize 6–8 cm of bowel (with its mesentery intact) through the circular opening in the abdominal wall, leaving its end securely clamped. Make sure that the mesentery is neither twisted nor tight and that the tip of the ileum remains pink.

3. After closing the main abdominal incision, remove the clamp and trim the crushed portion of ileum. Now suture the edge of the

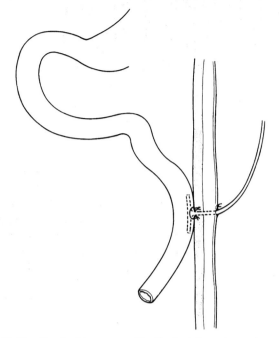

Fig. 10.19 Feeding jejunostomy. The T-tube is brought out through the abdominal wall, and the jejunum is stitched to the peritoneum around the margins of the stab incision.

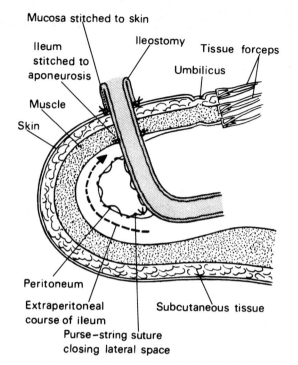

Fig. 10.20 Terminal ileostomy. Two methods of closing the lateral space are shown: a purse-string suture or taking the ileum along an extraperitoneal track. Alternatively, the lateral space can be left widely open. Tissue forceps on each layer of the wound edge prevent retraction of the layers while the ileostomy is being fashioned.

ileum directly to the skin, using catgut mounted on an atraumatic taper-pointed needle. Complete the circumferential sutures, producing a spout, which should project about 3 cm from the abdominal wall.

4. Carefully clean and dry the skin around the ileostomy and apply an ileostomy bag at once.

Loop ileostomy
1. A disc of skin and fat is excised (as above) and a loop of ileum is delivered on to the abdominal wall.
2. The bowel is opened not at the apex of the loop (as for a loop colostomy) but close to skin level.
3. The mucosa of the distal bowel is sutured to the skin.
4. The completed loop ileostomy looks very like a standard end ileostomy. As for loop colostomy, a plastic rod is used to prevent the bowel slipping back in, and a suitable appliance (with flange and clip-on bag) is fitted to the skin over the stoma.

FURTHER READING

Allison PR, da Silva LT 1953 The Roux loop. British Journal of Surgery 41: 173–180

Bradbury A 1995 Mesenteric ischaemia: a multidisciplinary approach. British Journal of Surgery 82: 1446–1459
Hesp WLEM, Lubbers EJC, de Boer HHM, Hendriks T 1988 Enterostomy as an adjunct to treatment of intra-abdominal sepsis. British Journal of Surgery 75: 693–696
Hill GL 1985 Massive enterectomy: indications and management. World Journal of Surgery 9: 833–841
Irwin ST, Krukowski ZH, Matheson NA 1990 Single layer anastomosis in the upper gastrointestinal tract. British Journal of Surgery 77: 643–644
Kirk RM 1985 Roux-en-Y. World Journal of Surgery 9: 938–944
Newman T 1998 The changing face of mesenteric infarction. American Surgeon 64: 611–616
Sansoni B, Irving MH 1985 Small bowel fistulas. World Journal of Surgery 9: 897–903
Williamson RCN 1991 Small intestine. In: O'Higgins NJ, Chisholm GD, Williamson RCN (eds) Surgical management, 2nd edn. Butterworth-Heinemann, Oxford, pp 562–593

Colonoscopy

R. J. Leicester

Appraise

1. Colonoscopy has revolutionized the diagnosis and treatment of colonic disease, allowing accurate mucosal visualization, biopsy and therapeutic polypectomy. Technological advances in instrumentation allow rapid and safe examination of the whole colon, provided the endoscopist has been adequately trained in the technique.

2. Use diagnostic colonoscopy to evaluate an abnormal or equivocal barium enema, particularly where diverticular disease or colonic spasm may often obscure a small mucosal lesion. In elderly patients, who often tolerate barium enema badly, colonoscopy should be the first-line investigation for unexplained rectal bleeding or anaemia and is the investigation of choice for all patients with a positive faecal occult blood test. Colonoscopy is the most accurate diagnostic tool for differential diagnosis and assessment of extent in inflammatory bowel disease, but should be avoided in acute disease, where technetium-labelled white cell scanning is a safer alternative.

3. Therapeutic colonoscopy has changed the surgical management of colorectal polyps, facilitating removal of all pedunculated and most sessile adenomatous lesions, thus providing an opportunity for colorectal cancer prevention. Diathermy coagulation or laser therapy of vascular abnormalities such as angiodysplasia may pre-empt laparotomy in acute colonic haemorrhage or cure anaemia due to chronic blood loss.

4. Relief of obstruction in colorectal cancer, either as an initial procedure prior to surgical resection or as long-term palliation, may be achieved using either laser vaporization or stent insertion.

5. Perform surveillance colonoscopy with multiple biopsies at least biennially in all patients with total ulcerative colitis, for more than 8 years, thus avoiding colectomy in over 80% of cases. Surgery is indicated only in those with definite dysplasia or carcinoma.

6. Following polypectomy or curative resection for colorectal cancer, carry out regular follow-up colonoscopy, initially after 3 years and thereafter 5-yearly if no new polyps are detected.

7. Commence screening of high-risk groups such as polyposis coli from age 15 (if gene-positive) and continue approximately 2-yearly until the age of 40. Hereditary non-polyposis coli families should undergo 1–2-yearly surveillance, commencing at least 10 years younger than the index case. If facilities exist, then screen subjects with a strong family history of colorectal cancer (i.e. one first-degree relative with onset before 40 years of age, or more than one first-degree relative of any age) in the hope of reducing the incidence of colorectal cancer by removing adenomatous lesions.

8. Carry out emergency colonoscopy in cases of acute, severe rectal bleeding after anorectal and upper gastrointestinal causes have been excluded by rigid proctosigmoidoscopy and gastroscopy. Bleeding usually ceases in up to 80% of patients, allowing colonoscopy within 24–48 hours, after bowel preparation. Even in the presence of active bleeding, while small mucosal lesions may be overlooked, you can obtain valuable clues as to the segment of colon from which the haemorrhage is arising, or note blood emerging through the ileocaecal valve, indicating a small-bowel lesion. When a diagnosis has not been reached and emergency laparotomy becomes necessary, you may perform colonoscopy under general anaesthetic with the peritoneal cavity exposed, following on-table lavage with saline or water introduced via a Foley catheter through a caecostomy.

Prepare

1. Accurate, rapid examination depends upon effective bowel preparation. Advise patients to discontinue any iron preparations or stool-bulking agents 1 week prior to endoscopy, and change to a low residue diet. 24 hours before examination restrict oral intake to clear fluids such as coffee or tea without milk, concentrated meat extract and glucose drinks. Give a purgative such as sodium picosulphate 12–18 hours before colonoscopy and repeat it 4 hours before examination. Alternatively, give balanced electrolyte solutions combined with polyethylene glycol, which have been shown to produce rapid preparation without the need for dietary restriction. Give oral metoclopramide 10 mg prior to ingestion of the 3–4 litres of solution, which enhances gastric emptying and reduces nausea and vomiting.

2. Obtain from all patients written, informed consent for the procedure. Give reassurance about the examination to allay fears, allowing minimal levels of sedation to be used.

3. Colonoscopy is usually performed under intravenous sedation with the addition of an analgesic. Do not give excessive sedation or analgesia, to avoid circulatory or respiratory depression. Additionally, it will dull appreciation of severe pain, which should occur only when a poor technique is used, causing dangerous overstretching of the bowel. For similar reasons do not perform colonoscopy under general anaesthesia, apart from as an intraoperative procedure in cases of acute colonic haemorrhage. Elderly patients in particular can suffer significant hypotension following pethidine, and this, combined with the synergistic effect of opiates and benzodiazepines, can also cause significant falls in oxygen saturation. In order to avoid these complications, use only small doses of analgesic and hypnotic such as intravenous pethidine 50 mg or pentazocine 30 mg plus midazolam 2.5–5 mg. Monitor all patients, during and after the procedure, by pulse oximetry, and give added inspired oxygen as appropriate. Always have available antidotes to benzodiazepines (flumazenil) and opiates (naloxone), together with full cardiorespiratory resuscitation equipment and trained staff to use it in case of emergency. Occasionally an antispasmodic, either

intravenous hyoscine butylbromide or intraluminal peppermint oil suspension, may be employed.

4. As a rule, examine the patient in the left lateral position or, alternatively, supine. Use a tipping trolley in case of cardiorespiratory problems. Have available at least two trained assistants: one to observe the patient's vital signs and the other to assist with the accessories for biopsy or snare polypectomy. Videoendoscopes are an essential tool to ensure accurate and safe polypectomy and also to maintain the interest of the assistants.

5. Check all equipment prior to intubation. The colonoscope must have been adequately cleaned and disinfected. The light source, endoscope angulation controls, air/water insufflation and suction facilities must be in full working order. Check the diathermy equipment for correct, safe operation. Ensure that all accessories such as biopsy forceps and polypectomy snares operate correctly.

Access

1. Modern colonoscopes are sophisticated precision instruments designed to enhance intubation of the colon in the most efficient manner. As well as a wide-angled lens to allow a greater field of vision, a graduated torque characteristic assists variability in the stiffness of the instrument.

2. During intubation, the instrument may be pushed forward or pulled back. Change of direction may be achieved by angulation of the distal end, up/down or left/right. Change of direction may also be achieved by up/down deflection, combined with rotation. Keeping the distal section of the instrument as straight as possible, restoring this to a neutral position as soon as possible after angulation around an acute bend helps to prevent loop formation. Avoid maximum up/down and left/right angulation, as this results in a J shape and rotation of the end of the instrument rather than change of direction. Advancement may also be achieved by the straightening of a loop using torque and withdrawal or by suction causing a concertina effect of the bowel over the endoscope.

3. Colonoscopy is made easier if the anatomy of the colon is properly understood. The rectum is fixed in a retroperitoneal position and consists of alternating mucosal folds forming the valves of Houston. The sigmoid colon is freely mobile on its mesentery and of variable length and configuration. The descending colon and splenic flexure are relatively fixed by their peritoneal attachments. At the splenic flexure, the direction of the colon is forwards and downwards to the transverse colon which, like the sigmoid, is of variable length and freely mobile on the transverse mesocolon. The bowel becomes fixed again at the hepatic flexure and the direction passes forwards and downwards into the ascending colon and caecum, which are usually fixed by peritoneal attachments, though less consistently than the descending colon. It is the mobile and variable-length sigmoid and transverse colon that cause the most difficulty through looping of the instrument.

4. The aim of colonoscopy is to achieve intubation from the anus to caecum with the minimum possible length of instrument (Fig. 11.1). Characteristically, the colonoscope, when straight and without loop formation, should be in a roughly U-shaped configuration with 70–80 cm of instrument inserted to the caecal pole (Fig. 11.2). Significantly greater insertion length indicates the presence of a loop.

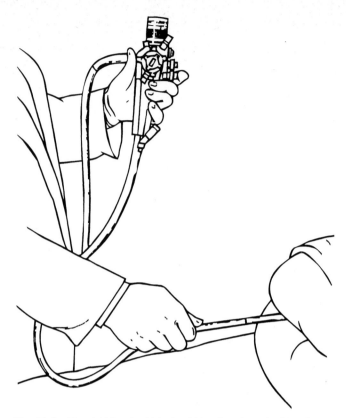

Fig. 11.1 The right hand, which should be gloved, manipulates the colonoscope shaft.

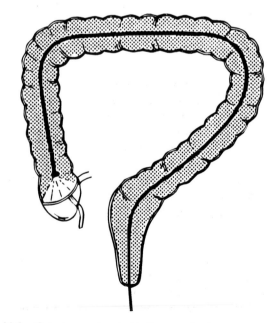

Fig. 11.2 Colonoscope inserted to the caecal pole.

Colon

A. Windsor, R. Phillips and P. Hawley

Contents

EXAMINATION OF THE LARGE BOWEL

Preoperative assessment

1. Obtain a full history and carry out a complete examination before any surgical procedure. Examine the abdomen, anus and rectum in every patient before undertaking surgery of the large bowel. This implies a thorough digital examination of the rectum and the passage of a rigid sigmoidoscope, which is an outpatient or bedside procedure. Carry out further investigations as necessary.

   a. *Fibreoptic sigmoidoscopy* – a simple outpatient procedure undertaken after one or two phosphate enemas. This reveals polyps or a carcinoma in the proximal sigmoid or descending colon.

   b. *Barium enema.* Carry out a barium enema on patients with suspected pathology above the reach of a sigmoidoscope. Use a double-contrast enema as this demonstrates much more pathology than the single-contrast technique.

   c. *Instant barium enema.* Barium is instilled into the rectum without any preparation. This is very useful in inflammatory bowel disease to demonstrate upper limit of disease during the outpatient visit.

   d. *Colonoscopy* (see Ch. 11). This has not taken the place of air-contrast barium enema but complements it. Carry out this investigation to evaluate equivocal findings on a barium enema. Pedunculated polyps can be removed by colonoscopic snaring and biopsies obtained from tumours and inflammatory bowel disease in the proximal colon. Carry out colonoscopy in the evaluation of gastrointestinal bleeding suspected to be from the colon. More advanced procedures such as endoscopic mucosal resection and stenting are available in specialist centres.

   e. *Other examinations.* These include: mucosal biopsy in inflammatory bowel disease to help in the differentiation of ulcerative colitis, Crohn's disease and infective colitis; stool microscopy and culture to differentiate bacterial and parasitic infection from inflammatory bowel disease; straight X-ray of the abdomen in suspected large bowel obstruction or perforation. Serial abdominal films are important in evaluating the progress of acute colitis and the onset of toxic megacolon. Imaging scans are of value in elucidating abdominal masses, abscesses and possible metastases. Ultrasonography is more readily available than computerized tomography but diagnostic accuracy is user-dependent. Computerized tomography (CT) scanning is increasingly used for the investigation of colonic pathology and, with the advent of spiral CT, the technique of CT colography or virtual colonoscopy is gaining clinical acceptance. Angiography helps to evaluate severe gastrointestinal haemorrhage and localizes haemangiomatous malformations.

2. Do not perform elective operation on the colon or rectum to establish a diagnosis. Diagnostic laparotomy is inappropriate to exclude a filling defect in the right colon on barium enema or to decide if an area of sigmoid diverticular disease hides a carcinoma. Skilled endoscopy will provide the answer.

ELECTIVE OPERATIONS

Key points

- Plan elective surgery carefully.

- When possible, use contrast radiology and cross-sectional imaging to determine the situation.

- Try to avoid 'laparotomy and proceed'.

- Always have X-ray films and results of other investigations available for study in the operating theatre.

Carcinoma

1. Examine the contents of the whole abdomen. Examine the whole of the colon from the appendix to the rectum. Small adenomatous polyps cannot be felt. Synchronous carcinomas occur in 4% of patients. Avoid handling the carcinoma; cover it with a swab soaked in dilute aqueous povidone-iodine solution. Feel for enlarged lymph nodes in the mesentery and in the para-aortic regions. Look for peritoneal metastases.

2. Estimate the resectability and curability of the tumour. Palpate

and visualize the liver to exclude metastases or biopsy them to confirm the diagnosis. Subsequent investigation will allow accurate assessment and partial hepatectomy may be planned in from 3–4 months time.

3. Treat potentially curable carcinoma of the right colon by one-stage right hemicolectomy, taking the ileocolic and middle colic vessels at their origin from the superior mesenteric vessels. If metastases are present perform a less extensive resection without wide mesenteric clearance.

4. Treat carcinoma of the transverse colon by extended right hemicolectomy or transverse colectomy, taking the hepatic and/or splenic flexure if the lesion is situated proximally or distally in the transverse colon. With a lesion at the splenic flexure and distal diverticular disease, an extended left hemicolectomy may be necessary; swing the right colon down on the right side of the abdomen to anastomose to the rectum (Fig. 12.1). Alternatively, perform an extended colectomy and ileosigmoid anastomosis.

5. Treat carcinoma of the descending and sigmoid colon by left hemicolectomy, taking the inferior mesenteric artery at its origin from the aorta and the inferior mesenteric vein at the same level.

6. Surgical management of rectal carcinoma has evolved rapidly in the last 5 years. Treat most cases of carcinoma of the rectum by anterior resection using either a sutured, stapled or peranal anastomosis. Only 15–20% should require abdominoperineal excision of the rectum because it is impossible to obtain a 2–5 cm distal clearance of the tumour. Sharp dissection is essential in the pelvis, allowing removal of the lymphovascular bundle (mesorectum) without breaching the fascial plane in which it is contained. Identify and preserve the hypogastric nerve plexus, if it is uninvolved with tumour. This avoids ejaculatory, erectile and urinary complications.

7. For rectal carcinoma with metastases carry out anterior resection if this can be safely done without having to perform a defunctioning colostomy, as many of these patients deteriorate and never have the colostomy closed. If the rectal carcinoma is low, if there is local extension to the side walls of the pelvis or if internal iliac nodes are involved, select a palliative abdominoperineal excision of the rectum or a Hartmann's operation.

Diverticular disease

1. Diverticular disease is very common and most elderly patients having operations for other abdominal conditions are found to have diverticula, mainly in the sigmoid colon. Although diverticular disease may be widespread in the colon, symptomatic disease is usually produced by the muscle hypertrophy, thickening and shortening of the sigmoid colon.

2. Even in elective resection, the disease may be associated with marked pericolic inflammation and oedema with pericolic abscess formation in the mesentery.

3. Indications for elective resection are not always definite, and with the introduction of high roughage diets and the addition of bran fewer operations are undertaken. However, offer operation to patients in good general health who have severe attacks of lower left-sided and suprapubic pain with marked diverticular disease on a barium enema X-ray, with muscle hypertrophy and narrowing of the colonic lumen which is unresponsive to dietary change and antispasmodic drugs. The barium enema findings and pathology do not always correlate and patients often wait too long before being offered surgical treatment. Definite indications for surgical treatment include:

a. male patients under the age of 50 years with symptomatic disease, since statistically over 80% eventually come to surgery, many with complications
b. patients with urinary infection associated with their attacks indicating adhesion to the bladder or ureter and an impending fistula, and indeed those with an established colovesical fistula
c. patients with two or more attacks of acute diverticular disease within a short period of time associated with a fever, mass and radiological signs of a pericolic abscess
d. recurrent bleeding in patients fit for operation. A single episode does not make surgery mandatory.

> ### 🔑 Key point
>
> - Avoid operation in patients with the irritable bowel syndrome and few diverticula; their symptoms will persist.

4. It is unnecessary to remove all the proximal diverticula. Resect all hypertrophied sections of bowel, usually including the whole of the sigmoid colon, with anastomosis between the middle or upper descending colon and the upper third of the rectum below the sacral promontory.

5. Operative treatment is always by resection and anastomosis.

Ulcerative colitis

1. Offer elective operation to patients with persistent or recurrent attacks of diarrhoea with the passage of blood, anaemia, weight loss and general ill health, which is unresponsive to treatment with corticosteroids and salazines. The majority of these patients have total or extensive colitis. Patients with purely distal disease, such as sigmoid or left-colon, do not usually require operation. Try to

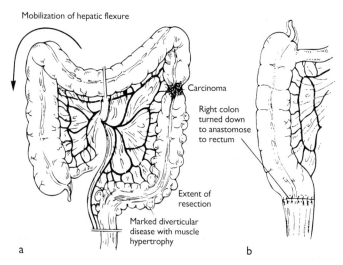

Mobilization of hepatic flexure

Carcinoma

Right colon turned down to anastomose to rectum

Extent of resection

Marked diverticular disease with muscle hypertrophy

a   b

Fig. 12.1 Management of carcinoma of the splenic flexure or distal transverse colon with significant diverticular disease. This is better than an ileorectal anastomosis in patients with a compromised sphincter.

operate on patients with several severe attacks of acute colitis during remission.

Total colitis of 10–15 years duration or longer may result in dysplastic epithelial changes and eventual carcinoma, even in the absence of any symptoms. Carefully follow these patients with colonoscopy and mucosal biopsy. If they eventually develop moderate or severe dysplasia, they require surgical treatment. Operate on patients with total colitis and strictures or filling defects on barium enema or colonoscopy. Steroid therapy is no contraindication to surgery as it makes no difference to the outcome, but these patients must have steroid cover during and after the operation.

2. In quiescent total colitis, the colon is slightly thickened, shortened and greyish white in colour. Even at elective operation, part of the colon may appear much more actively inflamed with thickening, oedema and marked hyperaemia. The paracolic and mesenteric nodes may be considerably enlarged.

3. The most straightforward operation to carry out is a procto-colectomy with a conventional Brooke ileostomy.

4. Consider alternative procedures.

a. If the patient comes to surgery early in the course of the disease when the rectum is still distensible and there is no dysplasia in rectal biopsies, consider performing a colectomy and ileorectal anastomosis.

b. Following proctocolectomy patients may wish to avoid a permanent conventional ileostomy; this is possible with a conservative proctocolectomy leaving the anal sphincters followed by an ileoanal reservoir.

c. If the patient is incontinent as a result of previous sphincter damage, you may construct a Kock reservoir ileostomy to avoid the patient having to wear an appliance.

4. If you are inexperienced in these operations, carry out a colectomy and ileostomy, retaining the whole rectum.

Crohn's disease

1. This can develop throughout the gastrointestinal tract. Primary treatment is always medical. Undertake surgical treatment if medical treatment fails to control the disease, or for complications such as stenosis causing obstructive symptoms, abscesses or internal or external fistula formation.

Key point

- Surgery is not curative so make sure you treat the patients and their symptoms, not appearances on radiological imaging.

---

2. The whole or part of the colon may be involved in Crohn's disease. Carefully examine the stomach and duodenum and the whole of the small bowel to exclude other sites of disease. Carefully measure the length of the small bowel and record the sites and extent of the disease; these patients often require multiple operations and may end up with 'short bowel syndrome' if surgery is not carefully planned.

3. When the disease affects the terminal ileum and/or caecum and ascending colon, carry out ileal resection with removal of the caecum or right colon as necessary. In a primary operation remove 5–10 cm of macroscopically normal ileum proximal to the lesion. If there is a chronic abscess cavity in the right iliac fossa, extend the right hemicolectomy so that the anastomosis lies in the upper abdomen away from the abscess cavity.

4. If the whole colon is severely involved and requires resection, perform a colectomy and ileorectal anastomosis or a total procto-colectomy and conventional ileostomy. Distal disease involving only the rectum may require an abdominoperineal excision with an end colostomy. Segmental colonic resection is rarely required.

Polyps and polyposis

1. Polyps in the rectum are often discovered on routine sigmoido-scopy when patients present with minor anal conditions. Remove one or more for histology. If the polyp proves to be an adenoma, carry out a colonoscopy to search for and treat proximal polyps. Sessile villous adenomas usually occur in the rectum and can be removed by endoanal local excision or in specialist centres with transanal endoscopic microsurgery.

2. If several large polyps are present in a patient with carcinoma, extend the resection to include these. In a patient with one or more carcinomas and several large polyps, consider colectomy and ileorectal anastomosis.

3. Perform anterior resection with coloanal anastomosis or a modified Soave procedure on circumferential villous tumours extending above 10 cm from the anal vent.

4. Familial adenomatous polyposis requires surgery to avoid inevitable malignant change. Options include colectomy and ileorectal anastomosis, or proctocolectomy and ileoanal pouch reconstruction. Following ileorectal anastomosis the rectum still carries the potential for malignant change, so plan to perform follow-up sigmoidoscopy every 6 months. Fulgurate rectal polyps if they are over 5 mm in diameter.

URGENT OPERATIONS

1. Urgent operations on the colon or rectum are carried out for obstruction, perforation, abscess formation, acute fulminating inflammatory bowel disease and acute haemorrhage.

2. Ensure that the patient is in the best possible condition before undertaking surgery. Replace blood, fluid and electrolyte loss and in major septic conditions commence antibiotic therapy with an amino-glycoside or a cephalosporin, together with metronidazole.

3. Decide on the best time for operation:

a. If the patient has severe bleeding, major abdominal sepsis or perforation operate as soon as the patient's condition allows;

b. Large bowel obstruction and inflammatory bowel disease rarely require emergency surgery; carry it out as soon as you, the anaesthetist and theatre staff are fresh.

c. Try to avoid operating in haste at night; in order to obtain good results.

Obstruction

1. Define the level of obstruction with a water-soluble contrast enema.

2. If an urgent resection is carried out, make sure it is as radical as would be achieved at an elective operation at the same site, provided cure is possible. If there are metastases, carry out palliative resection.

It is rare to find a proximal tumour that is not respectable but if you find yourself in this situation, carry out a bypass procedure. Remember that this will relieve the obstruction but not stop bleeding from the tumour and the consequent anaemia or pain and complications from the mass invading other structures. In an unresectable left-sided tumour carry out a proximal defunctioning colostomy.

3. Perform right hemicolectomy for carcinoma of the right colon causing acute intestinal obstruction. Left-sided obstruction is now rarely treated by a staged procedure with a defunctioning transverse colostomy, an interim resection and finally closure of the colostomy. More commonly, a carcinoma of the upper sigmoid or descending colon is treated by a one-stage colectomy with ileosigmoid or ileo-rectal anastomosis (Fig. 12.2). Treat carcinoma of the lower sigmoid or rectosigmoid junction by resection, peroperative irrigation of the obstructed colon and primary anastomosis. Alternatively perform a Hartmann's procedure (see later).

4. Acute obstructive diverticular disease is often complicated by paracolic abscess formation. The operation of choice is immediate resection with a Hartmann's procedure. It may be safe to carry out a resection and anastomosis with or without a defunctioning transverse colostomy, if the infection is localized and completely removed by resection, and if you carry out preoperative irrigation of the colon.

Perforation

Perforation of a carcinoma or diverticular disease requires resection and anastomosis with a covering colostomy or, in the presence of major contamination and abscess formation, a Hartmann's procedure. You may need to drain the abscess and create a defunctioning colostomy in a severely ill, debilitated patient. It is usually the less satisfactory alternative and will not preclude resection as soon as the patient's condition allows.

Acute inflammatory bowel disease

Treat acute fulminating colitis, with or without toxic megacolon, by colectomy and ileostomy with a mucous fistula. Do not excise the rectum and it is much safer to make a mucous fistula than to close the rectal stump. In order to avoid creating a second stoma, close the stump directly under the wound so that if it breaks down it will not contaminate the peritoneal cavity.

Excise a segment of acute ischaemic colitis and create a proximal and distal colostomy. Always leave the rectum and sigmoid colon as these usually recover sufficiently for anastomosis to be carried out later.

Acute massive haemorrhage

Determine if possible the site of bleeding by sigmoidoscopy, colonoscopy, upper gastrointestinal endoscopy and angiography. Remember that 50% of patients with episodes of haemorrhage and diverticular disease have another cause for the bleeding. If the site can be accurately determined it may be possible to stop it by interventional radiology (embolization). If not, carry out a limited resection. If you cannot determine the site and origin of colonic bleeding, it is wise to carry out a colectomy and ileorectal anastomosis.

SURGERY OF THE LARGE BOWEL

Appraise

1. Morbidity and mortality following colonic surgery is higher than following resections of the small bowel. The colonic blood supply is more tenuous and easily damaged. Tissue perfusion is often decreased postoperatively, resulting in a degree of ischaemic colitis. Infection is more common, resulting in abscess formation with potentiation of collagenase activity. Collagen undergoes lysis and may result in anastomotic dehiscence.

Prepare

1. Ensure that barium enema films and other imaging results are available at operation.

2. Ensure that the colon is empty before you undertake an elective operation. A variety of methods have been used to clean the colon mechanically: sodium picosulphate and magnesium citrate provides a stimulant preparation, polyethylene glycol is a mechanical preparation. Give adequate and fluids for 24 hours preoperatively. Intravenous fluids may be required in elderly patients. Enemas are not required.

3. Preoperative oral antibiotics are of little value. Give per-operative prophylactic antibiotics at induction of anaesthesia. Numerous regimens have been suggested; gentamicin and metronidazole, a cephalosporin and metronidazole or beta-lactamase inhibitor/broad-spectrum penicillin are popular. Give a further dose of antibiotics in the event of prolonged surgery (more than 2 hours) or significant intraoperative contamination. There is no evidence that routine use of more than one dose of prophylactic antibiotics reduces the risk of infection.

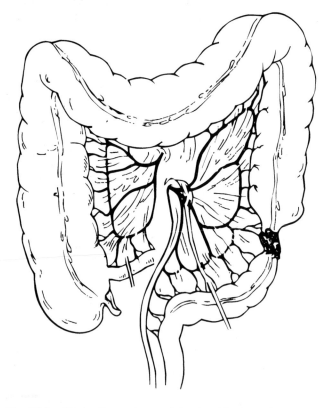

Fig. 12.2 Obstructing carcinoma of the sigmoid colon: colectomy followed by ileorectal or ileosigmoid anastomosis.

4. Catheterize the patient after induction of anaesthesia and monitor urinary output during and after surgery.

Action

1. Clamp the bowel to be resected with Parker–Kerr clamps. If the patient has been well prepared and the colon is empty, place no clamps on the ends to be sutured.

2. Clean the ends of the bowel to be sutured with moistened swabs wetted in 1:2000 aqueous chlorhexidine solution or aqueous 10% povidone-iodine solution.

3. Divide the colon at right angles to the mesentery. If there is disparity in size between the ends, particularly when carrying out a right hemicolectomy or an ileorectal anastomosis, slit up the anti-mesenteric border of the ileum or narrower colon until the two ends approximate in size. Alternatively carry out an end-to-side or side-to-side anastomosis. When a long length of mobilized colon is to be anastomosed to the rectum make certain there is not a 360° twist.

4. Carry out anastomosis of the colon end-to-end with the proximal bowel rotated 90° to the right, so that the mesenteric borders are not opposite each other, particularly when making a rectal anastomosis.

5. Suture the bowel in one layer with an appropriate absorbable suture such as polyglactin 910. This may be done in most instances as an interrupted or continuous stitch. Invert the edges but not so much as to produce a cuff that will cause an obstructive anastomosis. Ensure that the mucosa does not protrude from the suture line. Alternatively, there are a number of methods for carrying out a stapled anastomosis; apart from speed they add little to the more traditional approach and are significantly more expensive. Undertake rectal anastomosis using a circular stapling device such as the EEA stapler, using a 28 or 31 mm diameter device, particularly when forming an anastomosis low in the pelvis, when suturing is technically difficult.

6. Avoid contamination during the operation. If the colon is loaded, place a non-crushing clamp across the bowel 10 cm from the end before this is swabbed out and cleaned. If possible, screen the anastomosis from the peritoneal cavity and contents while it is being constructed. When it is complete, discard and replace the towels, gloves and instruments before closing the abdomen.

7. It is traditional for British surgeons to drain any colonic anastomosis. This is unnecessary. Drain an intraperitoneal abscess. Drain an extraperitoneal low anterior resection through the peritoneal cavity into the pelvis.

RIGHT HEMICOLECTOMY

Appraise

1. Perform this operation for carcinoma of the caecum and ascending colon and for the occasional benign tumour of the right colon. Undertake it for a perforated caecal diverticulum, so-called solitary ulcer of the caecum and carry out a limited resection for carcinoma of the appendix or a carcinoid tumour at the base of the appendix. Never carry out an ileocolic bypass for an extensive carcinoma, even if the operation is palliative. Try and carry out a right hemicolectomy.

2. Benign disease of the terminal ileum, particularly Crohn's disease, is treated by resecting an appropriate amount of ileum together with the caecum and 2–3 cm of the right colon. When Crohn's disease is associated with abscess formation in the right iliac fossa, extend the operation so that the anastomosis lies in the upper abdomen away from the abscess. This prevents fistula formation postoperatively.

3. Never make a small-bowel anastomosis close to the ileocaecal valve. Preferably remove the caecum and a small part of the ascending colon, and carry out an ileocolic anastomosis.

4. In obstruction, usually due to carcinoma of the ileocaecal region or the right colon, carry out an urgent right hemicolectomy, extending the operation distally as appropriate.

Action (Fig. 12.3)

Resect

1. Handle the tumour as little as possible. If the serosa and surrounding fat are infiltrated by carcinoma, cover it with a swab soaked in aqueous 10% povidone-iodine solution.

2. Leave the omentum adherent to the right colon.

3. Draw the caecum and ascending colon medially. Cut through the parietal peritoneum lateral to the colon from the caecum to the hepatic flexure. If the carcinoma infiltrates the lateral abdominal wall, excise a large disc of peritoneum and underlying muscle with the specimen.

4. Dissect the right colon from the posterior abdominal wall. Identify and preserve the right ureter, gonadal vessels and duodenum.

5. Mobilize the hepatic flexure and divide any ileal bands so that the whole of the right colon can be lifted from the abdomen.

6. Transilluminate the mesentery to identify the vessels; clamp and divide the ileocolic artery and vein close to the superior mesenteric vessels. Divide the right colic vessels and the right branch of the middle colic vessels close to their origin.

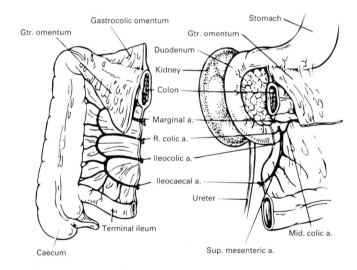

Fig. 12.3 Radical right hemicolectomy – the resected specimen is on the left and comprises the right half of the colon, the terminal ileum and the mesentery with vessels and nodes. Also included are the right halves of the gastrocolic and greater omenta. The ileocolic artery and vein are divided at their origins from the superior mesenteric vessels. The right branch of the middle colic artery is divided. The duodenum, pancreas and right kidney and ureter have been identified and protected from damage.

7. The extent of the resection depends to some degree on the size and site of the tumour but normally includes approximately 25 cm of terminal ileum to the middle third of the transverse colon.

8. Remove the right half of the greater omentum with the specimen. If the tumour is situated near the hepatic flexure remove the right side of the gastroepiploic arch of vessels to obtain a wider clearance.

9. Place a Parker–Kerr clamp across the ileum and transverse colon at the site of division. Unless the patient is obstructed and the colon is unprepared, do not clamp the ends to be anastomosed.

10. Divide the bowel and remove the specimen.

11. Hold the ends of the ileum and colon to be anastomosed in Babcock's forceps and clean them with mounted swabs wetted with aqueous 10% povidone-iodine solution.

Unite

1. Anastomose the terminal ileum end-to-end to the transverse colon, widening the ileum with an antimesenteric (Cheatle) slit if necessary. Mark the anastomosis with haemostatic clips if desired. Alternatively, divide the colon using a linear cutter stapling device and perform an end-to-side anastomosis, or construct a functional end-to-end anastomosis using the same linear cutter stapling device.

2. Suture the cut edges of the mesentery with a polyglactin 910 suture.

3. Cover the anastomosis with the remaining omentum.

Technical points

1. If the resection is for a benign condition such as Crohn's disease or a caecal diverticulum, it need not be extensive. The vessels can be divided in the middle of the mesentery rather than at their origin.

2. If the carcinoma is locally invasive but can be excised radically, widen the scope of the operation to include abdominal wall or part of the involved organs.

3. If the carcinoma is situated at the hepatic flexure or in the right side of the transverse colon, mobilize the splenic flexure as well. Divide the middle colic vessels close to their origin and anastomose the terminal ileum to the descending or sigmoid colon. If there are multiple metastases carry out a limited segmental resection rather than a bypass procedure.

Checklist

1. Make sure the bowel on each side of the anastomosis is viable and check that the anastomosis lies freely without twist or tension.

2. Examine the raw surfaces, particularly in the right flank, and stop any bleeding. Remove any blood collected above the right lobe of the liver and in the pelvis.

LEFT HEMICOLECTOMY

Appraise

1. Undertake left hemicolectomy for carcinoma of the left and sigmoid colon, and for diverticular disease.

2. If the operation is for an obstructed neoplasm, carry out an extended colectomy with an ileosigmoid or ileorectal anastomosis. Alternatively, carry out a resection with on-table irrigation of the obstructed proximal colon and create a primary anastomosis. Rarely, a Hartmann's operation or a staged procedure is necessary.

3. In diverticular disease, resect the sigmoid colon and as much of the ascending colon as is necessary. Leave isolated diverticula in the upper descending and transverse colon, providing the bowel wall is not thickened. Anastomose the proximal bowel to the upper third of the rectum below the sacral promontory and not to the sigmoid colon.

4. In any left hemicolectomy the splenic flexure and the left half of the transverse colon must be mobilized.

Prepare (Fig. 12.4)

Place the patient in the lithotomy Trendelenburg (Lloyd-Davies) position. Pass a catheter to empty the bladder and to monitor the urine flow during and after the operation.

Access

1. Stand on the patient's right side.

2. Make a long midline incision. You require access to the spleen when you mobilize the splenic flexure of colon, and in the pelvis when you construct the anastomosis.

Assess

1. If the operation is for a carcinoma, carefully palpate the liver bimanually, examine the colon and the whole of the small bowel, palpate the mesenteric and para-aortic nodes and the whole of the peritoneal cavity and pelvis.

2. Gently palpate the carcinoma to assess its mobility but touch it as little as possible. If the serosal surface is involved, cover it with a swab soaked in 10% aqueous povidone-iodine solution.

3. If you are performing partial colectomy for a benign condition, assess the diseased colon and decide the extent of resection, then explore the abdomen completely as in a case of carcinoma.

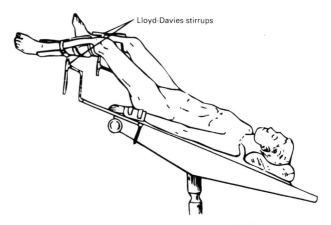

Lloyd-Davies stirrups

Fig. 12.4 Place the patient in the lithotomy Trendelenburg position of Lloyd-Davies for any operation on, or involving, the left side of the colon or the rectum. This allows simultaneous approaches to be made to the perineum or rectum and the abdomen without altering the patient's position.

- Carry out a radical resection of a carcinoma if possible. Tie the inferior mesenteric artery at its origin from the aorta and the inferior mesenteric vein below the inferior border of the pancreas.

- If the patient is very elderly and clearly unfit, and the blood supply to the colon is tenuous because of severe atheroma, undertake a less radical procedure, retaining the origin of the inferior mesenteric artery, and ligate the left colonic artery and sigmoid branches as appropriate.

- If the resection is for a benign condition, or a palliative resection for carcinoma, then the bowel resection need not be so wide and you may ligate and divide the vessels close to the bowel wall.

RADICAL RESECTION OF THE LEFT COLON

Action (Fig. 12.5)

1. Place damp packs over the wound edges. Suture the peritoneum overlying the bladder to the lower part of the skin wound and packs.

2. Exteriorize the small bowel to the right side and cover it with a moist pack. Never pack the small bowel into the wound as it severely restricts access.

3. Divide the congenital adhesions that bind the sigmoid colon to the abdominal wall in the left iliac fossa and then divide the adhesions between the descending colon and the lateral peritoneum. This is most efficiently achieved by following the plane of zygosis (true conjunction of posterior peritoneum and visceral peritoneum) or white line. Do not divide the peritoneum but stay on the mesenteric side of the white line to ensure that you remain in the correct plane.

4. Rotate the patient to the right side and then mobilize the splenic flexure by dividing the phrenocolic ligament. Ligate the few vessels in it. Avoid damaging the spleen and the tail of the pancreas. If the carcinoma is distal you may preserve the greater omentum by dividing the adhesions between the omentum and the colon as far proximally as the middle of the transverse colon and dividing the peritoneum along the end of the lesser sac. If the tumour is situated near the flexure, excise the left half of the greater omentum with the tumour by dividing the left side of the gastroepiploic arch and removing the lesser and greater omentum with the specimen.

5. Elevate the left colon on its mesentery and dissect it free from the duodenojejunal flexure, the left ureter and the gonadal vessels.

6. Incise the peritoneum overlying the aorta and mobilize the inferior mesenteric artery to its origin. Ligate and divide the artery and then identify the inferior mesenteric vein lying laterally and clamp, ligate and divide it a little below the lower border of the pancreas.

7. Mobilize the sigmoid colon if the anastomosis is to be made to the upper third of the rectum. Do not divide the sigmoid higher than about 10 cm above the rectum or its blood supply may be endangered.

8. Divide the mesentery and marginal vessels to the edge of the colon at the site chosen for resection in the transverse colon and rectum or sigmoid colon.

9. Place a Lloyd-Davies right-angled clamp across the rectum at the site of resection. Then irrigate the rectum by means of a catheter passed through the anus with povidone-iodine solution or a 1:2000 aqueous chlorhexidine solution until it is perfectly clean. Then swab the rectum dry.

10. While the rectal irrigation is being carried out prepare the proximal colon for division. Place a Parker–Kerr clamp across the bowel. If the colon is well prepared, do not clamp the proximal bowel to be used in the anastomosis. Divide the colon, hold the proximal end in Babcock's forceps and swab the bowel out with povidone-iodine solution or 1:2000 aqueous chlorhexidine solution.

11. Divide the rectum or sigmoid colon below the right-angled clamp and remove the specimen consisting of the left half of the colon, the inferior mesenteric artery and vein and the whole of the mesentery.

12. If it is necessary to mobilize the transverse colon or hepatic flexure to ensure a tension-free anastomosis, do this before dividing the colon.

Unite

1. Unite the bowel ends with one layer of seromuscular inverting sutures according to your preferred technique. Make the anastomosis end-to-end, with the proximal colon rotated 90° to the right so that the proximal mesentery lies opposite the cut edge of the peritoneum overlying the aorta.

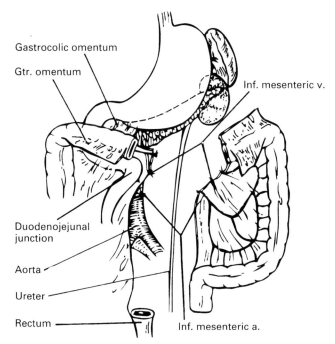

Gastrocolic omentum

Gtr. omentum

Inf. mesenteric v.

Duodenojejunal junction

Aorta

Ureter

Rectum

Inf. mesenteric a.

Fig. 12.5 Radical left hemicolectomy: the resected specimen is on the right and comprises the left half of colon, the mesocolon and the left halves of the gastrocolic and greater omenta. The left division of the middle colic artery and the origin of the inferior mesenteric artery have been ligated and divided. The duodenojejunal junction, left ureter and kidney, pancreas and spleen have been protected from damage.

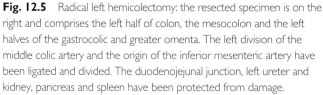

Key point

- Beware of using the EEA stapler at the top of the rectum. Introducing it around the rectal valves may tear the rectum. If you employ this technique, either resect more of the rectum or anastomose the colon end-to-side to the rectum.

2. Suture the cut edge of the transverse mesocolon to the cut edge of the peritoneum overlying the aorta.

1. Do not hesitate to involve another specialist if you are not experienced enough to deal with unfamiliar techniques.

2. If the tumour is situated in the left half of the transverse colon or at the splenic flexure, excise most of the transverse colon and unite the hepatic flexure or ascending colon to the lower descending or sigmoid colon. Alternatively, perform an extended right hemicolectomy with an ileo–descending anastomosis.

CARCINOMA OF THE RECTUM

Appraise

1. Assess all patients before operation by sigmoidoscopy, rectal biopsy and a barium enema or colonoscopy to evaluate the proximal colon.

2. Be willing to assess low, bulky tumours and those placed anteriorly, using computerized tomography or magnetic resonance imaging, to assess tumour stage.

3. Consider preoperative radiotherapy particularly for T3 and T4 lesions.

4. A few patients with small early carcinomas (assessed by transrectal ultrasound) are suitable for a peranal local excision.

ANTERIOR RESECTION OF THE RECTUM

Prepare

1. Place the anaesthetized patient in the lithotomy Trendelenburg (Lloyd-Davies) position.

2. Insert an indwelling Foley catheter.

3. Carry out an examination under anaesthetic to assess the fixity of low tumours (below the peritoneal reflection).

Access

1. Stand on the patient's right.

2. Make a long midline incision, as the splenic flexure will require mobilization and the rectal anastomosis may be deep within the pelvis.

Assess

1. Palpate and visualize the liver to establish if there are metastases.

2. Note any local or distant peritoneal metastases. Examine the omentum.

3. Palpate any nodes in the mesentery and note any para-aortic nodes.

4. Finally, palpate the tumour, note its size and position above or below the peritoneal reflection and decide whether it is mobile, adherent to other organs or fixed within the pelvis.

Do not be daunted to discover that a large rectal carcinoma lies in a small male pelvis. Determine not to compromise on the standard of radical resection by breaching the planes of direction. Take time and proceed in an ever-deepening circumferential manner. As you mobilize the rectum, dissection becomes progressively easier.

Action (Fig. 12.6)

1. Mobilize the left side of the colon from the peritoneum by dividing the congenital adhesions from the sigmoid colon to the splenic flexure.

2. Fully mobilize the splenic flexure and the left half of the transverse colon, preserving the omentum unless there are metastases present in it. Avoid damage to the spleen.

3. Mobilize the left colon, pull it to the right on its mesentery and separate and preserve the left ureter and gonadal vessels. Take care not to damage the duodenojejunal flexure or the tail of the pancreas.

4. To enter the 'mesorectal plane' lift the sigmoid loop vertically. Observe the arc of the inferior mesenteric artery as it leaves the aorta and enters the mesorectum. Divide the peritoneum on the right side just beneath the arc of the artery, follow it back up to its origin and down into the loose areolar tissue that denotes the beginning of the mesorectal plane. Push away the tissue deep to this arcing peritoneal incision, which contains the pelvic nerve plexus. Both branches of this plexus should be apparent as they divide around the rectum at the level of the sacral promontory.

Make a similar incision in the peritoneum of the left side to produce a window with artery above and nerves below from the origin of the inferior artery to the start of the mesorectal plane. Clamp, divide and ligate the inferior mesenteric artery at its origin from the aorta, but if

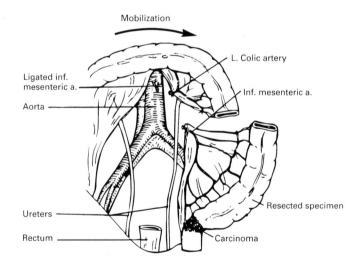

Fig. 12.6 Anterior resection of the rectum: the resected specimen is on the right and consists of the upper rectum, the sigmoid and part of the descending colon, together with the sigmoid mesocolon. The inferior mesenteric artery has been ligated and divided on the aorta and the inferior mesenteric vein at the lower border of the pancreas. The splenic flexure has been mobilized. Both ureters have been identified and preserved.

the patient is old and arteriosclerotic, preserve the left colic artery. Divide the inferior mesenteric vein at a slightly higher level, close to the lower border of the pancreas. Select a suitable area to transect the descending colon and divide the mesentery up to this point. Bowel transection at this stage facilitates the rectal dissection because the specimen can be pulled anteriorly while leaving the descending colon and small bowel packed up and out of the way in the upper abdomen.

5. The extent of rectal mobilization depends upon the level of the tumour. If it is retroperitoneal, you must completely mobilize the rectum and its mesorectum.

6. Move to the left of the patient. Pull the rectum forwards and dissect anteriorly to the sacral promontory and presacral fascia, as far down as the tip of the coccyx and the pelvic floor muscles. This is best done by holding a St Mark's lipped retractor in your left hand to pull the rectum forwards while carrying out sharp dissection with scissors or diathermy. Take care to visualize and preserve the presacral nerves.

7. As the posterior dissection deepens, divide the peritoneum over each side of the pelvis, close to the lateral wall. Eventually join the incisions anteriorly in the midline. The ideal site for this anterior division is about 1 cm above the most dependent part of the peritoneum. This usually corresponds to the bulge in the peritoneum overlying the seminal vesicles.

8. Hold the seminal vesicles forwards with a St Mark's lipped retractor and dissect between the vesicles and the rectum to uncover Denonvilliers's fascia. Incise this transversely and dissect down between the fascia and the rectum as far distally as necessary, and down behind the prostate to the pelvic floor. In a female dissect distally between the rectum and vagina as far down as necessary, even to the pelvic floor.

9. By traction on the rectum to one side and then the other side of the pelvis, identify the tissue described as the 'lateral ligaments'. This can be cauterized and divided without the need for formal clipping and dividing. Avoid tenting up and damaging the third sacral nerve root at this point.

10. Straighten out the rectum and draw the tumour upwards. Choose a suitable site for division of the rectum. If possible allow a 5 cm clearance below the lower edge of the carcinoma. If the tumour is low down, this degree of clearance may be impossible to achieve in a restorative procedure. Be willing to compromise but without jeopardizing a curative procedure. Obtain at least a 2 cm clearance. For lesions of the upper rectum, the mesorectum is present at the site selected for division of the rectum. Divide this perpendicularly to the rectal wall, taking care not to 'cone down' on to the rectum, getting so close that you risk leaving mesorectum containing tumour deposits. Apply a transverse stapler or right-angled clamp to the rectum at the site selected for division. Remember, if you intend using a stapled anastomosis, that the stapler removes an extra 8 mm of rectum.

11. Irrigate the rectum through the anus with povidone-iodine solution or 1:2000 aqueous chlorhexidine solution. If only a small cuff of sphincter and rectum remains, simply swab it out.

12. If you have not already divided it, select the site for division of the descending colon, place a Parker–Kerr clamp at right angles across the bowel and transect above it, holding the upper end of the colon with Babcock forceps so that it can be swabbed out.

13. Divide the rectum below the stapler or clamp with a long-handled knife. Remove the specimen containing the rectal carcinoma,

the complete mesentery and nodes up to the origin of the inferior mesenteric artery.

Unite

The anastomosis can be carried out in one of two ways, depending upon the level of anastomosis, the ease of access to the pelvis and the obesity of the patient.

Sutured anastomosis (Fig. 12.7)
Suture the bowel in one layer to produce an end-to-end inverted anastomosis. Insert vertical mattress sutures into the posterior layer and hold each suture with artery forceps until they have all been inserted. Now 'rail-road' the descending colon down to the rectum. The sutures are all held taut while the descending colon is pushed down until its posterior edge is in contact with the rectum, sometimes also called the 'parachute' technique. Tie the sutures with the knots within the lumen. Hold the two most lateral sutures and cut the others. Suture the anterior layer using interrupted seromuscular inverting stitches, inserting them all before they are tied. Place a haemostatic clip on each side of the anastomosis to mark it radiologically.

Stapled anastomosis (Fig. 12.8)
1. If the anastomosis is too low to suture conventionally, or if you prefer the technique, unite the bowel with the EEA circular stapling device. Carry out the operation exactly as described until the ends of the bowel have been prepared for anastomosis. Now insert the sizing heads into the colon to see if the stapling gun should be 25, 28 or 31 mm in diameter. For the colon it is best to select a 28 or 31 mm gun. Remember that the stapler removes an extra 8 mm of rectum and this can be taken into account when estimating the distal clearance below the tumour.

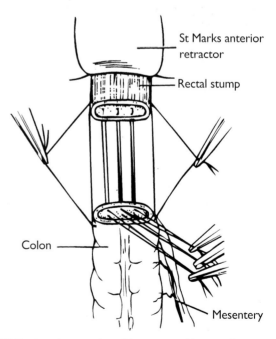

Fig. 12.7 Anterior resection of the rectum with sutured anastomosis. One-layer anastomosis, showing the insertion of sutures in preparation for the descending colon to be 'railroaded' down to the rectum.

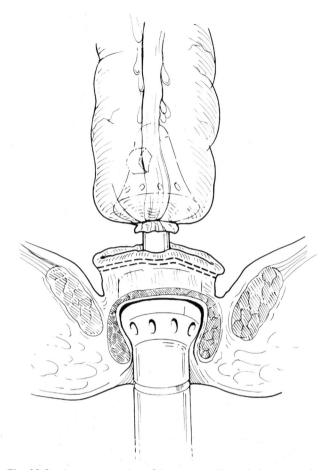

Fig. 12.8 Anterior resection of the rectum with stapled anastomosis, showing insertion of the circular stapling device through the anus with stapled rectal stump with the descending colon tied over the anvil.

2. Introduce the EEA gun through the anus and open it. Allow the spike of the gun to pass through the posterior aspect of the stapled rectal stump in the middle and just behind the staple line. Insert a purse-string suture into the end of the descending colon. Manipulate the end of the descending colon over the top of the anvil and tie the purse-string suture as tightly as possible. Connect the anvil and secured descending colon into the cartridge.

3. Have the assistant operating the gun approximate the anvil to the cartridge while you make sure that the gun is pushed firmly upwards and that the descending colon is pulled up tightly over the anvil. Ensure that no appendices epiploica and no part of the vagina are trapped between the ends of the bowel to be stapled. Rotate the descending colon 90° to the left so that the mesentery lies to the right side. Fire the staple gun to construct the anastomosis. Open the gun to separate the anvil from the cartridge, twist it to make sure the anastomosis is lying free, and then gently rock it and pull it free from the anus.

4. Check the integrity of the stapled anastomosis.

a. Examine the 'doughnuts' of colon and rectum removed from the gun. They should be complete. Identify the distal doughnut and send it for histological examination.

b. Feel the anastomosis digitally with a finger through the anus.

c. Pass a 1 cm sigmoidoscope to examine the anastomosis.

d. Place fluid in the pelvis and gently blow air into the colon through the sigmoidoscope. If no bubbles appear and the doughnuts are complete, the anastomosis is satisfactory.

Checklist

1. Make certain that there is no bleeding, particularly in the region of the splenic flexure and spleen.

2. Check that the anastomosis is under no tension and that the descending colon lies in the sacral hollow.

3. Ensure that the descending colon is viable.

4. Following a low anastomosis do not close the mesentery.

5. Drain the pelvis, preferably using a sump suction drain inserted through a stab wound in the left iliac fossa.

6. Replace and arrange the small bowel and cover it with omentum before closing the abdomen.

HARTMANN'S OPERATION

Appraise

After carrying out an anterior resection of the rectum or rectosigmoid it may be inadvisable to proceed with an anastomosis if:

1. the procedure is palliative and the anastomosis would demand the addition of a defunctioning colostomy
2. there is residual carcinoma in the lateral pelvic wall or internal iliac nodes.

Action

1. Close the distal rectum. If the rectum is cut off low down and the end is difficult to suture, leave it open and insert a drain through the anus into the pelvis.

2. Close the peritoneum over the rectal stump if possible. Bring out an end colostomy.

TRANSVERSE COLOSTOMY

Appraise

1. Carry out a transverse colostomy in the rare cases of distal obstruction in patients unfit to have an urgent resection carried out, or if you are too inexperienced to do this. It may be necessary as a preliminary operation in patients with severe distal sepsis with abscesses and fistula formation, for example in Crohn's disease or diverticular disease, or in vesicocolic fistula and severe urinary tract infection.

2. Site the stoma in the right upper quadrant of the abdomen, midway between the umbilicus and the costal margin.

3. Place the colostomy well to the right in the transverse colon since the next stage of the operation may require you to take down the splenic flexure and mobilize the distal transverse colon.

Access

1. Make a transverse incision 5–10 cm long centred on the upper right rectus muscle between the umbilicus and the costal margin so that an appliance can be fitted without encroaching upon either. Divide the

anterior and posterior rectus sheath, and the rectus muscle, transversely in the line of the incision. Through this locate the colon, explore the abdomen and feel the liver.

2. The abdomen may be already open when you make a decision to perform a colostomy. When a midline or left paramedian incision has been used, make a transverse incision as described above but only 6–7 cm long. If a right upper paramedian incision was used, bring the colostomy through the upper end of the incision, provided it is clear of the costal margin.

Assess

1. If the operation is undertaken to relieve a distal obstruction, examine the relevant structures and feel the obstructing mass in the distal colon. It may be impossible to determine if this is due to carcinoma or diverticular disease.

2. Palpate the liver for metastases.

3. Palpate the rest of the colon and the peritoneal cavity to determine if there are other metastases.

Action (Fig. 12.9a)

1. Draw the right side of the transverse colon and omentum out of the wound. Manipulate it so that a loop of proximal transverse colon lies in the wound without tension.

2. Separate the omentum from the colon and turn it upwards to expose the mesentery.

3. Pull the loop upwards through the incision and make a hole through the mesentery close to the bowel wall at the apex of the loop with a pair of long artery forceps, taking care not to damage the blood supply.

4. Pass a piece of narrow rubber tubing or a catheter under the mesentery. Pull the loop right out through the incision with the rubber tubing, making certain that the loop is not twisted and that the proximal opening is to the right and the distal opening to the left.

5. Pass a plastic colostomy device through the mesentery to form a bridge for the colostomy. Open the end of the colostomy device to keep it in place.

6. Do not insert any internal sutures.

7. If the colostomy is made to relieve obstruction, open it immediately by cutting across the apex of the bowel through half the circumference. Clean the contents away with mounted swabs wetted with 1:500 mercuric perchloride or povidone-iodine solution.

8. Turn back the edges of the opened colon and suture the whole thickness of the colon to the edge of the skin incision with interrupted 2/0 catgut sutures mounted on a cutting needle.

9. Insert a finger into each loop of the colostomy to make sure it is not too narrow and that the finger passes straight into the underlying colon.

10. Fix a suitable disposable appliance over the loop colostomy rod.

Aftercare

1. A transverse colostomy is a temporary defunctioning stoma made with a view to closure. Closure should be as easy as possible and not require excision of the colon and re-anastomosis.

2. Remove the colostomy device forming the bridge in about 7 days, depending on the obesity of the patient and the difficulty in bringing up the loop of colon.

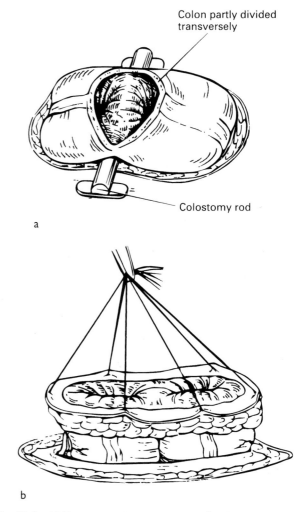

Colon partly divided transversely

Colostomy rod

a

b

Fig. 12.9 (a) Transverse colostomy: bring a loop of colon through the wound and keep it in place with a colostomy device or simple glass rod. Open the colostomy by a transverse incision. (b) Closure of colostomy: insert stay sutures to help mobilization.

Closure

Appraise

1. Do not close the colostomy until at least 1 month after it has been formed. This allows the oedema to settle down and makes the operation safer and easier.

2. Before closure ensure that the distal anastomosis is satisfactory following the definitive operation, as shown on sigmoidoscopy and/or Gastrografin enema X-ray. Prepare the proximal bowel as for colonic resection and anastomosis.

Action (Fig. 12.9b)

1. Make an incision in the skin close to the mucocutaneous junction.

2. Insert six 2/0 silk stay sutures into the mucocutaneous junction, each held in an artery forceps so that traction may be applied while dissecting.

3. Deepen the incision to reveal the colon and the external rectus sheath. Dissect the colonic loops from the abdominal wall until the whole of the loop is freed and can easily be drawn out from the abdominal cavity.

4. Excise the mucocutaneous junction and clean the edges of the colon with 1:2000 aqueous chlorhexidine solution and/or povidone-iodine solution prior to reanastomosis.

5. Close the colostomy transversely using one layer of 4/0 interrupted vertical mattress sutures of polypropylene or polyglactin 910 in one or two layers.

6. Replace the resutured colostomy in the peritoneal cavity, place the omentum over it and manipulate it so that it lies away from the abdominal incision.

7. Close the abdominal wound in one layer with a continuous or interrupted nylon suture. If the patient is obese, drain the subcutaneous space with a slip of corrugated latex sheet brought out through the end of the wound, or through a separate stab wound. Close the skin.

COLECTOMY FOR INFLAMMATORY BOWEL DISEASE

Appraise

1. Acute fulminating colitis, with or without toxic megacolon, usually occurs in idiopathic ulcerative colitis but may occur in Crohn's colitis.

2. The operation of choice is colectomy and ileostomy (Fig. 12.10). Emergency proctocolectomy carries a higher mortality and morbidity, and there is no opportunity to carry out a secondary ileorectal anastomosis.

3. Treat acute colitis medically with steroids. Correct anaemia with blood transfusion. Replace fluid and electrolyte loss.

4. Surgical treatment is usually indicated if:

a. the patient's condition does not improve within 72 hours
b. the patient does not improve in 24 hours and still has more than six bowel actions containing blood each day
c. there is a fever of more than 38°C and a tachycardia over 100.

5. Carry out daily plain X-ray of the abdomen to see if toxic dilatation develops.

6. If there is toxic dilatation or evidence of perforation carry out emergency surgery.

7. Beware of being lulled into a false sense of security, as the patient's condition is more critical than may be apparent.

FURTHER READING

Goligher JC 1984 Surgery of the anus, rectum and colon, 5th edn. Baillière Tindall, London

Keighley MRB, Williams NS 1999 Surgery of the anus, rectum and colon. 2nd edn. WB Saunders, London

Phillips RKS 1998 Colorectal surgery: a companion to specialist surgical practice. WB Saunders, London

Nicholls RJ, Dozois RR 1997 Surgery of the colon and rectum. Churchill Livingstone, Edinburgh

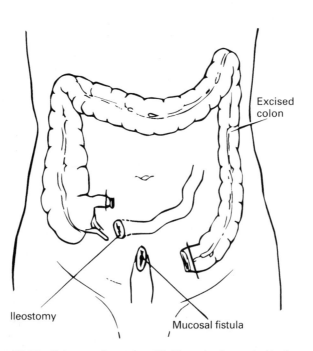

Fig. 12.10 Colectomy for acute colitis. The colon is resected to the mid-sigmoid colon, which is brought out as a mucous fistula through the lower part of the midline incision. An end ileostomy is constructed in the right iliac fossa.

Excised colon

Ileostomy

Mucosal fistula

Anorectum

R. Phillips, A. Windsor and J. Thomson

Contents

Introduction
Anatomy
Haemorrhoids
Clotted venous saccule evacuation (perianal haematoma)
Fissure
Anal abscess and fistula
Fistula
Pilonidal disease
Rectal prolapse

INTRODUCTION

Operations on the anal canal and perianal area are relatively simple but there is a need for finesse, meticulous attention to detail and carefully supervised postoperative care.

a. Make sure you have a sound understanding of the anatomy of the area, and precision in diagnosis is essential for effective treatment.

b. Always perform a full rectal examination, including inspection, palpation, sigmoidoscopy and proctoscopy, before carrying out any procedure.

c. Exclude serious diseases, such as neoplastic or inflammatory bowel disease, in appropriate cases with barium enema X-ray and colonoscopy.

ANATOMY

The anal canal extends from the anorectal junction superiorly to the anus below and is approximately 3–4 cm long. The lining epithelium is characterized by the anal valves midway along the anal canal. This line of the anal valves is often loosely referred to as the 'dentate line' (Fig. 13.1).

It does not represent the point of fusion between the embryonic hindgut and the proctoderm, which occurs at a higher level, between the anal valves and the anorectal junction. In this zone, sometimes called the transitional zone, there is a mixture of columnar and squamous epithelium.

Sphincters

The anal canal is surrounded by two sphincter muscles. The internal sphincter is the expanded distal portion of the circular muscle of the large intestine. It is composed of smooth muscle and is white in colour.

The external sphincter lies outside the internal sphincter. It is composed of striated muscle and is brown in colour.

Spaces

There are three important spaces around the anal canal – the intersphincteric space, the ischiorectal fossa and the supralevator space (Fig. 13.1). These spaces are important in the spread of sepsis and in certain operations.

1. *The intersphincteric space* lies between the two sphincters and contains the terminal fibres of the longitudinal muscle of the large intestine. It also contains the anal intermuscular glands, approximately 12 in number, arranged around the anal canal. The ducts of these glands pass through the internal sphincter and open into the anal crypts.

2. *The ischiorectal fossa* lies lateral to the external sphincter and contains fat. Abscesses may occur in this site as the result of horizontal spread of infection across the external sphincter.

3. *The supralevator space* lies between the levator ani and the rectum. It is important in the spread of infection.

Prepare

1. Familiarize yourself with the small range of essential instruments for examination of the patient, such as the proctoscope and the rigid sigmoidoscope. In patients with anal sphincter spasm, use a small paediatric sigmoidoscope.

2. Operating proctoscopes of the Eisenhammer, Parks and Sims type are essential for operations on and within the anal canal.

3. Use a pair of fine scissors, fine forceps (toothed and non-toothed), a light needle-holder, Emett's forceps and a small no. 15 scalpel blade for intra-anal work. Alternatively, for those familiar with diathermy dissection this creates a virtually bloodless field.

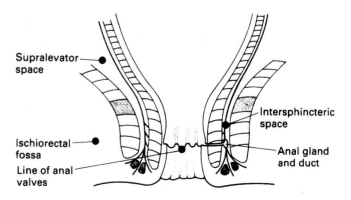

Fig. 13.1 A diagram to show the essential anatomy of the anal canal.

Supralevator space

Ischiorectal fossa

Line of anal valves

Intersphincteric space

Anal gland and duct

4. For fistula surgery have a set of Lockhart–Mummery fistula probes, together with a set of Anel's lacrimal probes.

5. Most patients require no preparation, or two glycerine suppositories to ensure an empty rectum before anal surgery. If for any reason the bowels need to be confined postoperatively, then carry out a full bowel preparation to empty the whole large intestine.

6. Take a blood sample from all patients for routine testing.

7. Minor operations can be performed under local infiltration anaesthesia; larger procedures demand regional or general anaesthesia.

8. For outpatient procedures use the left lateral position, or alternatively the knee–elbow position. For anal operations most UK surgeons favour the lithotomy position, although the prone jack-knife position (Fig. 13.2) has its advocates.

9. We favour shaving the whole area before starting any anal operation; this is best done in the operating theatre where there is good illumination.

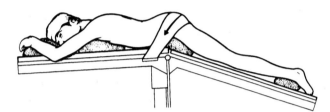

Fig. 13.2   The jack-knife position.

HAEMORRHOIDS

Appraise

1. Exclude pelvic tumours, large bowel carcinoma and inflammatory bowel disease.

2. Haemorrhoids do not always need treatment if the symptoms are minimal.

3. Small internal haemorrhoids can be treated by injection sclerotherapy, prolapsing haemorrhoids by rubber-band ligation and large prolapsing haemorrhoids, which are usually accompanied by a significant external component, by haemorrhoidectomy. Contrary to the views of many, with the advent of day-case diathermy haemorrhoidectomy and its high patient satisfaction and haemorrhoidal care, our threshold for advising surgery has fallen dramatically.

4. Haemorrhoidal treatment is usually contraindicated if the patient also has Crohn's disease.

Injection sclerotherapy

Although injection sclerotherapy is an outpatient procedure and does not require any anaesthesia, we shall describe it for completeness. It is most conveniently done after full rectal examination if no further investigation is required. The patient is usually in the left lateral position.

Action

1. Pass the full-length proctoscope and withdraw slowly to identify the anorectal junction – the area where the anal canal begins to close around the instrument.

2. Place a ball of cotton wool into the lower rectum with Emett's forceps to keep the walls apart (as it is not usually removed, the patients should be told they will pass the cotton wool with the next motion).

3. Identify the position of the right anterior, left lateral and right posterior haemorrhoids.

4. Fill a 10 ml (Gabriel pattern) syringe with 5% phenol in arachis oil with 0.5% menthol (oily phenol BP).

5. Through the full-length proctoscope, insert the needle into the submucosa at the anorectal junction at the identified positions of the haemorrhoids in turn. Inject 3–5 ml of 5% phenol in arachis oil into the submucosa at each site, to produce a swelling with a pearly appearance of the mucosa in which the vessels are clearly seen. Move the needle slightly during injection to avoid giving an intravascular injection.

6. After injecting, delay removal of the needle for a few seconds to lessen the escape of the solution. If necessary, press on the injection site with cotton wool to minimize leakage.

7. Warn the patient to avoid attempts at defecation for 24 hours.

Key points

- Avoid injecting the solution too superficially. This produces a watery bleb, which may ulcerate and subsequently cause haemorrhage.

- Avoid injecting the solution too deep. This produces an oleogranuloma with subsequent features of an extrarectal swelling. Too-deep anterior injection in male patients causes perineal pain and even haematuria from prostatitis. This is a serious problem. Halt the injection immediately. If there is any suggestion that the urinary tract had been entered, administer antibiotics. Do not hesitate to admit the patient, since septicaemia is common and may be severe.

Rubber-band ligation

Rubber-band ligation is also an outpatient procedure and does not need anaesthesia. There are several different designs of band applicator and the simplest is illustrated in Figure 13.3.

The suction bander, although relatively expensive, is convenient and easy to use. Have a pair of grasping forceps such as Patterson's biopsy forceps. There are two conceptually different strategies: one is to band (or inject) above the haemorrhoid in order to 'hitch' it back into its normal place; the other is to try to destroy the haemorrhoid itself. Whereas the latter is actually described here, the former can just as easily be achieved simply by grasping redundant mucosa proximal to the haemorrhoid and banding that instead.

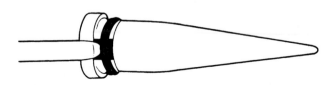

Fig. 13.3   A simple instrument with which to perform elastic-band ligation of haemorrhoids.

Action
1. Load two elastic bands on to the band applicator.
2. Pass the full-length proctoscope and withdraw it slowly to identify the anorectal junction. Position the end of the proctoscope midway between the anorectal junction and the dentate line.
3. Pass the tips of the grasping forceps through the ring of the band applicator, through the proctoscope and take hold of the selected haemorrhoid (or above it if employing the 'hitch-up' approach).
4. Pull the haemorrhoid through the ring of the band applicator while pushing the band applicator upwards. Establish whether or not the patient experiences any additional discomfort. If s/he does not, 'fire' the band on to the haemorrhoid. If s/he does, reposition the grip on the haemorrhoid slightly higher and retest before applying the band.
5. Any number of haemorrhoids can be banded on each occasion. Repeat banding may be necessary and should be delayed for 6–8 weeks.

Aftercare
1. Warn the patient to avoid attempts at defecation for 24 hours.
2. Warn the patient that there may be discomfort and that mild analgesics may be needed.

? Difficulty?

If the patient experiences severe pain the band may have been applied too low on to sensitive epithelium. If analgesics do not control the pain, remove the bands in the operating theatre under general anaesthesia, using an operating proctoscope.

3. Pain developing slowly in 1–2 days may be from ischaemia. Analgesics relieve the pain. Give metronidazole tablets 200 mg thrice daily, which may help reduce inflammation.
4. Warn the patient that the haemorrhoid and the band should drop off after 5–10 days. There may be a small amount of bleeding at this time.
5. Warn the patient of the risk of secondary haemorrhage – approximately 2%–and that it may occur any time up to 3 weeks after application. Report to hospital if this is severe since it may require transfusion and operative control of the bleeding.

Haemorrhoidectomy

Appraise
1. There are different methods of performing a haemorrhoidectomy, but we shall describe the diathermy technique, which has evolved out of the ligation and excision technique of Milligan and Morgan.
2. Haemorrhoidectomy should be a curative procedure and must be done very carefully and thoroughly.

Prepare
1. Start lactulose 30 ml twice daily 2 days preoperatively, which results in less postoperative pain.
2. Give oral metronidazole 400 mg tds for 5 days, which significantly reduces postoperative pain.

3. The anaesthetized patient is in the lithotomy position with some head-down tilt. Avoid caudal anaesthetic as it may provoke retention of urine.

Assess
1. Plan the operation by inserting the Eisenhammer retractor and establishing which haemorrhoids need removal and what is the state and size of the skin bridges.
2. Determine whether:

a. a three-quadrant haemorrhoidectomy will be sufficient
b. there is one additional haemorrhoid that needs removal, or
c. the situation is more complex than this.

3. In the circumstances of one additional haemorrhoid, the choices are:

a. Leave it. Return on another occasion if it proves troublesome.
b. Fillet it out by undermining the skin bridge.
c. Divide the skin bridge above the dentate line, reflect it out of the anus, trim the haemorrhoid with the back of a pair of scissors, excise redundant mucosa and stitch the trimmed flap back into position with 2/0 synthetic absorbable sutures (polyglactin 910).

4. In the circumstances of more extensive haemorrhoids than this, including circumferential:

a. Consider simple three-quadrant haemorrhoidectomy and returning on another occasion to tidy up any residual haemorrhoids.
b. If you are experienced in the technique, consider circumferential Whitehead haemorrhoidectomy with mucosal/cutaneous reanastomosis with polyglactin 910. But beware of the difficulty, avoiding Whitehead deformity (mucosal ectropion) and later stenosis.

Action
1. Inject bupivacaine 0.25% with adrenaline 1:200 000 into each skin bridge and into the external component of each haemorrhoid to be excised.
2. Wait, and gently massage away excess fluid from the injection with a moistened gauze.
3. Commence with the left lateral haemorrhoid. Place the Eisenhammer retractor in the anal canal and open it enough to put the internal sphincter under tension. This demonstrates the plane of the dissection.
4. Group the external component and excise it with electrocautery, using cutting diathermy on skin and coagulating diathermy for all other dissection.
5. Now extend the haemorrhoidal dissection up the anal canal, separating the haemorrhoid from the underlying internal sphincter.
6. Narrow the pedicle as you dissect up towards the apex, otherwise you risk encroaching on the skin bridge.
7. When you have encompassed the internal component of the haemorrhoid, simply transect the pedicle with diathermy.

8. Repeat the procedure on the right anterior haemorrhoid and then the right posterior haemorrhoid.

9. Ensure complete haemostasis and check each wound and apex.

🔑 Key point

● Remember that bleeding comes from what remains inside the patient, not from what has been removed.

---

10. Inspect the skin bridges and perform any further procedure as necessary and as earlier decided (see 'Assess') (Fig. 13.4).

11. Do not apply any anal canal dressing.

12. Insert a diclofenac suppository into the anus.

Aftercare

1. Allow the patient home after recovery from the anaesthetic.

2. Advise the patient that it is normal for there to be an early increase in pain from days 3–5 postoperatively.

3. Manage the bowels with lactulose 30 ml orally twice daily until comfortable.

4. Pain can usually be satisfactorily controlled with non-steroidal anti-inflammatory drugs.

5. 0.2% glyceryl trinitrate applied locally three times daily may help by creating a reversible chemical sphincterotomy.

6. Review in the outpatient clinic within 10–12 days.

Other procedures

1. *Closed haemorrhoidectomy*. The principle is much more limited removal of anoderm with immediate suturing. Randomized trials have failed to show advantage for this operation.

2. *Stapled haemorrhoidectomy*. Linear staples impinging on skin or the rectum are painful. Circular stapling above the dentate line has been advocated by Longo but has yet to be evaluated adequately by others.

CLOTTED VENOUS SACCULE EVACUATION (PERIANAL HAEMATOMA)

If the patient is seen within 24 hours of onset and the pain is very severe, evacuate the clot.

Action

1. Place the patient in the left lateral position and inject 5–10 ml 1% lignocaine hydrochloride with 1:200 000 adrenaline into and around the base of the swelling.

2. With scissors excise the top of the lesion and express the clot.

3. Close the wound with 000 chromic catgut and apply a pressure pad. Alternatively, pack it with haemostatic gauze. Otherwise postoperative haemorrhage may be severe, since a venous space is exposed.

FISSURE

Appraise

1. Most ulcers at the anal margin are simple fissures-in-ano, possibly associated with a sentinel skin tag and/or hypertrophied anal papilla or anal polyp.

2. Exclude excoriation in association with pruritus ani, Crohn's disease, primary chancre of syphilis, herpes simplex, leukaemia and tumours.

3. Treat superficial fissures with 0.2% glyceryl trinitrate (GTN) cream three times a day. When diltiazem 1% becomes available this may be preferable, as it avoids headache.

4. Reserve operative treatment failures, which are more common when there is a sentinel tag, an anal polyp, exposure of the internal sphincter or undermining of the edges (Fig. 13.5).

5. Anal dilatation, stretching the internal and external sphincters and lower rectum, increases the risk of incontinence and we do not use it.

6. The standard procedure is a lateral (partial internal) sphincterotomy.

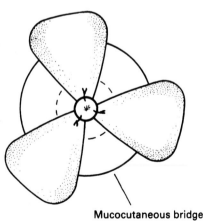

Fig. 13.4 Haemorrhoidectomy: it is essential to preserve three mucocutaneous bridges.

Mucocutaneous bridge

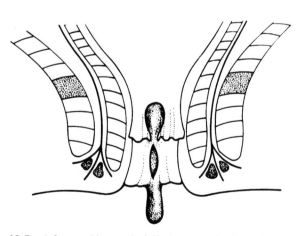

Fig. 13.5 A fissure with a sentinel skin tag, an anal polyp and undermining of the edges of the ulcer.

Lateral sphincterotomy

Appraise

1. This is very successful, curing more than 95% of patients.
2. To avoid exacerbating the pain, avoid preoperative preparation.
3. The operation can be carried out as a 'day-case' procedure.
4. Advise the patient of a 1 in 20 chance of permanent flatus incontinence.

Action

1. Have the patient in the lithotomy position, under general or regional anaesthesia.
2. Pass an Eisenhammer bivalve operating proctoscope. Examine the fissure to make certain there is no induration suggesting an underlying intersphincteric abscess. If there is, proceed to dorsal sphincterotomy.
3. Remove hypertrophied anal papillae or fibrous anal polyp and send for histopathological examination. Remove a sentinel skin tag.
4. Rotate the operating proctoscope to demonstrate the left lateral aspect of the anal canal. Palpate the lower border of the internal sphincter muscle. Insert a Parks instead of an Eisenhammer retractor, since it permits outward traction, making the internal sphincter more obvious.
5. Make a small incision 1 cm long in line with the lower border of the internal sphincter. Insert scissors into the submucosa, gently separating the epithelial lining of the anal canal from the internal sphincter, and into the intersphincteric space to separate the internal and external sphincters.
6. If you make a hole in the mucosa open it completely to avoid the risk of sepsis.
7. Clamp the isolated area of internal sphincter with artery forceps for 30 seconds. This will markedly reduce haemorrhage.
8. With one blade of the scissors on each side of it, divide the internal sphincter muscle up to the level of the top of the fissure (Fig. 13.6). Do not extend the division of the internal sphincter above the upper limit of the fissure and never above the line of the anal valves.
9. Press on the area for 2–3 minutes. The wound does not usually need to be closed.

10. Do not apply a dressing since it contributes to postoperative pain, unless there is bleeding that will be controlled by pressure from the dressing.
11. Apply a perineal pad and pants.

Aftercare

1. Prescribe a bulk laxative such as sterculia 10 ml once or twice a day.
2. Bruising under the perianal skin signifies a haematoma, but it requires no treatment.

ANAL ABSCESS AND FISTULA

Appraise

1. Most abscesses and fistulas in the anal region arise from a primary infection in the anal intersphincteric glands. Furthermore, they represent different phases of the same disease process. An acute phase abscess develops, when free drainage of pus is prevented by closure of either the internal or external opening of the fistula, or both, which is the chronic phase.
2. Other causes of sepsis in the perianal region include pilonidal infection, hidradenitis suppurativa, Crohn's disease, tuberculosis and intrapelvic sepsis draining downwards across the levator ani.
3. Once established, an intersphincteric abscess may spread vertically downwards to form a perianal abscess or upwards to form either an intermuscular abscess or supralevator abscess, depending upon which side of the longitudinal muscle spread occurs (Fig. 13.7). Horizontal spread medially across the internal sphincter may result in drainage into the anal canal, but spread laterally across the external sphincter may produce an ischiorectal abscess (Fig. 13.8). Finally, circumferential spread of infection may occur from one intersphincteric space to the other, from one ischiorectal fossa to the other and from one supralevator space to the other.
4. Once an abscess has formed surgical drainage must be instituted – antibiotics have no part to play in the primary management. As the tissues are inflamed and oedematous, it is best to do the minimum to ensure resolution of the infection. More tissue can be divided later to resolve the problem totally. Send a specimen of pus to the laboratory

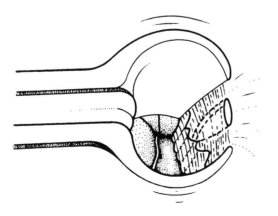

Fig. 13.6 Lateral partial internal sphincterotomy.

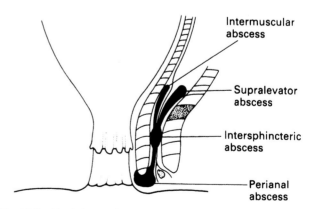

Fig. 13.7 Vertical spread upwards and downwards from a primary intersphincteric abscess.

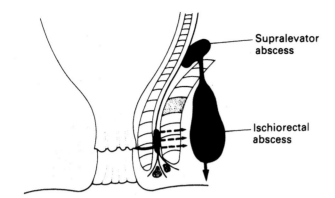

Fig. 13.8 Horizontal spread from infection medially across the internal sphincter into the anal canal, upwards into the supralevator space.

for culture. (The presence of intestinal organisms suggest that a fistula is present.)

5. Avoid preoperative preparation of the bowel as it causes unnecessary pain.

6. Have the anaesthetized patient in the lithotomy position and shave the patient on the table.

Perianal abscess

1. Recognize the abscess as a swelling at the anal margin.

2. Make a radial incision and excise overhanging edges. Allow pus to drain and send a sample to the laboratory.

3. Gently examine the wound to see if there is a fistula.

4. Insert a gauze dressing soaked in normal saline solution and surrounded by haemostatic gauze. Do not pack the wound tightly.

Ischiorectal abscess

1. Recognize this as a brawny inflamed swelling in the ischiorectal fossa.

2. As an ischiorectal abscess often spreads circumferentially from one side to the other, carefully examine the patient under anaesthesia to determine if this has occurred. Recognize the abscess by feeling the induration inferior to the levator ani muscle.

3. For the same reason, employ a circumanal incision to establish drainage. Excise the skin edges to create an adequate opening and send a specimen of pus to the laboratory.

> **Key point**
>
> - Be very careful when exploring the cavity with your finger. You may spread infection, damage the levator ani or injure the rectum itself. Never use a probe.

4. Gently insert a gauze dressing soaked in normal saline surrounded by haemostatic gauze to the upper limit of the wound. Do not pack the wound tightly.

Postoperative

1. Remove the dressing on the second postoperative day while the patient lies in the bath after having an intramuscular injection of pethidine 100 mg or papaveretum 20 mg.

2. Initiate a routine of twice-daily baths, irrigation of the wound and the insertion of a tuck-in gauze dressing soaked in physiological saline or 1:40 sodium hypochlorite solution.

3. If the patient has evidence of persistent local or systemic sepsis, administer systemic antibiotics guided by the culture report. Metronidazole is valuable against anaerobic organisms.

4. Assess the patient for the possible presence of a fistula detected at the time of abscess drainage, or a history of recurrent abscesses, or palpable induration of the perianal area, anal canal and lower rectum, or the presence of gut organism in the pus. If so, plan to re-examine the patient under anaesthesia and carry out the appropriate treatment.

FISTULA

Appraise

1. A fistula is an abnormal communication between two epithelial-lined surfaces. Therefore, in the context of fistula in-ano, there should be an external opening on the perianal skin, an internal opening into the anal canal and a track between the two.

2. There may be no external opening, or it may be healed over. Likewise there may be no internal opening as the sepsis arises in the area of the intersphincteric gland, which is the primary site of infection. It may not drain across the internal sphincter into the anal canal. Finally, the track may follow a very complicated path.

3. The presence of infection is characterized by the physical sign of induration, detected by palpation with a lubricated, covered finger.

> **? Difficulty?**
>
> Accurate definition of a complex fistula can be difficult. Do not be tempted to risk causing incontinence by dividing the external sphincter. Insert a loose seton and order a magnetic resonance imaging scan to clarify the situation; you can then plan effective and safe definitive treatment.

Superficial fistula

Assess

1. Have the anaesthetized patient in the lithotomy position. Perform sigmoidoscopy in all cases, especially looking for inflammatory bowel disease.

2. Palpate the perianal skin, anal canal and lower rectum thoroughly for induration. This will be confined to the distal anal canal and localized to one area, as superficial fistulas are really fissures covered with skin and lower anal canal epithelium (Fig. 13.9).

Action

1. Insert a bivalve operating proctoscope and pass a fine probe along the track.

2. Lay open the fistula using a no. 15 bladed knife or electrocautery.

3. Curette the granulation tissue and send a specimen for histopathology.

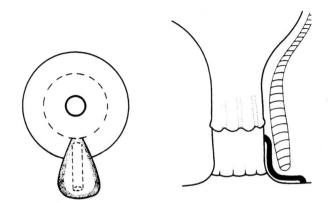

Fig. 13.9   A diagram to show a superficial fistula and the pear-shaped wound required to treat it.

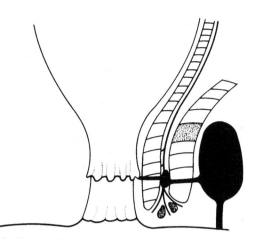

Fig. 13.10   Trans-sphincteric fistula.

4. If there is no induration deep to the internal sphincter, fashion the external skin wound so that it becomes pear-shaped and perform a lateral sphincterotomy (see above).

5. Insert a gauze dressing soaked in normal saline solution and surrounded by haemostatic gauze to the upper limit of the wound.

🔑 | **Key point**

- Never force a probe or you may create false passages.

Trans-sphincteric fistula

In a trans-sphincteric fistula, the primary track passes across the external sphincter from the intersphincteric space to the ischiorectal fossa. The infection may also have drained across the internal sphincter into the anal canal, where you will find the internal opening of the fistula, which is usually at the level of the anal valves (Fig. 13.10).

Assess

1. Have the anaesthetized patient in the lithotomy position with the buttocks well down over the end of the table. Perform sigmoidoscopy in all cases, especially looking for inflammatory bowel disease.

2. Palpate carefully for induration. The external opening(s) are usually laterally placed and indurated, but there is not usually any induration extending towards the anus subcutaneously in a trans-sphincteric fistula. Palpation may reveal induration within the wall of the anal canal, the site of the primary anal gland infection. Induration will also be detected under the levator ani muscles and is often circumferential. Palpate between a finger (in the lower rectum) and thumb (on the perianal skin) for a large area of induration. This is especially obvious if circumferential spread has not occurred and the contralateral side is normal.

Action

1. Pass a bivalve operating proctoscope in order to try and identify the internal opening.

2. Pass a Lockhart–Mummery probe into the external opening. It may extend several centimetres and be felt very close to a finger in the

---

🔑 | **Key points**

- Remember that there may be no internal opening – the infection has not crossed the internal sphincter.

- If there is an internal opening at the level of the anal valves, the level at which the primary track crosses the external sphincter may not be the same – it may be lower or higher (Fig. 13.11).

- Infection can spread vertically in the intersphincteric space and open into the rectum, in addition to spreading across the external sphincter.

- Circumferential spread of infection and other secondary tracks may also develop.

---

rectum. Do not force the probe, and do not pass it into the rectum, as this is never the site of the internal opening.

3. If there is spread of infection towards the midline posteriorly, direct the probe previously inserted into the external opening posteriorly towards the coccyx. With a scalpel (no. 10 blade) in the groove

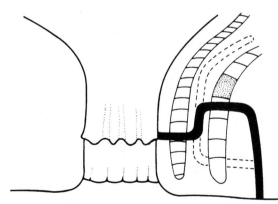

Fig. 13.11   The level at which the primary track crosses the external sphincter is not necessarily at the same level as the internal opening into the anal canal. It may be higher or lower; furthermore there may be an upward intersphincteric extension.

of the probe divide the tissue between the skin and the probe (skin and fat only – no muscle should be divided). Apply tissue-holding forceps to the skin edges and secure any major bleeding points. Alternatively, perform the laying open with electrocautery.

4. Curette away granulation tissue (send some for histopathological examination) and look for a forward extension from the site of the external opening. Lay it open.

5. Seek any extension of the sepsis to the opposite side by palpation, probing and looking for granulation tissue pouting from an opening in the previously curetted track. Use a no. 10 bladed knife or electrocautery to divide skin and fat to lay open any further tracks.

6. Insert the bivalve proctoscope again and re-identify the internal opening. It may or may not be possible to pass a probe either through the internal opening into the previously opened tracks or from the previously opened tracks into the anal canal.

7. Divide the anal canal epithelium and the internal sphincter to the level of the internal opening (if present) with a no. 15 bladed knife or electrocautery, thus opening up the intersphincteric space. If there is no internal opening, open the intersphincteric space in a similar way to the level of the anal valves. Curette any granulation tissue.

8. The primary track across the external sphincter should now be identifiable. If it is at or below the line of the anal valves, divide the muscle. If it is higher, as it often is, it may be possible to divide the muscle, but determining this requires considerable experience. It is often safer to drain the track by inserting a length of fine silicone tubing (1 mm diameter) or a braided suture material (1). Such a piece of material is called a seton. Monofilaments such as nylon are often uncomfortable for the patient because of the sharp knot ends.

9. Once all the septic areas have been drained, fashion the wound so that drainage can continue and the wound can heal from its depth. Skin and fat will almost certainly need to be trimmed.

10. Insert gauze dressings soaked in normal saline surrounded by haemostatic gauze into the wounds and the anal canal. Do not pack the dressings tightly.

11. Apply a perineal pad and pants.

Postoperative

1. Remove the dressing on the second or third postoperative day after giving an intramuscular injection of pethidine 100 mg or papaveretum 20 mg. Carry out the first dressing in the operating theatre under general anaesthesia if the wound is very extensive.

2. Initiate a routine of twice-daily baths, irrigation of the wound and insertion of gauze soaked in physiological saline.

3. Inspect the wound at regular intervals until healing is complete.

4. Encourage the bowel movements to coincide with these dressing times by giving laxatives. If they do not coincide, arrange bath–irrigation–dressing routines as necessary.

5. If voluminous pus discharges, review the wound in theatre under general anaesthesia after 10–14 days. In patients with large wounds, this may need to be repeated. Lay open any residual tracks and curette away the granulation tissue.

6. Administer antimicrobial agents such as erythromycin 250 mg 8-hourly and metronidazole 400 mg 8-hourly for up to 28 days, to assist in the elimination of the sepsis.

7. A seton does not complicate the postoperative routine. Allow the wound to heal around it; this may take 3 months. Then, under general anaesthesia, remove the seton and curette its track free of granulation tissue. Spontaneous healing occurs in approximately 40% of patients. If healing does not occur, lay open the residual track. The advantage of this staged division of the external sphincter is that healing occurs around the 'scaffolding' of the external sphincter. When it is subsequently divided, and this is not always necessary, its ends separate only slightly. This gives a better functional result than if it were divided at the outset.

Complications

1. Failure to heal may be from inadequate or inappropriate drainage of intersphincteric abscess of origin, or of secondary tracks, or of the primary track. Make sure that the nurses are given clear instructions and advice about the dressings. If not, there is danger that inadequate postoperative dressings will allow bridging of the wound edges and pocketing of pus. If there is excessive growth of granulation tissue, cauterize it with silver nitrate or curette it away under general anaesthetic.

🔑 Key points

Slow healing?

● Is the patient malnourished or suffering from zinc deficiency?

● Hairs growing into the wound? Shave the area.

● Have you missed a specific cause for the fistula, such as Crohn's disease?

---

2. Secondary haemorrhage may occur from any potentially septic open wound, healing by second intention.

3. Anal incontinence of varying degrees may follow division of the sphincter muscles. If all the sphincter complex has inadvertently been divided, consider repairing it once the sepsis has been eradicated and healing has occurred.

4. Successful fistula surgery depends upon accurate definition of the pathological anatomy, drainage of the intersphincteric abscess of origin, the primary and secondary tracks, and excellent postoperative wound care.

Other procedures

1. A tight seton is designed to cut through the fistula track slowly with hopefully less separation of muscle ends. Apply firmly but not tightly. Replace at monthly intervals.

2. Advancement flaps avoid sphincter division but, along with the intersphincteric approach and core-out fistulectomy, they are probably best left to specialist colorectal surgeons. Only about 50% are successful. Considered particularly in high trans-sphincteric fistulae, especially when situated anteriorly in women (whose anal canal is short).

PILONIDAL DISEASE

A simple pilonidal sinus detected as a chance finding during routine examination probably does not require treatment. Operate only if it is painful or infected, producing a pilonidal abscess.

Prepare

Place the anaesthetized patient in the left lateral position with the right buttock strapped to hold it up. Elastic adhesive strapping is adequate and adheres better if the skin has been sprayed with compound tincture of benzoin. Carefully shave the area.

Action

1. Determine the extent of sepsis by palpation for induration and by using probes.
   2. Completely excise the skin of the septic area.

RECTAL PROLAPSE

Appraise

1. The symptom of prolapse, i.e. tissue slipping through the anus, may result from causes other than complete rectal prolapse. Distinguish haemorrhoids, anal polyps, mucosal prolapse and rectal adenomas.
   2. Treatment consists of control of the prolapse, re-education of the bowel habit and improvement, if necessary, of sphincter function.
   3. First control the prolapse. While an internally intussuscepted rectum lies in the lower third of the rectum (the first phase of prolapse) sphincter function is inhibited, as it will be as a complete prolapse passes through the anal sphincter and keeps it open. Many operations have been described to achieve control. In the UK complete rectal prolapse is usually treated either by abdominal rectopexy or by perineal mucosal sleeve resection (Delorme's procedure).
   4. Abdominal rectopexy is associated with unpredictable post-operative constipation, which in some patients can be severe. There are claims that concomitant sigmoid resection (resection rectopexy, also known as the Frykman–Goldberg operation) reduces this risk.
   5. After rectopexy only a few patients have sphincter dysfunction severe enough to produce significant incontinence. Pelvic floor physiotherapy, faradism and electrical stimulators give little long-term benefit. The problem is anatomically the result of pelvic floor neurogenic myopathy producing a shortened anal canal with widening of the anorectal angle. Postanal pelvic floor repair reduces the anorectal angle and lengthens the anal canal, restoring satisfactory continence in some patients.
   6. All abdominal pelvic dissection in male patients has the potential to cause either erectile or ejaculatory dysfunction. Because of this it is now required that the aspect has been mentioned and recorded when obtaining informed consent.

FURTHER READING

Goldberg SM, Gordon PH, Nivatvongs S 1980 Essentials of anorectal surgery. J B Lippincott, Philadelphia, PA

Goligher JC 1984 Surgery of the anus, rectum and colon, 5th edn. Baillière Tindall, London

Keighley MRB, Williams NS 1999 Surgery of the anus, rectum and colon. 2nd edn WB Saunders, London

Nicholls RJ, Dozois RR 1997 Surgery of the colon and rectum. Churchill Livingstone, Edinburgh

Phillips RKS 1998 Colorectal surgery: a companion to specialist surgical practice. WB Saunders, London

Open biliary operations

R. C. N. Williamson and V. Usatoff

Contents

INTRODUCTION

1. This chapter will concentrate on open operations for gallstones, since until lately these have been by far the commonest indication for 'open' biliary surgery. Introduced as recently as 1987, laparoscopic cholecystectomy has rapidly been taken up by many centres throughout the world. At the present time the majority of elective cholecystectomies are carried out by the laparoscopic route, which is described in Chapter 15, but open operation is still commonly performed in developing countries and also in difficult or complicated cases.

2. When operating on the biliary tract, always ensure that the patient is positioned on the operating table so that the upper abdomen overlies a radiolucent tunnel. Alert the radiographer in advance that an operative cholangiogram may be required.

3. Routine antibiotic prophylaxis is a wise precaution in biliary surgery. Choose a broad-spectrum agent excreted in bile, such as one of the cephalosporins. A single parenteral dose given shortly before operation may suffice, unless the bile is obviously infected.

4. Thromboprophylaxis should be carried out as a routine unless there is a specific contraindication. We use subcutaneous low-dose heparin and below-knee compression stockings.

OPEN CHOLECYSTECTOMY

Appraise

1. Whether symptomatic or 'silent', gallstones are the overwhelming indication for cholecystectomy. Their prevalence makes cholecyst-ectomy the second commonest intra-abdominal operation in western countries (after appendicectomy). Cholecystectomy is occasionally indicated for acalculous cholecystitis, gallbladder carcinoma or chole-cystoses (cholesterosis, adenomyosis) or during the course of partial hepatectomy or pancreatoduodencetomy. A diseased gallbladder encountered incidentally at operation should usually be removed, provided there is adequate access and an additional procedure would not be inappropriate.

2. Although cholecystectomy can safely be performed by the laparoscopic route in many patients, certain situations will make it safer to convert to open operation. Difficulties can arise when: (a) the pathology encountered is difficult, such as Mirizzi syndrome; (b) the anatomical anomalies are not clearly understood or, finally; (c) the ex-perience of the surgeon is insufficient to deal with a problem, such as bleeding. To persist with laparoscopic removal in such circumstances is to risk injury to the bile duct.

3. Dissolution therapy with cheno- or ursodeoxycholic acid is a reasonable alternative to cholecystectomy in very elderly or infirm patients with a functioning gallbladder and a limited number of small, radiolucent calculi.

4. The earlier lists of absolute contraindications to laparoscopic cholecystectomy have mostly been reduced to relative contraindica-tions as surgical expertise and equipment have improved. Nevertheless, some consideration should be given to open cholecys-tectomy in cases of previous upper abdominal operations, acute chole-cystitis, cirrhosis, pregnancy and cholecystoenteric fistula. Currently, one of the remaining contraindications to laparoscopic cholecys-tectomy is when a strong suspicion of gallbladder carcinoma exists preoperatively.

5. Acute cholecystitis will generally settle when the patient is treated with rehydration and antibiotics, allowing operation to be delayed for a few days or weeks according to policy (see below). Persistence of fever and local tenderness or evidence of spreading peritonism are indications for urgent operation because of the risk of gangrene or perforation (see also the section on cholecystectomy below). About 10% of patients with acute cholecystitis have acalculous disease, and these patients are at particular risk of perforation.

6. The timing of operation after an acute attack of cholecystitis or biliary colic is disputatious. Our preference is to confirm the diagnosis at an early stage by ultrasonography (or contrast radiology) and to put the patient on the next 'cold' operating list.

7. Transient jaundice is compatible with stones confined to the gallbladder. Continuing jaundice suggests obstruction of the bile duct and requires further investigation, including an 'invasive' cholangiogram (either percutaneous transhepatic or endoscopic retrograde).

8. Half the population have some variation from 'normal' in the arterial supply of the gallbladder or the disposition of the bile ducts. Therefore, do not embark upon cholecystectomy without learning the common anatomical variations.

Prepare

As described above, ensure that the operating table will allow operative cholangiography (if needed) and 'cover' the operation with prophylactic antibiotic therapy.

Access

1. Choose between a right upper paramedian, an oblique subcostal or a transverse incision, according to your experience and the shape of the patient's abdomen.

2. In a paramedian incision it is simpler to split the fibres of rectus abdominis than to mobilize and retract the muscle belly. In practice, no harm ensues from denervation of the medial portion of the rectus. The incision starts at the costal margin 5 cm from the midline and runs down to just below the umbilicus.

3. Some surgeons prefer Kocher's oblique subcostal incision, which extends parallel to the costal margin for about 15 cm. If the incision is taken further to the right, isolate and preserve the ninth thoracic nerve. The muscles are divided by diathermy in the line of the skin incision. A transverse incision provides a better cosmetic scar at the expense of slightly limited access.

4. 'Minicholecystectomy' can be carried out through a short (5 cm) transverse incision with careful retraction (in favourable cases). It gives an excellent cosmetic result but has probably been superseded by laparoscopic cholecystectomy.

Assess

1. Examine the gallbladder to see if it is inflamed, thickened or contains stones. With the patient supine, stones sink to the neck of the gallbladder. If the organ is hard and adherent to the liver, consider the possibility of carcinoma.

2. Gallstone symptoms can mimic those of other diseases. Explore the rest of the abdomen, looking in particular for hiatus hernia, peptic ulcer, diverticular disease of the colon and diseases of the liver, pancreas and appendix.

3. Examine the (common) bile duct. It should not exceed 6–8 mm in diameter. Insert the left index finger through the epiploic foramen (of Winslow) and feel the duct between finger and thumb. Is it thickened, does it contain stones? The lower duct may be felt after splitting the peritoneum in the floor of the foramen with the edge of the finger.

4. Examine the head of pancreas between finger and thumb, again with the left index finger passed through the epiploic foramen and down behind the gland. Normal pancreas has a nodular feel, but with experience you will learn to detect the induration that denotes chronic inflammation or neoplasia.

Action

1. Place your hand over the liver and gently manipulate the right lobe downwards into the wound.

2. Ask the anaesthetist to empty the stomach by aspirating the nasogastric tube. Divide any omental adhesions to the undersurface of the gallbladder.

3. Place one pack in the subhepatic space to retract the intestines and another just covering the duodenal bulb.

4. Decide whether to commence gallbladder dissection at the fundus or in the region of the cystic duct. We generally prefer to display the structures in Calot's triangle (Fig. 14.1) and to ligate and divide the cystic artery before proceeding to the fundus and working back towards the cystic duct. If chronic inflammation is severe, it is safer to start at the fundus; some surgeons advocate this approach routinely.

5. Cholecystectomy may be performed with the surgeon standing on the right- or left-hand side of the operating table. Try both positions on different occasions and see which you find more comfortable.

6. If the gallbladder is very distended, it should be aspirated before proceeding (Fig. 14.2).

The empty gallbladder is easier to grasp for dissection and less likely to contaminate the peritoneal cavity if accidentally entered. Pack off the fundus and insert an Ochsner trocar, which is connected to the sucker tubing. Alternatively, use a syringe and wide-bore needle. Afterwards, seal the defect by grasping it with tissue-holding forceps.

'Duct-first' technique

1. The first assistant's left hand draws the duodenal bulb downwards, while a retractor draws the liver upwards. Grasp the neck of the gallbladder with sponge-holding forceps and draw it to the patient's right. This three-way traction provides good exposure (Fig. 14.1).

2. Incise the peritoneum over the neck of the gallbladder and continue for a short distance along its superior border. With blunt dissection gently open the space between the gallbladder and the liver at this point and expose the cystic artery. Follow the vessel on to the gallbladder wall and confirm that it is the cystic artery and not the right

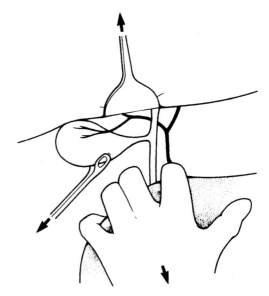

Fig. 14.1 Cholecystectomy. Traction in three directions displays Calot's triangle, which is bounded by the cystic duct, common hepatic duct and inferior border of the liver. The triangle has been extended by mobilization of the neck of the gallbladder. The cystic artery normally arises from the right hepatic artery within Calot's triangle.

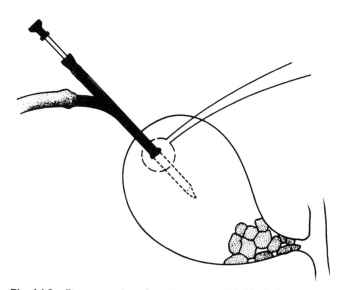

Fig. 14.2 Decompression of an obstructed gallbladder before cholecystectomy (or cholecystostomy). The side-arm of the Ochsner trocar is connected to the sucker tubing.

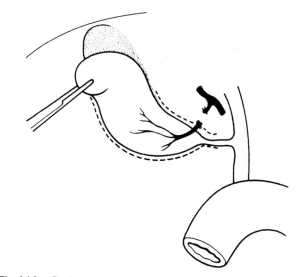

Fig. 14.3 Cholecystectomy: separation of the fundus of the gallbladder from the liver. The lines of peritoneal division are shown. The fundal dissection may be carried out after ligation and division of the cystic artery (as shown) or as the first stage of cholecystectomy.

hepatic artery. Ligate the vessel twice in continuity and divide it between the ligatures.

3. Prior division of the cystic artery helps to straighten out the cystic duct. The duct is now exposed by a combination of sharp and blunt dissection, and it is traced to its junction with the common hepatic duct to form the bile duct. It is vital to display this three-way junction before dividing the cystic duct.

4. Perform an operative cholangiogram via the cystic duct (see next section). Take a swab of the bile for bacteriological culture on opening the duct.

5. While awaiting the X-ray films (this is avoided if the cholangiogram is performed with real-time fluoroscopic images), proceed to dissect the gallbladder from its liver bed. Leave the cholangiogram catheter in situ but complete the division of the cystic duct, grasping its gallbladder end with Moynihan's cholecystectomy forceps. Incise the peritoneum along the anterior and posterior aspects of the gallbladder, proceeding either towards or away from the fundus. Traction on the fundus assists the dissection (Fig. 14..3).

Numerous small vessels and occasionally accessory bile ducts traverse the areolar tissue between the liver and the gallbladder. Diathermy can be used to secure these vessels, but it may be simpler to ligate leashes of tissue on the hepatic side and then divide with scissors. Remove the gallbladder, preserving it for subsequent gross and histological examination.

6. It should be routine practice to open the gallbladder, inspect its contents and submit any suspicious nodule or ulcer to urgent frozen-section examination to exclude carcinoma.

7. If the cholangiogram pictures are technically satisfactory, withdraw the catheter and ligate the cystic duct close to the origin of the bile duct. Try and avoid leaving too long a cystic duct stump but do not struggle to place the ligature exactly flush with the bile duct. Avoid tenting or narrowing the bile duct while tying the ligature. We use an absorbable suture material for the ligature, such as 2/0 or 3/0 polyglactin 910. If the cystic duct is large, use a transfixion suture.

8. Use diathermy to stop any residual oozing from the liver bed. Often the application of a surgical pack to the gallbladder fossa (with or without the aid of a haemostatic agent) for a few minutes will stop most bleeding. If you observe a leak of bile from a small cholecysto-hepatic duct, close the duct with a catgut stitch. Do not attempt to close the raw area of liver with sutures.

9. Remove the packs and aspirate any blood.

'Fundus-first' technique

1. Grasp the fundus of the gallbladder with tissue-holding forceps. Incise the peritoneum between the fundus and the liver, using frequent diathermy to secure the many fine vessels. Larger vessels can be ligated on the hepatic side and divided.

2. Extend the peritoneal incision along the anterior and posterior aspects of the gallbladder (Fig. 14.3).

Open up the plane between the liver and the gallbladder, and proceed towards the neck of the organ, staying close to the gallbladder. Identify the cystic artery. Ligate and divide the artery close to the gallbladder wall.

3. The advantage of the 'fundus-first' technique is that it brings you directly on to the cystic duct from the safe side and lessens the risk of bile-duct injury. Trace the cystic duct to its junction with the common hepatic duct. Perform a cholangiogram. Ligate and divide the cystic duct and remove the gallbladder.

4. Secure haemostasis in the liver bed. Remove the packs.

Key point

- Usually straightforward, cholecystectomy can sometimes (unpredictably) be a major technical challenge. Under such circumstances great care is needed to avert future disaster. The golden rule is never to cut any major structure (whether duct or artery) until the crucial anatomy has been displayed, notably the entry of the cystic duct into the bile duct.

☒ Difficulty?

1. *Is the gallbladder stuck to the duodenum or transverse colon and obscured by inflammatory adhesions?* The organ can usually be freed by gentle digital dissection, but remember that calculi may have fistulated into the adherent viscus.

2. *Can you not identify the cystic artery or the three-way union of ducts?* Perhaps the tissues are fibrotic or bleed too easily. The liver may be enlarged and stiff; the gallbladder may be inaccessible because the costal margin is low or the patient obese. Do not proceed until you have improved the view. Enlarge the incision if necessary. Have the light adjusted. Use the sucker. Make sure the assistants are usefully employed or summon further assistance.

3. *Can you still not safely progress?* Adopt the 'fundus-first' technique. Seek senior help. If the dissection is very difficult, consider an alternative procedure, either cholecystostomy or subtotal cholecystectomy.

4. *Are you proceeding with the dissection, but the anatomy is anomalous or confusing?* In these circumstances do not divide any structure until the anatomy of the area is fully displayed and understood. Remember the common variations, summon a textbook of surgical anatomy or seek assistance from a senior surgeon. If the cystic duct can be identified with confidence, cholangiography may clarify the remaining ductal anatomy.

5. *Do you suspect damage to the common hepatic duct or the bile duct?* If the possibility exists, you must declare the issue and not just hope for the best. Enlist the help of the most experienced surgeon available. Cholangiography may be helpful. Partial division of the main duct should be repaired immediately, using fine absorbable sutures and placing a T-tube across the anastomosis through a separate stab incision. Complete transection and particularly resection of a length of duct is often better dealt with by performing a hepaticojejunostomy repair using a Roux loop of jejunum. Resolve to make accurate notes, with drawings to display the exact situation.

6. *Severe bleeding?* Do not panic and apply haemostats blindly or use inappropriate diathermy; the situation is almost certainly recoverable. Control the bleeding by local pressure. Arrange for blood to be available, for arterial sutures, tapes and bulldog clamps. Summon further advice and assistance if necessary.

   a. If the bleeding is arterial, compress the free edge of the lesser omentum between finger and thumb or apply a non-crushing intestinal clamp just tightly enough to control bleeding (Pringle's manoeuvre, Fig. 14.4).

   Dissect out and control the hepatic artery, which normally lies on the left-hand side of the bile duct. Remember that accessory hepatic arteries arising from the left gastric or superior mesenteric arteries will not be controlled by occluding the main hepatic artery. Expose the damaged vessel. If large, repair it with arterial sutures; if small, ligate each end. You may find that you have pulled the cystic artery off the right hepatic artery. If so, suture the defect in the parent vessel. In the absence of jaundice or hypotension, ligature of the right hepatic or common hepatic artery (though best avoided) will not lead to infarction of the liver.

   b. If the bleeding is venous, control it by compression for 5 minutes timed by the clock, then explore, evaluate and repair the damage as necessary.

7. *Can the gallbladder not be separated from the liver?* Suspect carcinoma, and consider frozen-section examination if the diagnosis is equivocal. Carcinoma of the gallbladder should be removed if a curative resection can be achieved. This usually necessitates resection of the gallbladder bed and the nodes at the porta hepatis. This decision is often guided by the depth of tumour invasion into the gallbladder wall. Alternatively, some surgeons favour partial hepatectomy, but operative treatment is invariably palliative once carcinoma has spread into the adjacent liver. If severe (benign) fibrosis makes it extremely difficult to develop a safe plane of dissection, it is permissible to leave the back wall of the gallbladder attached to the liver and to diathermy the exposed mucosa.

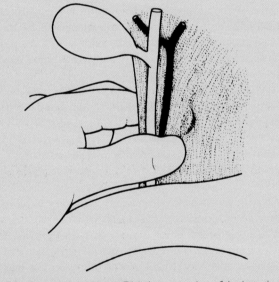

Fig. 14.4 Pringle's manoeuvre. Digital compression of the hepatic artery within the free edge of the lesser omentum controls haemorrhage from branches of the vessel beyond that point.

Checklist

1. Review the clinical and radiological criteria for continuing to exploration of the bile duct (see below).

   2. Examine the gallbladder bed, the common duct and the ligatures on the cystic duct and cystic artery.

Closure

1. Place a tube drain or fine-bore suction drain to the subhepatic pouch.

   2. Close the abdominal wall in layers as for a standard laparotomy incision (see Ch. 4).

Aftercare

1. The nasogastric tube can usually be removed at 12–24 hours and the drain at 48 hours. In straightforward cases a light diet can be reintroduced at 24–36 hours and patients are ready for discharge at 3–8 days.

   2. A small amount of bile may drain at first from the raw surface of the liver but will cease spontaneously within a few days. A larger leak (e.g. more than 100 ml bile per day) or a persistent fistula must be regarded as a complication and managed accordingly.

Key point

● In the setting of postoperative biliary ascites and sepsis, it is important first to control the bile leak and treat the sepsis. This goal can often be achieved by positioning a percutaneous drain. Before reoperation and repair is contemplated, imaging of the bile ducts is imperative and this may be undertaken either from above (percutaneous transhepatic cholangiography) or from below (endoscopic retrograde cholangiography) and often both.

Complications

1. Copious bile drainage through the wound or drain site suggests unrecognized injury to the bile duct or a slipped ligature on the cystic duct. Under these circumstances a retained calculus in the bile duct may be associated with persistence of the biliary fistula. Damage to the main duct is often accompanied by jaundice. The diagnosis is confirmed by cholangiography, obtained either by transhepatic needling or by retrograde cannulation of the ampulla. Re-operation will be needed. A small defect in the bile duct may be amenable to repair over a T-tube (after ensuring that there are no ductal calculi), but a larger defect or complete transection requires Roux-en-Y hepaticojejunostomy.

2. Wound infection is uncommon unless the bile duct is explored or there is severe acute cholecystitis.

3. Subhepatic abscess occasionally results from an undrained collection of blood or bile; management is considered in Chapter 7. True subphrenic abscess is rare, likewise septicaemia.

4. The mortality rate of cholecystectomy is well under 1%. Most deaths occur in the elderly, those with gangrene or perforation of the gallbladder or those with concomitant ductal stones. Most post-cholecystectomy symptoms result from unrecognized intercurrent disease.

OPERATIVE CHOLANGIOGRAPHY

Appraise

1. Cholangiography is an integral part of cholecystectomy and should be carried out at an early stage of the operation, unless pre-operative visualization of the ducts (e.g. by retrograde cholangiography) has been excellent and they are normal. This policy of routine cholangiography has been challenged in the laparoscopic era (see Ch. 15) but, as most cases performed with open operation are likely to represent the more difficult cases, we still believe that this traditional teaching holds true during open cholecystectomy.

2. The justification for this policy of routine cholangiography is that it will detect ductal stones that have been missed by inspection or palpation of the bile duct. However, a slick technique is required to obtain X-rays of good quality and to avoid artefacts such as air bubbles that can lead to negative exploration of the duct. In experienced hands a selective policy is acceptable, in which cholangiography is reserved for those patients with a history of jaundice or recent acute pancreatitis and those with laparotomy findings suggestive of ductal stones (e.g. a dilated bile duct or a short, wide cystic duct with multiple gallbladder stones).

3. Whatever your policy, always obtain an operative cholan-giogram to display the ductal anatomy if there is any suspicion of an anomalous arrangement. If necessary, a check film can be obtained by cannulating the gallbladder without the need for formal exposure of the cystic duct.

4. Warn the X-ray department preoperatively. Ensure that the patient is correctly placed on the operating table, with the upper abdomen overlying a radiolucent tunnel. An image intensifier can facilitate visualization of the biliary tree, but it is still best to obtain 'hard-copy' X-rays for record purposes (unless video records are available).

5. Cholangiograms should normally be obtained via the cystic duct. Alternatively, contrast material can be injected directly into the common hepatic or bile ducts. If ductal stones are obviously present at operation, it may still help to discover their number and size and the state of the duct before proceeding to exploration.

6. After choledocholithotomy, it is always sensible to check that all stones have been removed by repeating the cholangiogram.

Action

1. Fill a 20 ml syringe and attached fine plastic cannula with saline, making sure no air bubbles remain in the syringe or tubing. Prepare a second syringe filled with 25% sodium diatrizoate (Hypaque) and clearly marked.

2. Isolate 2 cm of cystic duct and ligate on the gallbladder side. Pass a second ligature around the duct, but do not tie. Partly divide the cystic duct between these ligatures about 2 cm from its entry into the main duct (Fig. 14.5).

3. Pass the cannula down the cystic duct for about 2 cm and ligate in situ. If difficulty is encountered from spiralling of the ductal mucosa (Heister's valve), withdraw the cannula, gently pass a probe and try again.

4. Check the patency of the cannula when it is tied in place. Inject a small quantity of saline, or detach the syringe and observe bile pass back up the tubing.

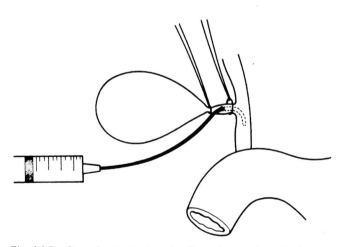

Fig. 14.5 Operative cholangiography. Through a small opening in the cystic duct, a fine polythene cannula is passed into the bile duct and secured in position by tightening a ligature around the cystic duct.

5. Remove instruments and swabs from the field. Cover the wound with a sterile towel and allow the radiographer to position the X-ray machine. Spectators, assistants and nursing personnel should now leave the theatre or take their place behind a lead screen. The anaesthetist remains for the moment to control the patient's respiration.

6. Inject 3–4 ml of contrast medium and have an X-ray film exposed. Insert a further 5–10 ml and obtain a second film.

7. Other techniques are convenient in particular circumstances. The contrast material can be injected directly into the main duct through a fine 'butterfly' needle. Alternatively, the neck of the gallbladder may be clamped and contrast is injected immediately beyond this point. When duodenotomy has been performed, a retrograde cholangiogram may be obtained by cannulation of the papilla.

8. Postexploratory films are obtained via a T-tube inserted into the bile duct. Care must be taken to clear the tube and the ductal tree of air. The T-tube is repeatedly irrigated during closure of the choledochotomy incision, the last stitch being inserted and tied under water. One or two films are obtained after injection of 10–20 ml of 25% Hypaque.

9. If the films are technically unsatisfactory, do not hesitate to repeat them. Use further contrast material to try and clear any air bubbles or to obtain better filling of the hepatic ducts.

Interpretation

1. Inspect the films carefully. Make sure that the right and left hepatic ducts are displayed together with their tributaries. The bile duct usually overlies the spine, and occasionally this can obscure certain features. If necessary, obtain further films with the operating table rotated 15° to the right to throw the bile duct clear of the spine (some surgeons adopt this precaution routinely). In some patients it may be difficult to demonstrate the intrahepatic bile ducts and in this situation, a degree of head-down tilt will facilitate contrast flowing into the proximal ducts. Care must be taken to study the film closely, as many anomalies can occur.[1]

2. On the pre-exploratory films, exclude the following features: filling defects, obstruction of a major hepatic radicle, dilatation of the bile duct (> 10 mm), failure of contrast to enter the duodenum. Remember that the bile duct normally tapers before smoothly entering the duodenum. If you suspect spasm rather than organic obstruction of the papilla, consider obtaining a further X-ray after an intravenous injection of hyoscine hydrobromide or glucagon.[2]

3. On the postexploratory films the most important feature is the presence or absence of a filling defect, consistent with a residual calculus. It is quite common for contrast not to enter the duodenum at this stage, especially after instrumentation of the papilla.

REFERENCES

1. Puente SG, Bannura GC 1983 Radiological anatomy of the biliary tract: variations and congenital abnormalities. World Journal of Surgery 7: 271–276
2. Al-Jurf A 1990 A simplified technique to relax the sphincter of Oddi during intraoperative cholangiography. Surgery, Gynecology and Obstetrics 170: 163–164

EXPLORATION OF THE BILE DUCT

Appraise

1. Absolute indications for exploration of the bile duct at laparotomy are stones unequivocally shown on a preoperative or operative cholangiogram, stones that can be palpated within the bile duct and stones causing obstructive jaundice. Preoperatively detected stones should probably be treated by endoscopic retrograde cholangiopancreatography (ERCP) and stone extraction unless the patient is to be subjected to open operation anyway. The detection of duct stones during laparoscopic cholangiography is usually not an indication to convert to an open procedure as in most cases the duct can be cleared by laparoscopic duct exploration or postoperative ERCP. In the latter case, a transcystic duct drain can be left in situ to provide adequate drainage until the ERCP can be organized. This strategy may be appropriate in the elderly patient, although the mortality rate of open common bile duct exploration is low at 1%.

2. Relative indications for choledochotomy are any abnormalities shown on operative cholangiography apart from obvious stones. If the radiological criteria are doubtful, the following clinical factors would tend to favour exploration of the duct: a history of jaundice or acute pancreatitis, dilatation and opacification of the wall of the bile duct, multiple small calculi in the gallbladder and a short wide cystic duct.

3. If narrowing of the terminal bile duct is the only abnormality, it is sometimes possible to rule out appreciable stenosis by passing a soft Jacques catheter (no. 8F) through the cystic duct stump and into the duodenum. Ultra-thin choledochoscopes are becoming available for passage through the cystic duct.

4. If doubt remains, explore the duct. Negative exploration is safer than ignoring disease (usually stones but conceivably tumour).

5. Remember that a jaundiced patient needs proper perioperative precautions taken.

6. Endoscopic papillotomy may avoid the need for laparotomy in selected patients with bile duct stones, especially those without a gallbladder (see next section).

ALTERNATIVES TO CHOLECYSTECTOMY

Appraise

1. Cholecystostomy is a temporary expedient for draining an obstructed or infected gallbladder to the exterior. It should be considered when gross disease of the gallbladder or intercurrent illness make cholecystectomy unsafe. In the very elderly or infirm with empyema of the gallbladder or necrotizing cholecystitis, open cholecystostomy under local anaesthetic can be life-saving. If cholecystectomy is planned, but obesity and/or severe inflammation cause serious technical difficulties, cholecystostomy is a reasonable option, especially for an inexperienced surgeon. A second operation may well be needed at a later date, however.

2. Cholecystostomy is sometimes performed to relieve obstructive jaundice before proceeding to resection of a periampullary cancer or to drain an obstructed biliary tree, or if gallstones are encountered during laparotomy for severe acute pancreatitis.

3. Subtotal cholecystectomy may be a better option than cholecystostomy if difficulty is encountered in removing the entire gallbladder for stones. It avoids the need for further surgery.

4. Percutaneous cholecystostomy may be a better option than open cholecystostomy in a patient with severe acute cholecystitis (especially the acalculous type) who is unfit for operation and occasionally in a child who develops acute dilatation (hydrops) of the gallbladder.

PERCUTANEOUS CHOLECYSTOSTOMY

Access

This technique is carried out by an interventional radiologist in the X-ray department, using local anaesthetic with or without intravenous sedation. Under ultrasound guidance a fine needle is inserted into the gallbladder, using the transhepatic route to reduce the risk of bile leakage.

Action

1. Once access has been gained to the gallbladder, a sample of bile is aspirated for bacteriological culture.

2. A guide-wire is placed through the needle, which is then removed, and dilators are used to dilate the track and allow insertion of a cholecystostomy catheter.

3. A catheter cholecystogram is performed at 24–48 hours to evaluate the cystic duct and confirm the presence of gallstones. Once the patient improves, a choice can be made whether to proceed to cholecystectomy or attempt percutaneous extraction of the stones.

? Difficulty?

In difficult cases the transperitoneal route can be used to puncture the gallbladder, but loss of access and bile leakage are greater risks by this route.

Complications

There is a small risk of a vasovagal response and cardiac arrest. Bile leakage can occur if the catheter becomes dislodged.

OPEN CHOLECYSTOSTOMY

Access

Planned cholecystostomy should be carried out through a short transverse incision in the right upper quadrant. The incision is placed over the fundus of the gallbladder, when this is palpable.

Action

1. Protect the margins of the wound and pack off the area of the gallbladder to prevent contamination by infected bile. Free adhesions sufficiently to expose the fundus of the gallbladder.

2. Aspirate the fluid contents of the gallbladder by suction through an Ochsner trocar and cannula or syringe and wide-bore needle.

3. Grasp the partly-collapsed fundus with tissue-holding forceps to control the organ and prevent its retraction. Make a short incision in the fundus and obtain a culture of the bile. Suck out residual bile.

4. Explore the lumen of the gallbladder with a finger and extract all the stones. Saline irrigation may help or insertion of a gauze swab

to trap small calculi. If the patient's condition allows, try and determine the presence or absence of gangrene, perforation and obvious calculi in the cystic duct or Hartmann's pouch, which could be gently disimpacted and milked towards the fundal incision.

5. After the gallbladder has been cleared of stones, insert a large Foley or Malecot catheter into the lumen and secure it with catgut sutures to effect a watertight closure (Fig. 14.6).

The Foley catheter will need to be brought through the abdominal wall via a separate stab incision immediately over the gallbladder before placement. A corrugated drain should be inserted to the subhepatic space if there has been quite an extensive dissection.

? Difficulty?

1. *Is the gallbladder friable or necrotic and does it tear during the dissection?* Excise devitalized segments and close the remnant around the tube. If the cystic duct is cleared of stones and bile flow is re-established, subtotal cholecystectomy without external tube drainage is a reasonable alternative in unfavourable circumstances (see below).

2. *Cannot calculi easily be disimpacted from the depths of the gallbladder?* The options are to remove as much debris as possible and insert a tube as before or proceed to subtotal or complete cholecystectomy despite the patient's poor condition.

Aftercare

1. Record the amount of cholecystostomy drainage and replace electrolytes as needed. Obtain a tube cholecystogram at 7–10 days. If there are no residual stones and contrast enters the bile duct, clamp and then remove the tube. Consider elective cholecystectomy at a later date.

2. Residual stones are a clear indication for reoperation when the patient's condition allows.

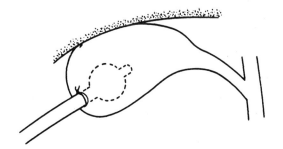

Fig. 14.6 Cholecystostomy. A large Foley catheter is sutured into the gallbladder, taking care not to puncture the balloon when inserting the stitches.

SUBTOTAL CHOLECYSTECTOMY

Assess

1. This procedure should be considered during an attempted cholecystectomy when gross oedema and fibrosis in Calot's triangle make recognition of the surgical landmarks very difficult. To persist with

total cholecystectomy in such circumstances would risk injury to the hepatic artery and the bile duct.

2. By leaving the posterior wall of the gallbladder in situ, subtotal cholecystectomy may reduce the severity of haemorrhage in a cirrhotic patient with gallstones. It may also be appropriate when a gangrenous gallbladder is discovered during planned cholecystostomy.

Action

1. No attempt is made to dissect the cystic artery in Calot's triangle. The gallbladder contents are aspirated and then the organ is opened. It is removed piecemeal leaving part of the posterior wall attached to the liver. Bleeding vessels are under-run with sutures, and the retained mucosa can be diathermied if it is oozy.

2. It may be possible to obtain a cholangiogram by cannulating the cystic duct via the neck of the opened gallbladder, but in the absence of jaundice this step can be abandoned if necessary. The orifice of the cystic duct is closed with a purse-string suture inserted within the gallbladder lumen.

Aftercare

A drain is left to the subhepatic space, and this is removed when appropriate. It should not be necessary to perform any further procedure (unless ductal stones have been left behind).

FURTHER READING

Blumgart LH 1994 Surgery of the liver and biliary tract, 2nd edn. Churchill Livingstone, Edinburgh

Williamson RCN 1990 Acute cholecystitis, calculous and aculculous. In: Williamson RCN, Cooper MJ (eds) Emergency abdominal surgery. Churchill Livingstone, Edinburgh, pp 110–127

Laparoscopic biliary surgery

CHAPTER

15

J. N. Thompson and S. G. Appleton

Contents

LAPAROSCOPIC CHOLECYSTECTOMY

Appraise

1. Laparoscopic cholecystectomy is now the treatment of choice for patients with symptomatic gallstones. Because of the decreased morbidity and improved convenience of the technique the total number of cholecystectomies performed has increased. Additional indications for the operation include selected patients with gallstones who have no symptoms but are at risk of severe complications and those who have no stones but suffer severe 'biliary' symptoms.

2. There are few absolute contraindications to laparoscopic cholecystectomy. Cirrhosis with portal hypertension is dangerous because of the substantial risk of uncontrollable bleeding during the operation, which may also precipitate hepatic failure. Sustained CO_2 pneumoperitoneum can cause significant cardiovascular changes in patients with ischaemic heart disease and significant hypercarbia in patients with respiratory disease. In the unusual event that carcinoma of the gallbladder is diagnosed preoperatively, avoid laparoscopic excision.

3. Contraindications to the laparoscopic technique may become apparent during the procedure. These include:

a. discovery of a different pathology from that expected
b. an inability to identify the anatomy safely – usually because dense adhesions make safe dissection impossible
c. uncontrollable bleeding and damage to adjacent structures or organs.

> **Key point**
>
> ● In the face of these findings convert to an open procedure sooner rather than later. Conversion to an open cholecystectomy is not a failure of surgical technique but safe practice.

4. Some centres now perform laparoscopic cholecystectomy as a day-case procedure, though this requires appropriate facilities and good postoperative support.

5. Laparoscopic cholecystectomy has rendered virtually obsolete non-operative treatments of gallstones such as lithotripsy or dissolution therapy.

6. Minicholecystectomy performed through a 5 cm right upper quadrant incision is an alternative to laparoscopic cholecystectomy and has comparable results. However, as with the laparoscopic procedure, special instruments and training are required.

Prepare

1. Obtain informed consent for laparoscopic cholecystectomy including discussion of:

a. the possibility of conversion to an open operation during the procedure, which varies from unit to unit but is of the order of 5%
b. the possibility of finding common bile duct stones (10%) and their management.

2. Institute thromboprophylaxis (subcutaneous heparin and compression stockings) because the reverse Trendelenburg position together with a positive pressure pneumoperitoneum encourages the development of deep venous thrombosis.

3. General anaesthesia is required, with endotracheal intubation and muscle relaxation.

4. Biliary tract surgery rarely involves anaerobic microorganisms and satisfactory prophylaxis is achieved with a cephalosporin alone. Give prophylactic antibiotic (cefuroxime 1.5 mg i.v.) as a single dose at the induction of anaesthesia. If there is leakage of bile during the operation, give a further two postoperative doses.

5. Place the patient supine on a radiolucent operating table that allows on-table cholangiography. The patient's upper abdomen and lower chest lie over the radiolucent section. There should be room for the C-arm of the image intensifier both above and below the table.

6. Pass a nasogastric tube to deflate the stomach. This decreases aspiration associated with the pneumoperitoneum, reduces the risk of accidental perforation by a trocar and improves visibility during the procedure. Similarly, pass a catheter to empty the urinary bladder and avoid accidental perforation, a risk that occurs only when the initial trocar and cannula are inserted 'blind' using the closed laparoscopy method.

7. Most surgeons stand on the patient's left with the first assistant opposite (see Fig. 5.1, Ch. 5). Alternatively the patient may be placed in the Lloyd-Davies position with the surgeon operating from the foot of the table between the patient's legs.

8. Prepare the skin of the abdomen from the nipples to the suprapubic region using 10% povidone-iodine in alcohol or other cleansing

agent. Ensure the skin is prepared up to the posterior axillary line on the patient's right side, for the lateral port. Similarly, ensure that the drape at the top end extends above the level of the xiphisternum and that the right drape is as lateral as possible.

9. Arrange the various leads and piping that may be required before establishing the pneumoperitoneum; these include the gas tubing, diathermy lead, light source and irrigation/suction tubing. Secure them with clips or tape to the surgical drapes around the operating field, to minimize tangling.

Access

1. We use an 'open' laparoscopic technique to access the peritoneal cavity, insert the primary subumbilical cannula and establish a pneumoperitoneum. An alternative is to use the Veress needle to establish the pneumoperitoneum and then insert the initial trocar and cannula blind (see Ch. 5). Insert all subsequent trocars under direct vision. Maintain an intra-abdominal pressure of 10–14 mmHg throughout the procedure.

2. A 30° laparoscope is best for 'looking down' on to Calot's triangle and obtaining 'angled' views, but a 0° scope is often used.

3. Four ports are required initially (Fig. 15.1): a 10 mm umbilical port for the camera; a 5 mm lateral port to retract the fundus of the gallbladder; a 5 mm right upper quadrant port, placed in the midclavicular line, to manipulate the neck of the gallbladder and a 10 mm cannula with a 5 mm reducer (or a 5–12 mm disposable port) in the epigastrium just to the right of the midline and 2–5 cm below the xiphisternum.

The epigastric port should enter the abdominal cavity through or just to the right of the ligamentum teres and is the main port for dissecting instruments, diathermy, clip applicators, suction and irrigation.

4. A large or floppy left lobe of the liver occasionally obstructs the view of Calot's triangle. This can be overcome using a liver retractor placed through an additional 5 mm port in the left upper quadrant.

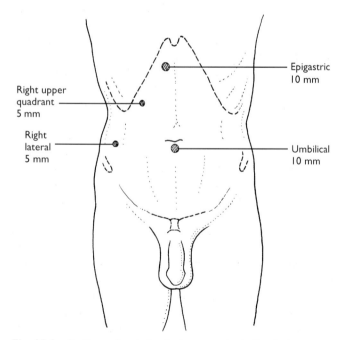

Right upper
quadrant
5 mm

Right
lateral
5 mm

Epigastric
10 mm

Umbilical
10 mm

Fig. 15.1   Positions of port sites for laparoscopic cholecystectomy.

Assess

1. As in a laparotomy, the initial task is to examine the abdominal cavity. Carry out a systematic inspection of the contents of the four quadrants and pelvis. This is equivalent to the exploratory laparotomy in open biliary surgery. Note common disorders of a benign nature – colonic diverticular disease, pelvic adnexal disease in the female, etc. – but these do not preclude the performance of laparoscopic cholecystectomy. More serious findings, particularly if considered to be neoplastic in nature, may necessitate conversion to open laparotomy or postponement of the surgical treatment pending further investigations and preparation of the patient.

2. Assessment of the subhepatic region is best achieved with the operating table tilted 25–35° head up and 10–15° sideways to the left, which encourages the abdominal contents to fall away from the area.

3. *Assess feasibility of laparoscopic cholecystectomy.* This is an assessment of the technical difficulty and safety of gallbladder excision using the laparoscopic method. To a large extent, the decision is influenced by your experience of laparoscopic surgery. The situations that may be encountered are:

   a. *Easy cases.* The patient is thin and the intraperitoneal fat is minimal. The gallbladder is floppy and non-adherent. When the gallbladder is lifted and retracted upwards by a grasping forceps, the cystic pedicle (fold of peritoneum covering the cystic artery, duct and lymph node) is readily identified as a smooth triangular fold between the neck of the gallbladder, the inferior surface of the liver and the common bile duct. These patients are undoubtedly better served by laparoscopic than by open cholecystectomy.

   b. *Feasible but more difficult cases.* These include obese patients in whom the cystic pedicle is fat-laden. A gallbladder containing a large stone load may be difficult to grasp and this can cause problems with retraction and exposure. The gallbladder may be distended by cholecystitis or because of a stone impacted in the neck. Difficulties may also be encountered because of adhesions from previous surgery. Provided you are experienced and prepared to proceed carefully, laparoscopic cholecystectomy can be accomplished with safety and a good outcome.

   c. *Cases of uncertain feasibility – trial dissection.* This group includes patients with dense adhesions, those in whom the cystic pedicle cannot be visualized and patients with contracted fibrotic gallbladders where the neck or Hartmann's pouch appears to be adherent to the common bile duct. If you are experienced, it is reasonable to perform a careful trial dissection. The feasibility or otherwise of the operation becomes apparent as the dissection proceeds. In adopting this approach, common sense must prevail; trial dissection does not equate with a long hazardous procedure. If you cannot for any reason clearly identify and expose the structures of the cystic pedicle in Calot's triangle, convert to an open procedure.

   d. *Unsuitable cases.* These include patients with the following findings:

   i.   severe acute cholecystitis with gangrenous patches or a gross inflammatory phlegmon obscuring the structures of the porta hepatis
   ii. chronically inflamed gallbladder when the neck is adherent to the common hepatic duct, indicative of a Mirizzi syndrome
   iii. cirrhosis with established portal hypertension and large high-pressure varices surrounding the gallbladder and cystic pedicle.

In patients with severe acute cholecystitis that precludes safe dissection, a laparoscopic cholecystostomy may be performed, with interval cholecystectomy at a later date (see later). It is foolhardy to attempt laparoscopic cholecystectomy in patients in whom the gallbladder neck/Hartmann's pouch is densely adherent or fistulated into the common hepatic duct, since the risk of damage to the bile duct is considerable. These patients are best served by open operation (see Ch. 14).

4. If the gallbladder is not visible then use blunt-tipped grasping forceps or a probe in the lateral port to gently sweep away omentum, colon or small bowel. Alternatively, insert grasping forceps under the edge of the liver and gently lift it to expose the fundus of the gallbladder.

5. Grasp the fundus of the gallbladder with self-retaining toothed grasping forceps inserted through the lateral port. Gently push the gallbladder up over the liver towards the diaphragm as far as it will comfortably go and have your assistant hold it in this position.

6. It is difficult to grasp a distended and tense gallbladder so decompress it with a Veress needle or a 16G Abbocath® passed through the abdominal wall just below the costal margin in the midclavicular line. Aspirate bile using a 20 ml syringe or suction tubing put in the barrel of a 10 ml syringe with the plunger removed. Send the bile to microbiology for culture and sensitivity. Withdraw the Veress needle or Abbocath® and place the grasping forceps over the puncture site in the gallbladder to limit further bile spillage.

7. If the gallbladder has been previously inflamed, adhesions are commonly found to its serosal surface. Flimsy adhesions may pulled off with fine non-toothed grasping forceps while thicker more vascular adhesions require diathermy division close to the gallbladder wall. Take care to avoid the hepatic flexure of the transverse colon laterally, and the duodenum medially, which may be closely adherent to the gallbladder.

Action

Dissecting Calot's triangle

1. Grasp the neck of the gallbladder with grasping forceps, fairly close to the origin of the cystic duct, if visible. This is probably the most important instrument in the initial dissection, as it allows the structures in the cystic pedicle to be exposed under tension and the gallbladder neck can be moved up and down so you can see both superior and inferior surfaces of Calot's triangle. Some surgeons manipulate the grasping forceps with their left hand while others delegate it to an assistant so they can use two hands for dissection.

2. A stone impacted in the neck of the gallbladder may be massaged back into the body with forceps. If this fails, the grasping forceps may be positioned just behind the stone and still permit adequate movement of the gallbladder. Alternatively, replace the 5 mm port in the right upper quadrant with a 10 mm port and use heavy grasping forceps to hold the stone within the gallbladder.

3. Begin the dissection by using the diathermy hook or scissors to make a small hole in the peritoneum overlying the cystic duct close to the gallbladder neck.

4. Dissection of Calot's triangle (Fig. 15.2) may then proceed one of three ways.

a. Grab the free edge of peritoneum just created with fine-tipped, straight or curved grasping forceps and peel the peritoneum medially to

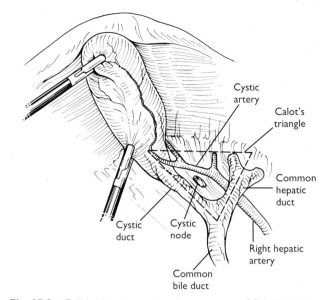

Fig. 15.2 Gallbladder retracted to show anatomy of Calot's triangle.

expose the structures of the cystic pedicle. Sometimes the peritoneum peels back easily to reveal the cystic duct and cystic artery but if you feel any resistance it is safer to proceed to one of the following methods.

b. With the diathermy hook divide the peritoneum on the undersurface of Calot's triangle, aiming posterolaterally towards the junction of gallbladder wall and liver. Remember to keep the peritoneum under tension using the grasping forceps on the neck of the gallbladder and to keep close to the gallbladder wall. When you reach the sulcus between the body of the gallbladder and the liver, continue dividing the peritoneum along the inferior border of gallbladder and liver for about 1–2 cm laterally. Move the neck of the gallbladder down and divide the peritoneum over Calot's triangle in a similar manner laterally towards the junction of gallbladder and liver, again taking care to keep close to the gallbladder wall. Continue the dissection for 1 to 2 cm laterally along the gallbladder/liver junction to open out Calot's triangle and improve the view.

c. Employ a similar approach to (b) but using dissecting scissors attached to diathermy instead of the hook. This technique requires care, to be sure you know what is between the blades of the scissors before you cut.

5. The aim of the dissection is to identify and clear the cystic duct and cystic artery so they may be clipped and divided safely. Frequently, this requires a disjointed dissection that alternates between the superior and inferior aspects of Calot's triangle, which is why the grasping forceps on the neck of the gallbladder is so important.

6. The cystic duct and artery usually run parallel to each other. The peritoneum overlying them will have been divided at right angles to these structures but create the window between them by inserting the tips of the scissors or dissecting forceps and opening them parallel to the duct and artery.

7. Diathermize any small bleeding vessels immediately; blood quickly obscures the view of Calot's triangle. It also absorbs the light from the camera, so darkening the view considerably. Remove clots with the suction/irrigation device.

8. Clear and skeletonize the cystic duct close to the neck of the gallbladder for 1–1.5 cm if possible. Ensure that the structure you think is cystic duct is entering the gallbladder and has no 'branches' or other connections. There is no advantage in dissecting out the junction of cystic duct and common hepatic duct; you are more likely to injure the bile duct if you attempt to identify the T-junction.

> **Key point**
>
> - To ensure it is the cystic artery that has been identified, and not the right hepatic artery, follow the vessel to the gallbladder wall.

9. Sometimes the cystic artery can be seen to divide into its terminal anterior and posterior branches; this may occur more medially than anticipated and require distal clips on each of the branches before dividing the artery. To confirm a structure as an artery, observe it carefully and closely, to detect visible pulsation both before and after division.

10. When clipping either artery or duct, ensure that both tips of the clip applicator can be seen behind the structure being clipped in order to avoid inadvertently clipping important adjacent structures such as the common hepatic or common bile duct. When there is a short cystic duct avoid placing clips close to the junction with the common duct– instead divide the neck of the gallbladder and use an Endoloop suture ligature.

Peroperative cholangiogram
1. The necessity and indications for peroperative cholangiogram during laparoscopic cholecystectomy are fiercely debated. Peroperative cholangiography may be performed routinely, selectively or rarely.

a. *Routinely.* Some surgeons always perform a cholangiogram during laparoscopic cholecystectomy. They argue that it allows for the detection of bile duct stones and, by identifying the anatomy of the biliary tree, guards against damage to the extrahepatic ducts. It may also be useful training.

b. *Selectively.* A cholangiogram is performed if there is a preoperative suggestion of bile duct stones (history of jaundice, dilated common bile duct on ultrasound or abnormal liver function tests). Any identified ductal stones may then be dealt with at the time of the operation (either by laparoscopic or open bile duct exploration) or postoperatively by ERCP.

c. *Rarely.* Surgeons who rarely or never perform cholangiography depend on a pre- or postoperative ERCP to deal with bile duct stones and argue that identifying the anatomy does not alter the incidence of bile duct injury.

2. Close the medial end of the cystic duct in one of three ways.

a. *Clips.* Use metal (titanium) clips or absorbable polydioxanone (Ethicon) clips to close the cystic duct stump. Apply these at right angles to the duct and check that they occlude the whole width of the duct. Failure to do this could result in a postoperative bile leak. Most surgeons use two clips on the medial cystic duct stump for added safety. Do not squeeze the clips too tightly – a particular hazard with re-useable instruments – because they may 'cut through' the duct.

b. *Endoloop.* Apply a 2/0 chromic catgut or 2/0 polyglactin 910

endoloop once the cystic duct has been divided. This is particularly useful for a wide, oedematous or inflamed cystic duct where clips are liable to slip or cut through. Pass the endoloop through the epigastric port. Pass the tips of dissecting forceps through the endoloop and pick up the cystic duct stump. Apply enough tension on the cystic duct to slide the endoloop down over it without tenting up the bile duct. Tighten the endoloop securely around the cystic duct stump and then cut the ligature.

c. *Ligate in continuity.* Pass a length of 2/0 chromic catgut or 2/0 polyglactin 910 thread behind the intact cystic duct. The duct can then be ligated in continuity using intra- or extracorporeal knotting techniques.

When the medial end of the cystic duct has been secured the duct can be divided using scissors. The gallbladder is now detached from the structures of the porta hepatis.

Dissection of the gallbladder off the liver
1. This step can be relatively straightforward in a non-inflamed gallbladder; especially one attached to the liver by a mesentery. However, more often than not, the gallbladder is chronically inflamed, contracted, adherent or partially buried in the liver bed.

2. Keep the gallbladder on the stretch using grasping forceps attached to the fundus and neck respectively. Divide the serosa along the upper and lower junctions of gallbladder and liver using scissors or the hook attached to diathermy. Coagulate any obvious vessels before dividing the peritoneum.

3. Retract the gallbladder neck laterally (Fig. 15.3).

This raises the neck of the gallbladder from the liver bed and reveals

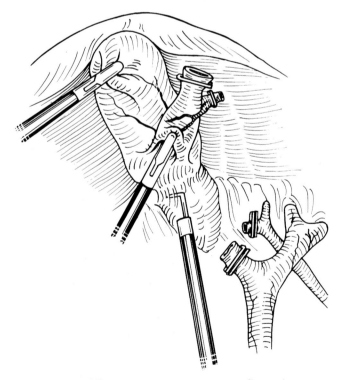

Fig. 15.3 Retraction of gallbladder neck to expose fibrous tissue connecting gallbladder to liver.

the loose fibrous tissue plane that separates the gallbladder wall from the liver parenchyma. Divide this fibrous tissue using a combination of blunt and sharp dissection (scissors) and diathermy (scissors and/or hook; Fig. 15.4).

Stay close to the gallbladder wall; if the dissection is carried out too close to the liver parenchyma then considerable bleeding can occur. If bleeding does occur push the gallbladder back into the gallbladder fossa to compress the area for a few minutes until the bleeding has stopped or has slowed enough for bleeding points to be identified and diathermied.

4. Midway through dissection of the gallbladder from the liver bed move the grasping forceps from the neck of the gallbladder to its undersurface (liver aspect). This allows better control of dissection for the lateral half of the gallbladder.

5. Occasionally a small cystohepatic bile duct (duct of Luschka) is found entering the gallbladder directly from the liver parenchyma. If you recognize it clip it to avoid a troublesome postoperative bile leak.

6. Before the gallbladder is completely detached, push it up over the liver towards the diaphragm. This retracts the liver edge and exposes the gallbladder fossa, allowing thorough inspection for coagulation of residual bleeding points. Pay particular attention to the cut peritoneum at the edge of the gallbladder fossa. Irrigating the gallbladder fossa with saline under pressure helps to identify bleeding points, which may occasionally need clipping. This manoeuvre also allows inspection of the cystic pedicle to check the clips on the cystic duct and artery.

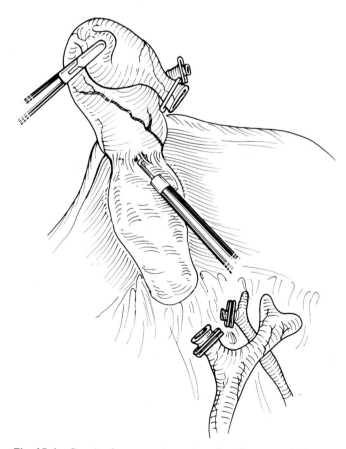

Fig. 15.4 Grasping forceps on the undersurface (liver aspect) of the gallbladder to aid dissection of the fundus from the liver.

7. Dissecting the fundus of the gallbladder can be difficult, particularly if the gallbladder is large or embedded in the liver. Techniques that may be helpful include:

a. Retract the fundus of the gallbladder medially and the undersurface laterally to reverse the usual position of the gallbladder

b. Remove the grasping forceps from the fundus and place them on the undersurface of the gallbladder to push it upward over the liver edge. Frequently a combination of manoeuvres is required to detach the fundus completely.

8. Once detached, place the gallbladder out of the way on the superior surface of the liver.

9. Use blunt-tipped grasping forceps or a probe to lift up the liver edge to allow a final inspection of the gallbladder fossa and cystic pedicle for any bleeding or bile leaks. Aspirate any remaining blood or clots from the subhepatic fossa, over the right lobe of the liver and the right paracolic gutter.

Extracting the gallbladder

1. The gallbladder may be removed via the epigastric or umbilical port sites.

2. *Gallbladder removal through the epigastric port.* This is suitable for small, non-distended gallbladders. Insert a pair of heavy, self-grasping, toothed (alligator) forceps through the epigastric port. Bring the gallbladder into view and grasp the clipped (cystic duct) end. Under direct vision, gently withdraw the gallbladder into the epigastric cannula as far as it will go. Slide the cannula and alligator forceps out of the abdominal cavity. Grasp the exteriorized neck of the gallbladder on the abdominal surface with a pair of Kocher's forceps or a heavy arterial forceps to prevent retraction back into the abdominal cavity. Release the alligator forceps and, with a combination of gentle rotation and traction, extract the gallbladder. Avoid excessive traction as this may cause gallbladder perforation with intraperitoneal spillage of bile and stones.

3. *Gallbladder removal through the umbilical port.* Remove the laparoscope from the umbilical port and replace it in the epigastric port. Insert alligator forceps into the umbilical port and under direct vision follow them up to the liver. Grasp the clipped end of the gallbladder and withdraw it through the umbilical port in the manner described above.

4. If the intraperitoneal portion of the gallbladder is distended with bile, grasp the exteriorized neck between two clips. Cut between them to enter the lumen of the gallbladder and insert the suction device to aspirate the bile and allow extraction of the gallbladder.

5. If the gallbladder has a large stone load that prevents extraction, open the exteriorized neck, aspirate the bile and insert a Desjardins or Spencer–Wells forceps into the gallbladder lumen to crush or extract the stones. The disadvantages of this technique include the risk of perforating the fundus of the gallbladder, stone spillage and wound contamination.

6. Large forceps (Spencer–Wells) can be inserted down the outside of the partially extracted gallbladder. When you see the tips laparoscopically in the abdominal cavity, open the forceps. This may stretch the port site sufficiently to allow removal of the gallbladder.

7. A cutdown may be required for larger stones (> 3 cm) that are heavily calcified or impacted. Take care to suture-repair the defect in the linea alba to prevent subsequent herniation.

8. Some surgeons routinely place the gallbladder in a retrieval bag before removal. We particularly recommend it if the gallbladder has been perforated during the procedure or is very distended with bile or stones, as it minimizes the risk of perforation and spillage during extraction. A number of bags are available, some attached to introducing instruments – we use a Bert bag. Moisten a fabric bag with saline to ease its manipulation. Insert fine grasping forceps into the base of the bag and then twist it around the shaft of the forceps. Insert the bag and forceps through the epigastric port and place it on top of the liver. Unfurl the bag and have your assistant grab one edge of the open end with grasping forceps in the lateral port while you grab the other edge to open out the bag. Using the forceps in the right upper quadrant port, guide the gallbladder into the bag fundus first. Grab the edges of the retrieval bag in alligator forceps and extract both the bag and gallbladder in the manner described above; increased traction may now be safely applied as bags are made of very strong material.

Checklist

1. Re-establish the pneumoperitoneum after extracting the gallbladder, and insert the laparoscope to make a final check for bleeding or bile leak.

2. Check there is no previously unnoticed damage to other organs, including the liver (lacerations or tears), transverse colon and duodenum (diathermy burns), and small bowel (trocar injuries).

Closure

1. *Drains*. Many surgeons do not use a subhepatic drain after routine laparoscopic cholecystectomy unless there is concern about bleeding or bile leakage. Routine drainage overnight has the advantage of detecting the occasional postoperative bile leak at an early stage, thus avoiding inappropriate early discharge from hospital. A drain (suction or non-suction) can be inserted through the lateral or right upper quadrant port and placed in the subhepatic space with grasping forceps in the epigastric port. Secure the drain to the skin with a suture.

2. Remove the cannulas under vision and ensure there is no bleeding from the abdominal wall puncture sites.

3. Deflate the pneumoperitoneum as much as possible to reduce postoperative referred pain to the shoulder.

4. Close wounds greater than 1 cm in the linea alba under direct vision with 0 polyglactin 910 or PDS to avoid subsequent hernia formation.

5. Infiltrate the skin wounds with long-acting local anaesthetic (bupivacaine) and approximate the edges using subcuticular absorbable sutures, skin tapes or staples.

Postoperative

1. Remove the nasogastric tube at the end of the operation.

2. Following reversal of muscle relaxation and extubation, insert an oropharyngeal airway. Administer oxygen by mask for the first 3 hours.

3. Remove the drain, if inserted, on the day following surgery if there is no bile in it and minimal blood loss (< 50 ml/24 h) has occurred.

4. The majority of patients are ready for discharge from hospital on the day following operation.

? Difficulty?

1. Convert to an open operation if laparoscopic cholecystectomy proves to be too difficult, if bleeding cannot be controlled or if visceral damage occurs.

2. If a thin-walled gallbladder is perforated during the procedure, bile and often also small stones spill into the peritoneal cavity. Insert the suction device into the perforation to aspirate the gallbladder to dryness before aspirating as much of the escaped bile as possible. Multiple small stones may be more easily aspirated using a 10 mm suction device. Prevent further escape of stones by closing the perforation with grasping forceps or metal clips. Try to locate and remove all stones from the peritoneal cavity. Larger stones may be placed in a retrieval bag (with the gallbladder) for extraction.

3. *Retrograde (fundus first) cholecystectomy*. This may be a useful technique in experienced hands when the gallbladder is acutely inflamed or when dense adhesions distort Calot's triangle. Use it with caution and not as an alternative to conversion to open operation, if this appears necessary. Insert a retractor through the lateral port. Position it under the liver to the left of the gallbladder and lift up the liver edge. It is then possible to start the dissection at the fundus of the gallbladder and work down towards its neck. Mobilize the gallbladder fully. Retract the mobilized gallbladder laterally and in a caudal direction to open out Calot's triangle, which assists in identification of the anatomy. Heavier bleeding than usual may occur during dissection of the gallbladder, since the cystic artery is patent.

4. *Partial cholecystectomy*. In chronic fibrotic cholecystitis, when the gallbladder is very adherent to the liver, dissection of the gallbladder can result in significant bleeding and damage to the hepatic parenchyma. In this situation, it is acceptable to perform an incomplete cholecystectomy. After dividing the cystic duct, use scissors to open the gallbladder close to its border with the liver. Aspirate the gallbladder to dryness and remove any stones with grasping forceps or suction. Cut along the gallbladder wall close to its junction with the liver. Follow this all the way round so leaving the back wall of the gallbladder in situ. Diathermize the mucosal surface of the residual gallbladder with coagulating diathermy to prevent mucus production.

5. *Subtotal cholecystectomy*. If Calot's triangle is obliterated or considered hazardous to dissect, divide the gallbladder with scissors at the level of Hartmann's pouch. Extract stones and place them in a retrieval bag, and aspirate bile. It is usually possible at this stage to dissect out a short length of Hartmann's pouch/cystic duct, which can be ligated with an endoloop or alternatively oversewn. Dissect the body and fundus of the gallbladder from the liver in the usual way and place it in a bag for extraction.

Complications

1. *Bile leak*. If a drain has been placed then this complication is usually recognized by the presence of bile in the drain bottle on the day following surgery. In the absence of a drain the patient may be discharged from hospital only to return unwell 3–5 days following operation with pain and tenderness in the right upper quadrant of the abdomen and jaundice. Biliary leaks may arise from the cystic duct stump, divided cystohepatic duct (of Luschka) in the gallbladder bed or injury to a major bile duct (see below).

An ultrasound or CT scan will determine the size and position of any intra-abdominal collections, which can also be drained under imaging control. If a significant bile leak continues after drainage, undertake early ERCP to demonstrate the site of the leak and determine if any significant bile duct injury has occurred. The majority of minor biliary leaks will seal in time with external drainage alone; however, a temporary biliary stent inserted endoscopically will decompress the biliary system, hasten closure of the leak and shorten hospital stay.

2. *Major bile duct injury*. The incidence of bile duct injury was initially higher following laparoscopic cholecystectomy than after open surgery, but the incidence is now comparable at 1 in 300–500 operations. Major bile duct injuries include complete transections and clipping the common duct.

Key point

- The management of major bile duct injuries is complex and best dealt with in a unit specializing in their treatment.

FURTHER READING

Gallegos N 1998 Biliary tract and gallbladder: laparoscopic cholecyst-ectomy. In: Hobsley M, Treasure T, Northover J (eds) Laparoscopic surgery. The implications of changing practice. Edward Arnold, London

Nathanson LK, Easter DW, Cuschieri A 1991 Laparoscopic cholecystectomy: the Dundee technique. British Journal of Surgery 78: 155–159

Pancreas

R. C. N. Williamson and V. Usatoff

Contents

Introduction
Laparotomy for acute pancreatitis
Principles of surgery for pancreatic cancer
Laparotomy for islet cell tumour

INTRODUCTION

Operations on the pancreas are some of the most challenging in abdominal surgery for the following reasons.

1. The pancreas is relatively inaccessible in its retroperitoneal position. The neck, body and tail of pancreas lie behind the lesser sac while the head is obscured by the greater omentum and transverse colon. Thus the approach to the pancreas requires a good deal of mobilization (Fig. 16.1).

2. The pancreas is intimately related to major blood vessels, notably the splenic and superior mesenteric veins, which unite to form the portal vein behind its neck. Adherence to the superior mesenteric vessels can make for a difficult dissection in inflammatory or neoplastic diseases of the pancreas. The pancreas has a rich arterial supply: the right pancreas (head) receives blood from the pancreatico-duodenal arcades and the left pancreas (body and tail) from the splenic artery. Its venous drainage to the portal system is by a number of quite large but thin-walled veins.

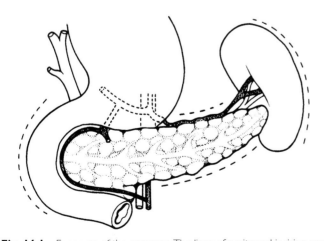

Fig. 16.1 Exposure of the pancreas. The lines of peritoneal incision are shown. The head and neck of pancreas and uncinate lobe are supplied by the superior and inferior pancreaticoduodenal arteries, and the body and tail by the splenic artery.

3. Shared blood supply and a close anatomical relationship mean that adjacent organs are routinely removed as part of a pancreatic resection. Thus the spleen is generally included in a distal pancreat-ectomy. More importantly, the duodenum and lower bile duct are excised during proximal pancreatectomy, necessitating a complex reconstruction thereafter.

4. Resection of the head of the pancreas is followed by anastomosis between the pancreatic stump (a solid organ) and a hollow tube, gener-ally the jejunum. If this anastomosis leaks, powerful digestive enzymes are liberated in active form and can cause severe tissue destruction.

5. Acute and chronic pancreatitis are some of the most difficult inflammatory conditions to manage anywhere in the body. Likewise, pancreatic cancer is often advanced by the time of diagnosis and its surgical eradication requires an extensive operation.

6. Diseases of the head of pancreas commonly present with obstructive jaundice. The function of many of the body's systems is impaired in deeply jaundiced patients, notably the kidney, the reticulo-endothelial system and coagulation pathways, as well as the liver itself. Thus special precautions are required when undertaking major procedures on such patients.

LAPAROTOMY FOR ACUTE PANCREATITIS

Appraise

Diagnostic laparotomy may be undertaken to determine the cause of generalized or upper abdominal peritonitis. Perhaps acute peritonitis has not been suspected, or the elevation of serum amylase is not enough to be pathognomonic. Other surgical emergencies such as perforated peptic ulcer, small bowel infarction and leaking aortic aneurysm can also cause a raised serum amylase level.

Prepare

1. Hypovolaemia is a consistent feature of acute pancreatitis and may be profound. Make sure that the fluid depletion has been fully corrected by intravenous administration of colloid and crystalloid solutions before embarking on the operation. Monitor the central venous pressure and urine output during resuscitation in the elderly or those with severe fluid loss.

2. Look for and treat early complications such as hypoxaemia, hypocalcaemia and incipient renal failure.

3. Cover the operation with broad spectrum antibiotics.

Access

1. If the cause of peritonitis was uncertain, the patient is likely to have had a midline or right paramedian incision performed for abdominal

exploration. If necessary extend the incision upwards to permit examination of the biliary apparatus and pancreas.

2. When operating for established pancreatitis use a transverse ('gable') incision.

Assess

1. Bloodstained free fluid is usually present in the abdominal cavity in acute pancreatitis. Whitish plaques of fat necrosis are visible on serosal surfaces, especially in the region of the pancreas.

2. Lift up the greater omentum and transverse colon. There is oedema and blackish discoloration of the retroperitoneal tissues. The pancreas itself is swollen and may be haemorrhagic or even necrotic.

3. Examine the gallbladder and, if possible, the bile duct to determine if these organs are diseased. A more thorough examination is required if the patient has obstructive jaundice.

4. In a case of infected pancreatic necrosis, the full assessment requires an extensive exploration is the retroperitoneal tissues (see below).

Action

For diagnostic laparotomy

Once the diagnosis has been made, do nothing unless there is a definite indication. Attempts at debridement of the pancreas at this stage can be disastrous. Formal exploration of the pancreas is usually unnecessary to obtain a diagnosis and may be meddlesome.

For infected pancreatic necrosis

1. Enter the lesser sac by dividing the greater omentum. Often the lesser sac is obliterated by the inflammatory process and one quickly enters a large cavity containing pus and necrotic debris. Although the pancreas itself can undergo haemorrhagic infarction in a severe case of pancreatitis, more often the gland is viable and there is peripancreatic necrosis affecting the retroperitoneal fat.

2. Digitally explore the necrotic cavity, remove dead tissue. Send samples of fluid and necrotic material for bacteriological examination.

3. Check the viability of the small and large intestine.

4. Irrigate the large retroperitoneal cavity thoroughly with warm saline and secure haemostasis.

5. Choose between closing the abdomen with generous drainage and leaving it open as a 'laparostomy' (see pp. 41, 42).

PRINCIPLES OF SURGERY FOR PANCREATIC CANCER

Appraise

1. Ductal adenocarcinoma of the pancreas is both common and difficult to treat. Its cause is largely unknown. Most tumours are irresectable by the time they are diagnosed, and this is particularly so for cancers of the body and tail of pancreas, where early symptoms are scarce and non-specific. A few are treatable by distal pancreatosplenectomy (Fig. 16.2). When the tumour is within the head of pancreas, the patient may present with obstructive jaundice while the tumour is still relatively small and localized.

2. Most patients with cancer of the head of pancreas require laparotomy to confirm the diagnosis, determine the potential

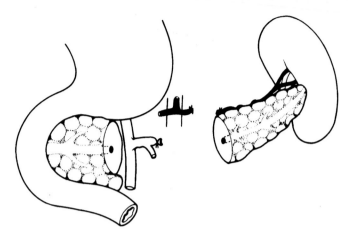

Fig. 16.2   Conventional distal pancreatectomy including splenectomy. Transection just to the right of the portal vein removes about 60% of the gland.

resectability of the tumour and allow a choice to be made between resection and bypass. Despite the scale of the operation required, resectable tumours should be resected in those of reasonable general health, since this policy offers the only chance of cure (Figs 16.3, 16.4).

3. Staging laparoscopy, possibly in combination with laparoscopic ultrasound, will allow detection of peritoneal deposits, small liver metastases and even portal venous invasion, but the number of patients in which this will add extra information above that obtained from conventional imaging is controversial.

4. Most patients with cancer of the body or tail of pancreas do not require laparotomy because the tumour either metastasizes or encases

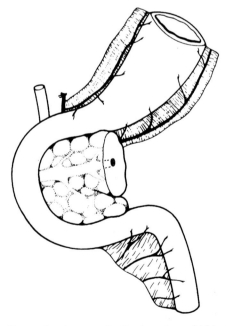

Fig. 16.3   Conventional pancreaticoduodenectomy (Whipple's operation). The resection specimen is shown and includes the distal half of the stomach, the duodenal loop and duodenojejunal flexure, the terminal bile duct and the head and uncinate process of the pancreas.

the superior mesenteric vessels at an early stage and is therefore seldom resectable. Moreover, jaundice and duodenal obstruction occur late if at all.

5. It is debatable whether non-operative stenting or surgical bypass (Fig. 16.5) is the better option for irresectable cancer of the pancreatic head.

Prepare

1. Patients with prolonged obstruction of the extrahepatic biliary tree tolerate major resectional procedures very poorly. The following specific problems should be anticipated and countered:

a. Coagulopathy
b. Hepatorenal syndrome
c. Sepsis
d. Malnutrition
e. Wound failure.

2. Preoperative decompression of the obstructed biliary tree is controversial.

Access

A right subcostal incision will suffice for cholecystojejunostomy alone. If (as usual) further bypass procedures or pancreatectomy are indicated, extend the incision across the midline, dividing both recti to complete a gable incision.

Assess

1. *The gallbladder is distended and there is such diffuse metastatic spread that the patient is unlikely to live very long.* Relieve obstructive jaundice by the simple expedient of cholecystojejunostomy (see Ch. 14). If you are in doubt about the patency of the cystic duct, consider obtaining an operative cholecystogram via a Foley catheter inserted into the fundus. Cholecystojejunostomy is generally best avoided. Patients with carcinomatosis are better served by non-operative stenting, whereas for those with a better prognosis (but irresectable tumours) the use of the common hepatic duct for anastomosis prevents recurrence of jaundice from encroachment of tumour on the cystic duct.

2. *The tumour is clearly irresectable but not as advanced as the above*; alternatively, the gallbladder is collapsed or contains calculi. Do not use the gallbladder for anastomosis. More lasting biliary diversion is achieved by choledochojejunostomy Roux-en-Y (see Ch. 10), dividing the bile duct above the 'leading edge' of tumour to limit upward spread. Cholecystectomy generally facilitates the operation and is certainly advisable if the gallbladder is obstructed.

3. *The tumour could be resectable and there is no overt metastasis.* Embark on a trial dissection.

4. *You have decided against resection.* Be sure that you obtain a positive tissue diagnosis by appropriate biopsy with frozen-section confirmation. Palliative procedures should be considered to relieve jaundice, vomiting and pain. Carry out biliary diversion as described in 1 and 2 above.

5. In *younger patients with locally advanced disease*, palliative resection may provide the best solution for control of jaundice and pain.

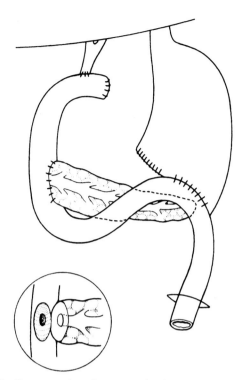

Fig. 16.4 Reconstruction after conventional pancreaticoduodenectomy with an end-to-side pancreaticojejunostomy. To create the pancreatic anastomosis (inset), the pancreatic duct is sutured directly to the jejunal mucosa; the anastomosis can be splinted by a fine polythene tube.

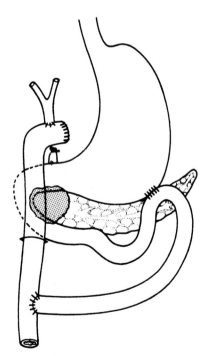

Fig. 16.5 Bypass procedures for an irresectable carcinoma of the head of pancreas. The bile duct is transected well above the tumour, cholecystectomy is performed and biliary drainage is achieved by hepaticojejunostomy Roux-en-Y. An antecolic gastroenterostomy is included.

Aftercare

1. Watch the patient closely for the first 48 hours after this major procedure. Check the postoperative haemoglobin levels and correct any anaemia promptly. Monitor the serum amylase level also, together with urea and electrolytes.

2. Keep a close eye on the drain output. Brownish fluid may indicate a developing pancreatic fistula and a high amylase level in the effluent will confirm this fact.

3. Pancreatic stents should drain a variable quantity of clear juice but if they slip out into the jejunum the fluid becomes bile-stained. Consider performing an X-ray down the tube after 5–7 days. Thereafter it may well be possible to clamp the tube before removing it at 10–12 days.

4. Some surgeons give octreotide routinely for 5–7 days postoperatively (100 µg tds s.c.), starting immediately before operation. Others reserve the drug for 'high-risk anastomoses', i.e. those with a soft pancreas and a tiny duct, which are especially prone to leak.

LAPAROTOMY FOR ISLET CELL TUMOUR

Appraise

1. *Insulinoma* is the commonest islet cell tumour. It is usually solitary and benign. It presents with episodic hypoglycaemia and the diagnosis is confirmed by finding a low blood sugar and an inappropriately high serum insulin either spontaneously or after provocation by fasting. Most insulinomas are sufficiently vascular to be localized as a 'blush' on selective pancreatic arteriography. Local excision is sufficient.

2. *Gastrinoma* can arise in the pancreas, the duodenal wall or sometimes further afield. It presents with the Zollinger–Ellison syndrome of intractable peptic ulceration and diarrhoea. The best surgical treatment is to identify and resect all tumour tissue, but subtotal or even total gastrectomy is sometimes required.

3. Glucagonoma, somatostatinoma and other hormone-secreting tumours are rare entities, but a commoner condition is the *nonfunctioning neuroendocrine tumour* of the pancreas.

FURTHER READING

Aldridge MC, Williamson RCN 1991 Distal pancreatectomy with and without splenectomy. British Journal of Surgery 78: 976–979

Boyle TJ, Williamson RCN 1994 Bypass procedures. Current Practice in Surgery 6: 154–160

Bradley EL III 1987 Management of infected pancreatic necrosis by open drainage. Annals of Surgery 206: 542–550

British Society of Gastroenterology 1998 United Kingdom guidelines for the management of acute pancreatitis. United Kingdom guidelines for the management of acute pancreatitis. Gut 42 (Suppl 2): S1–S13

Cooper MJ, Williamson RCN 1984 Drainage operations in chronic pancreatitis. British Journal of Surgery 71: 761–766

Grant CS 1998 Insulinoma. Surgical Clinics of North America 7(4): 819–844

Keighley MRB, Moore S, Thompson H 1984 The place of 'fine needle' aspiration cytology for the intraoperative diagnosis of pancreatic malignancy. Annals of the Royal College of Surgeons of England 66: 405–408

Kozarek RA, Taverso LW 1996 Pancreatic fistulas: etiology, consequences and treatment. Gastroenterologist 4(4): 238–244

Merchant NB, Conlon KC 1998 Laparoscopic evaluation in pancreatic cancer. Seminars in Surgical Oncology 15(3): 155–165

Poston GJ, Williamson RCN 1990 Surgical management of acute pancreatitis. British Journal of Surgery 77: 5–12

Schoenberg MH, Rau B, Beger HG 1999 New approaches in surgical management of severe acute pancreatitis. Digestion 60 (Suppl S1): 22–26

Trede M, Schwall G 1988 The complications of pancreatectomy. Annals of Surgery 207: 39–47

Watanapa P, Williamson RCN 1992 Surgical palliation for pancreatic cancer: developments during the past two decades. British Journal of Surgery 79: 8–20

Williamson RCN, Cooper MJ 1987 Resection in chronic pancreatitis. British Journal of Surgery 74: 807–812

Liver and portal venous system

K. E. F. Hobbs and S. Bhattacharya

Contents

INTRODUCTION

The liver is considered by many surgeons to be a hallowed organ, and one that presents them with insurmountable problems. They fear massive haemorrhage after any violation of the capsule and dread the thought of attempting any elective procedure. These are unfounded myths – the liver is as amenable to surgery as any other organ, providing certain principles are respected.

TRAUMA

The most frequent and frightening procedure you are called upon to perform on the liver is to arrest haemorrhage following trauma or spontaneous rupture of a tumour. Injuries to the liver can occur as a result of penetrating trauma such as stab or gunshot injuries (which usually result in liver laceration, though high-velocity bullets can cause significant contusion as well), or of blunt trauma, often sustained in road traffic accidents (this is usually associated with contusions and haematomas). Contusion carries a very high mortality rate, which is directly related to the severity and number of other affected organs. For recent reviews of the management of liver trauma refer to the papers by Watson[1] and Krige.[2]

Appraise

1. A patient may well present in a shocked state with an obvious history. Concentrate your initial attention on maintaining the patient's airway, breathing and circulation, in keeping with advanced trauma life support (ATLS) principles. Then turn your attention to the patient's internal bleeding.

2. If you are in doubt about possible intra-abdominal bleeding in a severely shocked patient, obtain a contrast-enhanced computed tomography (CT) scan, if it is available and can be done without undue delay – it will provide an accurate demonstration of liver parenchymal injury. An emergency portable abdominal ultrasound (US) can also demonstrate a ruptured liver.

3. Treat penetrating injuries in general, and gunshot wounds in particular, by laparotomy. Only a small number of selected patients with stab injury who are haemodynamically stable and in whom no hollow viscus perforation is suspected can be treated conservatively. On the other hand, treat conservatively those patients with blunt trauma who are haemodynamically stable, even if there is demonstrable liver injury on CT or US. Only the shocked patient who does not respond adequately despite aggressive initial fluid replacement requires urgent laparotomy. The conservative approach, however, requires repeated clinical assessment and repeated scans. If the patient develops haemodynamic instability or signs of developing peritonitis, proceed to a laparotomy.

> **Key point**
>
> - A patient with an occult liver tumour that ruptures spontaneously may present with shock and a distending abdomen, or an 'acute abdomen of unknown cause', and require urgent laparotomy.

Exploration of a damaged liver

Prepare

1. You are about to embark on a major surgical procedure, which carries a high mortality rate. As far as possible, ensure you have an experienced anaesthetist, a good assistant and an experienced scrub nurse. Have an intensive care unit bed available for the patient should it be needed postoperatively.

2. Pass a bladder catheter. To avoid the complication of hepato-renal failure it is important to ensure that urine flow continues during major liver surgery. This is done by giving adequate fluid volume replacement. An infusion of dopamine 2.5 µg/kg/min through a central venous catheter may help.

3. Place a central venous line and, if facilities permit, an arterial catheter to allow constant measurement of arterial pressure.

4. Ensure there is plenty of blood available (at least 12 units) together with fresh frozen plasma (FFP) and platelets to replace lost clotting products.

Access

1. If the diagnosis is suspected preoperatively, then use a right subcostal incision 3 cm below the costal margin. If necessary the incision can be extended across the midline 3 cm below the left costal margin as an inverted 'V' or vertically upwards as a low sternal split. If you need to gain access above the liver, make another incision in

the 10th rib bed from the anterior axillary line to the original subcostal incision, joining it at right angles. This allows you to open the chest, divide the costal margin and so gain control of the inferior vena cava above the diaphragm.

2. If you discover the rupture at diagnostic laparotomy through a midline incision, extend this to the costal margin to gain access and assess the need for further extensions.

3. If you discover the rupture through a totally inappropriate lower abdominal incision, close it and re-explore through a more appropriate incision.

4. The use of a self-retaining retractor that can be fixed to the operating table and provides forcible upward retraction of the costal margins, e.g. a Thompson's retractor (Rocialle Medical), can make a crucial difference. Such retraction reduces the need for manual assistance, greatly improves access and usually eliminates the need for thoracic extensions. If you have a Thompson's (or similar) retractor available, use it.

Assess

1. There is usually much blood clot in the peritoneal cavity and probably some fresh bleeding. Remove clot with your hands and with the help of a sucker.

2. Look systematically for damage to the liver, the gut from oesophagus to rectum, the spleen, the pancreas, the anterior and posterior abdominal wall and the diaphragm.

Action

1. If there is obvious damage and haemorrhage from other intra-abdominal viscera, surround the bleeding area of the liver with large sterile packs and have an assistant apply gentle pressure to control the bleeding. Attend to the lesions in the other organs first.

2. Remove blood and blood clot to gain adequate exposure of the bleeding area of the liver. Control the haemorrhage. Most patients do not require major surgical procedures. Attempt only the minimum surgery necessary to control haemorrhage. Avoid exploration and rough handling of injuries that are not bleeding at the time of exploration despite a normal blood pressure.

⚷ Key point

- Your primary aims are – in this order – to stop the bleeding, remove obviously devitalized liver tissue and stop bile leaks.

---

3. Explore the tear of the liver locally and remove any avascular tissue. If the laceration is still bleeding and extends deeply into the liver parenchyma, gently explore the depth of the wound but avoid creating further damage. This procedure is very important in contusion injuries, for major branches of the liver vessels may be ruptured, producing large areas of devascularized tissue. Do not be tempted to explore tears that are not bleeding – you only encourage further bleeding.

4. Identify bleeding points and apply fine haemostats. Ligate with fine synthetic absorbable material such as polyglactin 910 or polydioxane sulphate (PDS) or use titanium clips. Suture-ligate larger vessels with PDS or polyglactin 910.

5. If there is vascular oozing from a large raw area of liver, cover this with one layer of absorbable haemostatic gauze and apply a pack. Avoid using deep mattress sutures to control such bleeding, for they may produce areas of devascularized tissue which will predispose to subsequent infection.

❓ Difficulty?

1. Is there uncontrolled haemorrhage from a torn liver? If haemorrhage is massive, attempt to control it by inserting a finger through the opening into the lesser sac behind the hepatic hilar structures and apply a Satinsky or other vascular clamp across them (if vascular clamps are not available in a real emergency, use a non-crushing intestinal clamp with great care). This is called the Pringle manoeuvre and it will stop bleeding from branches of the hepatic artery or portal vein. Try to identify any large vessels crossing the tear in the liver and ligate them or suture any tears in their walls. If bleeding persists despite the Pringle manoeuvre, either the patient has an aberrant arterial supply (an accessory left hepatic artery to the left lobe, or an aberrant right hepatic artery arising from the superior mesenteric), or – more commonly – the bleeding is from the hepatic veins or the inferior vena cava. Injuries involving the major hepatic veins or the inferior vena cava are very difficult to treat and even in the hands of experienced liver surgeons these are associated with a high mortality rate. After clamping the liver hilar vessels, remember that, although a normal liver can tolerate normothermic ischaemia for up to 1 hour, the hilar clamping is best released every 15 minutes. Have an operating room attendant 'clock watch' for you. Before releasing any vascular clamps following prolonged clamping, warn the anaesthetist, who may wish to take measures against the effects of massive acidosis and potassium release, which can cause cardiac arrest.

2. Packing. If you cannot achieve control using these techniques, do not attempt a major resection as an emergency procedure without the assistance of an experienced hepatic surgeon. In these circumstances it is better to obtain control of the bleeding by packing around the liver with gauze rolls. Do not insert gauze into the depths of the laceration in the liver. Place the packs above, behind and below the liver to gently compress the bleeding areas. Then close the abdomen. This gives you time to assess the next move and possibly to carry out a contrast-enhanced CT scan and a hepatic angiogram. You may then choose to re-explore in 48-72 hours to remove the packs and re-assess, or transfer the patient to a specialist surgery unit.

Check

1. When you have gained control of the bleeding from the liver, carry out a full, careful and gentle exploration for other intraperitoneal injuries if you have not done so already. Explore the entire gut from the oesophagus to rectum and pay special attention to the retroperitoneal duodenum. Explore the pancreas and the spleen carefully.

2. When you are certain that haemorrhage is controlled and that other lesions have been attended to in the appropriate manner, unless you have had to pack the liver to control haemorrhage, inspect it again. If there are devascularized areas, they will need to be removed to prevent infection but if you have had no experience of liver resection operations it is safer to close the abdomen and either transfer the patient to an experienced colleague or seek advice before re-exploring the liver yourself after a few days when the patient's condition is

stable. If you find bile leaking from damaged intrahepatic bile ducts, ligate or suture them. Carry out a gentle, large-volume saline lavage of the peritoneal cavity to help reduce subsequent infection.

Closure

Close the abdomen 'en masse' in a standard fashion. The insertion of a peritoneal drain is controversial. If you have operated on any part of the biliary tract then insert a drain, preferably a closed-system drain. If there is only liver parenchymal damage then a drain is probably unnecessary unless there is an obvious biliary leak.

Aftercare

Admit the patient to an intensive care unit or high-dependency nursing area. If further surgery is going to be needed (e.g. because you have had to employ packing to control haemorrhage), arrange for transfer to a unit experienced in handling major liver trauma if possible.

> **Key point**
>
> - If you are in any doubt about further bleeding or sepsis, re-exploration is safer than waiting. If you fail to recognize and treat it, the patient may die.

REFERENCES

1. Watson CJE, Calne RY, Padhani AR, Dixon AR 1991 Surgical restraint in the management of liver trauma. British Journal of Surgery 78: 1071–1075
2. Krige JE, Bornman PC, Terblanche J 1997 Liver trauma in 446 patients. South African Journal of Surgery 35(1): 10–15

PRINCIPLES OF ELECTIVE SURGERY

Appraise

> **Key point**
>
> - Complex hepatic surgery should, as far as possible, be carried out in specialist units.

1. Do not undertake an elective operation on the liver without complete preoperative investigation and a fairly certain working diagnosis. Occasionally, an isolated hepatic lesion may be identified during a scan carried out for another reason or during a laparotomy. In this last case consider carefully before trying to excise or biopsy the lesion. You could run into serious problems if you have no idea of its nature. Operation on a patient with a severely impaired liver can be very hazardous and accompanied by a high morbidity and mortality.

2. Before undertaking any operative procedure on a patient with a liver disease, check the blood film, platelet count and clotting profile. Correct these if possible by giving blood products. Rarely are platelet infusions necessary, but all patients undergoing liver surgery, especially if jaundiced or with severe biochemical dysfunction, benefit from injec-

tions of vitamin K_1. If the clotting profile is badly deranged, the patient may need an infusion of FFP and occasionally cryoprecipitate.

OPERATIVE LIVER BIOPSY

Prepare

This is rarely carried out as an isolated procedure. Check the patient's blood group. If you anticipate a more major procedure than a simple biopsy, cross-match an adequate quantity of blood and platelets and have available some FFP for replacement therapy during surgery.

Action

1. Always take the liver biopsy at an early stage during any laparotomy. Prolonged trauma to the liver during laparotomy can produce changes that make histological interpretation of the specimen difficult.

2. Select an area of diseased liver or an edge that presents easily through the incision.

3. Place two mattress stitches using 3/0 polyglactin 910 or PDS on an atraumatic round-bodied needle to form a V, the apex of this pointing towards the hilum of the liver (Fig. 17.1a).

4. Gently but firmly tie these stitches (Fig. 17.1b) and remove the wedge of tissue between them with a sharp knife (Fig. 17.1c). The cut edges of the liver should be dry. Insert another suture of similar material if haemostasis is not complete or use diathermy coagulation to establish haemostasis.

5. You may also use a Tru-cut® needle to take a liver biopsy. If you are not used to the needle, rehearse your movements before you actually insert the needle into the liver. After removing the needle, check that you have an adequate core of tissue. Gently shake or tease the core of tissue into a pot of formalin, taking care not to crush it. The puncture site occasionally requires a figure-of-eight or Z stitch with 4/0 polyglactin 910 or PDS to obtain haemostasis

6. Complete your examination of all abdominal structures.

7. Close the incision in the standard way.

NEOPLASMS

Appraise

1. Neoplastic lesions in the liver can be solid or cystic, benign or malignant. The latter can be primary or secondary and all can be single or multiple.

2. Not every neoplasm requires excision once it can be proved that it is benign, unless it is causing symptoms. However, patients with malignant, suspected malignant or symptomatic benign disease should be considered for laparotomy.

3. Wedge excision of solitary liver lesion.

4. Right or left hepatectomy.

SURGICAL MANAGEMENT OF HAEMORRHAGE FROM OESOPHAGEAL VARICES

The most life-threatening complication of portal hypertension that requires surgical treatment is bleeding from oesophageal varices.

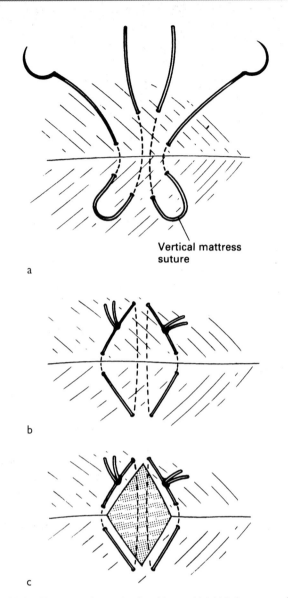

Vertical mattress
suture

a

b

c

Fig. 17.1 Technique for wedge liver biopsy: (a) initial placement of two mattress stitches; (b) tie each firmly; (c) remove the wedge of tissue between them.

While the majority of patients do stop bleeding spontaneously, the in-hospital mortality from the first bleed is in the region of 50%. Management is complex and should ideally be undertaken by a team that includes a medical hepatologist, a specialist radiologist and a surgeon. A good review of this is to be found in a paper by Stanley.[1] For extensive overviews of portal hypertension and its management, refer to the recent editions of textbooks of hepatology by Bircher et al[2] and Sherlock.[3]

Management

1. Aim to resuscitate the patient, find the cause of the bleeding and stop it. These three processes must be carried out in parallel.

2. Endoscope a patient admitted to hospital with massive upper gastrointestinal haemorrhage. This is the most certain way of discovering if bleeding is from ruptured oesophageal varices.

3. If variceal bleeding is confirmed at endoscopy, perform sclerotherapy

4. If this fails, control bleeding for up to 24 hours maximum by

> **🔑 Key point**
>
> • Although a previous history and clinical examination may suggest variceal bleed, direct visualization of the bleeding area is mandatory before undertaking treatment, since some patients, especially alcoholics with known varices, bleed from other gastrointestinal lesions.

oesophagogastric tamponade using an orogastric triple lumen balloon tube (Sengstaken–Blakemore tube).

5. If variceal bleeding persists despite the measures outlined above, next consider performing a TIPSS, i.e. a transjugular intrahepatic porta-systemic shunt, provided the necessary expertise is available.

6. If TIPSS is not available, after resuscitation and full assessment, decide if a surgical procedure is required. This can be either a 'veno-occlusive' procedure designed to stop the venous haemorrhage, such as oesophageal disconnection or oesophagogastric devascularization, or a 'portal decompression' procedure, namely a porta-systemic shunt.

Oesophagogastric disconnection

This is best achieved using a circular stapling device. The head of the stapling instrument is introduced through an incision in the anterior stomach wall and opened in the lower oesophagus. An encircling ligature is tied incorporating the oesophagus and veins within the opened jaws of the device, between the staple cartridge and the anvil. The device is closed and activated, transecting the lower oesophagus and the veins. Simultaneously the ends are re-anastomosed with two concentric rows of staples.

Portal decompression

Portacaval shunt was formerly the most frequently performed procedure. The portal vein is ligated and divided close to its entrance into the liver. The distal cut end is anastomosed end to side into the inferior vena cava. This allows portal vein blood to bypass the liver. More frequently other forms of shunt are created. These are:

1. *Mesocaval shunt* is created by inserting a graft joining the superior mesenteric vein to the inferior vena cava.
2. *Proximal splenorenal shunt.* The spleen is removed and the distal end of the splenic vein is joined into the left renal vein.
3. *Distal splenorenal (Warren) shunt.* The splenic vein is ligated and transected without removing the spleen and the distal cut end is anastomosed to the left renal vein.

REFERENCES

1. Stanley AJ, Hayes PC 1997 Portal hypertension and variceal haemorrhage. Lancet 350(9086): 1235–1239
2. Bircher J, Benhamou J-P, McIntyre N et al (eds) 1999 Oxford textbook of clinical hepatology, 2nd edn. Oxford University Press, Oxford
3. Sherlock S, Dooley J 1997 Diseases of the liver and biliary system, 10th edn. Blackwell Scientific Publications, Oxford

Spleen

R. C. N. Williamson and A. K. Kakkar

Contents
Elective splenectomy
Emergency splenectomy
Conservative splenic surgery

ELECTIVE SPLENECTOMY

Appraise

1. The spleen is an important organ and should not lightly be removed. It has haematological functions in the maturation of red blood cells and the destruction of effete forms. Of greater importance in surgical practice, it has certain immunological functions, notably production of opsonins (tuftsin, properdin) for the phagocytosis of encapsulated bacteria. Where possible, conservation of at least part of the spleen, as opposed to total splenectomy, may protect against serious postsplenectomy sepsis (see below). *Streptococcus pneumoniae* is the commonest infecting organism and less commonly *N. meningitidis* and *H. influenzae*.

2. Elective splenectomy may be indicated for certain lymphomas and leukaemias, for haemolytic anaemias (e.g. acquired autoimmune, hereditary spherocytosis), for idiopathic thrombocytopenic purpura, for other types of splenomegaly with hypersplenism and occasionally for conditions such as cyst, abscess, haemangioma or splenic artery aneurysm.

3. Splenectomy is sometimes carried out as a part of other operations, such as total gastrectomy, radical proximal gastrectomy, distal pancreatectomy and 'conventional' splenorenal shunt.

4. An alternative to elective open splenectomy is laparoscopic splenectomy.

Prepare

1. Patients with hypersplenism, anaemia, thrombocytopenia and coagulopathies require preoperative correction. Immunocompromised patients should receive prophylactic antibiotic cover.

2. Risk of postsplenectomy sepsis necessitates prophylactic immunization against *Streptococcus pneumoniae*, *Haemophilus influenzae* type b and meningococcal strains A and C. Vaccination should be given 3–4 weeks before operation, except in children under the age of 2 years or those who are immunocompromised (e.g. patients with Hodgkin's disease who have received extensive chemotherapy).

3. Consent of the patient should include advice on the risks of postsplenectomy sepsis.

Access

1. An upper midline, left upper paramedian or left subcostal incision is usually appropriate.

2. Occasionally a left thoracoabdominal approach facilitates the removal of a very large spleen.

3. Staging laparotomy requires a long midline incision.

Assess

1. Explore the whole abdomen, particularly noting the liver and any enlarged lymph nodes and taking appropriate biopsies.

2. Make a careful search for accessory spleens (splenunculi). These are usually to be found near the splenic hilum, in the gastro-splenic ligament or greater omentum. Remove all splenunculi if splenectomy is being undertaken for a blood dyscrasia.

Action

1. If the spleen is enormous, first tie the splenic artery in continuity (Fig. 18.1).

Enter the lesser sac by dividing 8–10 cm of greater omentum between ligatures, keeping to the colic side of the gastroepiploic vessels. Divide the adhesions between the back of the stomach and the front of the pancreas. Palpate along the superior border of the body of pancreas for arterial pulsation. Incise the peritoneum at this point, mobilize the vessel with right-angled forceps and ligate it with 0 or 1 silk. Injection of 1 ml of 1:10 000 adrenaline into the splenic artery

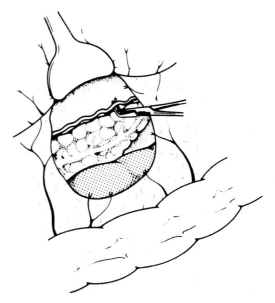

Fig. 18.1 Ligation of the splenic artery at the superior border of the body of pancreas. Part of the greater omentum has been divided, allowing access to the lesser sac.

immediately before ligating it can shrink the size of a massive spleen and facilitate the subsequent dissection.

2. Pass the left hand over the top of the spleen to draw it medially, and retract the left side of the abdominal wall. Coagulate and divide any adhesions between the convex surface of the spleen and the parietal peritoneum.

3. Swab any blood out of the groove behind the spleen, then cut through the peritoneum just lateral to the spleen (left leaf of the lienorenal ligament), slitting it upwards and downwards (Fig. 18.2).

4. Gently mobilize the spleen forwards and medially, using the fingers of the left hand. Identify the left colic flexure and free it from the spleen. Identify the tail of pancreas as it turns forwards into the splenic hilum, and dissect it gently free. Place a pack in the splenic bed while completing the splenectomy.

5. Proceed to free the spleen from its attachments to the diaphragm (avascular) and greater curvature of the stomach (containing the vasa brevia). Carefully incise the anterior peritoneal leaf of the gastro-splenic ligament. Identify, ligate and divide the short gastric vessels, taking care not to include any of the stomach wall in the ligatures. Sometimes it is easier to delay this manoeuvre until you have dealt with the splenic artery and vein.

6. Control the vascular pedicle of the spleen between fingers and thumb and dissect away the fatty tissue to expose the splenic artery and vein.

Doubly clamp, ligate and divide each vessel. Be careful not to injure the tail of pancreas at this point. After dividing the remaining peritoneal attachments (right leaf of the lienorenal ligament) the spleen can be removed. Platelet transfusions may now be given in thrombocytopenic patients.

7. Place a pack in the splenic bed, then remove the pack and obtain haemostasis.

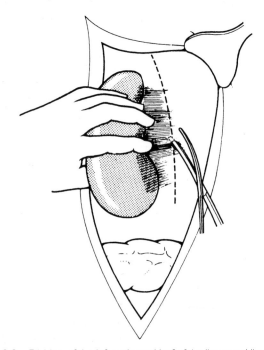

Fig. 18.2 Division of the left peritoneal leaf of the lienorenal ligament as a preliminary to mobilization of the spleen.

🔑	**Key point**

- In dividing and ligating the short gastric vessels during splenic mobilization, care must be taken not to include any of the stomach wall within the sutures. This may otherwise lead to gastric fistula formation.

Closure

1. Remove the pack, inspect the splenic bed and coagulate any oozing vessels.

2. Examine the ligatures on the main vascular pedicles. Make sure that the adjacent viscera are undamaged.

3. Place a suction drain to the splenic bed. If there is an enormous cavity or if the stomach or pancreas have been wounded, a wide-bore tube drain may be preferable.

4. Consider nasogastric intubation for 24–28 hours.

Aftercare

1. Remove the nasogastric tube when gastric aspirates diminish and the drain when it stops draining much.

2. Check the haemoglobin, white cell and platelet counts post-operatively. Leucocytosis and thrombocythaemia nearly always ensue, with peaks at 7–14 days. Persistent leucocytosis and pyrexia may suggest a subphrenic abscess. Consider some form of prophy-lactic anticoagulation if the platelet count exceeds 1000×10^9/l.

3. Immunization with antipneumococcal vaccine should be given if previously overlooked. Children should receive prophylactic penicillin for 2 years to prevent postsplenectomy sepsis. Adults should be advised to take an antibiotic such as amoxycillin at the first sign of any infective illness. Immunocompromised patients should receive either penicillin V (250 mg bd) or amoxycillin (250 mg od) as routine prophylaxis against postsplenectomy sepsis.

Complications

1. *Respiratory*. Chest infection may result from splinting of the left diaphragm causing atelectasis. Vigorous physiotherapy may avoid the need for antibiotics. Occasionally a left pleural effusion requires aspiration.

2. Subphrenic abscess should be suspected if there is fever and leucocytosis. Ultrasonography will confirm the diagnosis and permit percutaneous drainage.

3. Reactive haemorrhage may be caused by a slipped ligature and necessitate reoperation.

4. Gastric or pancreatic fistula is rare. It may close with conser-vative management including parenteral nutrition, but otherwise repeat laparotomy will be needed.

EMERGENCY SPLENECTOMY

Appraise

1. Emergency splenectomy may be indicated for traumatic rupture. Enlarged spleens are at increased risk of rupture, which can even occur spontaneously. Most cases of ruptured spleen follow road traffic accidents. Classically patients are shocked, with pain in the

left hypochondrium and shoulder-tip and evidence of left lower rib fractures. Diagnostic paracentesis may confirm a haemo peritoneum, and urgent laparotomy is normally required after initial resuscitation.

2. Some minor splenic injuries can be managed conservatively with vigilant clinical observation and blood transfusion. Appropriate patients are less than 60 years of age, haemodynamically stable, with a blood transfusion requirement not exceeding 3–4 units and CT scan evidence that the spleen has not been fragmented. Failure of conservative treatment is indicated by renewed evidence of bleeding or spreading peritonism; laparotomy is then required forthwith.

3. Accidental splenic injury sustained during operations such as vagotomy or left hemicolectomy used to be an indication for splenectomy, but the bleeding can usually be controlled by lesser means.

Access

Use a midline upper abdominal incision. Do not hesitate to make a T-shaped extension towards the left costal margin if access is difficult and the patient is exsanguinating.

Assess

1. First check that a ruptured spleen is the source of bleeding. It is often easier to feel than to see whether the spleen is intact.

2. Remove or repair a ruptured spleen without further ado, postponing exploration of the rest of the abdomen until later.

3. Particularly in young children try to avoid total splenectomy if at all possible, because they are at particular risk of postsplenectomy sepsis. If the spleen is shattered or bleeding profusely, however, you have no alternative but to remove it promptly to save life.

Action

1. Quickly but carefully mobilize the spleen and bring it forwards into the abdominal wound. In ruptured spleen it is often possible to break down the left peritoneal leaf of the lienorenal ligament using your fingers. If splenic repair is at all likely, however, try to avoid further injury to the spleen during this manoeuvre.

2. Once the spleen has been brought up into the wound, compress its vascular pedicle between finger and thumb to control the bleeding. Inspect the organ thoroughly and assess the extent of damage.

3. If total splenectomy is inevitable, proceed as for an elective operation, securing the splenic artery and vein at an early stage. Consider placing thin slices of splenic tissue in omental pockets at the end of the operation to encourage splenic regeneration (splenosis). Conservative splenic operations are sometimes indicated.

Key point

- In emergency splenectomy a good view is essential. The left costal margin must be lifted by a retractor, and you should scoop and suck blood and clot from the left hypochondrium. Control the splenic hilar vessels with your hand if necessary to stop bleeding.

Difficulty?

1. The patient is bleeding to death from the spleen, but you cannot identify the precise source of haemorrhage. There may not be time to summon senior help. Consider extending the incision as described above. Place your hand over the top of the spleen, break down its posterior attachments and deliver it into the wound as quickly as possible. Now compress or clamp the pedicle, and you will bring the situation under control.

2. You have inadvertently injured the stomach or pancreas during splenectomy, usually because of inadequate mobilization of the spleen. Remove the spleen and place a pack in the splenic bed. Inspect the damage carefully. Repair a gastric defect in two layers. Repair or resect the tail of pancreas, using non-absorbable sutures. Ask the anaesthetist to insert a nasogastric tube, and drain the splenic bed.

Closure, aftercare and complications

These are essentially the same as for elective splenectomy. Give triple vaccine immunization during the recovery period plus prophylactic penicillin as an additional precaution in children or the immuno-compromised.

CONSERVATIVE SPLENIC SURGERY

Appraise

Following splenectomy there is a 1.0–2.5% risk of developing overwhelming septicaemia from encapsulated bacteria (especially the pneumococcus), usually within 2 years of operation. The mortality rate of postsplenectomy sepsis is high. The risk is higher in young children and after splenectomy for haematological disease, but fatal cases have occasionally been reported in adults after removal of a ruptured spleen.

Non-operative management may be appropriate for lesser degrees of splenic injury, especially in children. Embolization therapy has been attempted in hypersplenism. With these exceptions, alternatives to total splenectomy can only be assessed at laparotomy, but they may be feasible in at least 40% of patients with blunt splenic trauma.

Assess

When a fragmented, avulsed spleen must be removed, consider placing thin slices in omental pockets at the end of the operation to encourage splenic regeneration.

Capsular tears and other minor injuries seldom necessitate splenectomy. If necessary extend the incision in order to inspect the spleen without the need to mobilize it. Application of a haemostatic agent will usually suffice, with or without suturing.

FURTHER READING

Büjükünal C, Danismend N, Yeker D 1987 Spleen-saving procedures in paediatric splenic trauma. British Journal of Surgery 74: 350–352
Clarke PJ, Morris PJ 1994 Surgery of the spleen. In: Morris PJ, Malt RA (eds) Oxford textbook of surgery. Oxford University Press, Oxford, pp 2121–2130

Cooper MJ, Williamson RCN 1983 Splenectomy: indications, hazards and alternatives. British Journal of Surgery 71: 173–180

Gilchrist BF, Trunkey DD 1990 Injuries to the spleen and pancreas. In: Williamson RCN, Cooper MJ (eds) Emergency abdominal surgery. Churchill Livingstone, Edinburgh, pp 36–51

Longo WE, Baker CC, McMillen MA et al 1989 Nonoperative management of adult blunt splenic trauma. Criteria for successful outcome. Annals of Surgery 210: 626–629

Wilhelm MC, Jones RE, McGehee R et al 1988 Splenectomy in hematological disorders. The everchanging indications. Annals of Surgery 207: 581–589

Breast

M. Baum and C. Saunders

Contents

MANAGEMENT OF BREAST SYMPTOMS

Appraise

1. Before describing operative techniques for breast problems it is important to have a scheme of management in mind for patients presenting with a breast complaint to the clinic (Fig. 19.1).

2. Common symptoms include lumps, lumpiness, nipple changes (including inversion, bleeding and discharge) and breast pain. Lumps and nipple changes are discussed below. New nipple inversion, especially in an older woman, is always suspicious of carcinoma. Lumpiness and breast pain are managed medically after exclusion of a carcinoma or other pathology.

3. At the first stage you must make up your mind whether or not a truly discrete lump is present. If, after careful examination, you cannot detect a lump but a diffuse nodularity, then re-examine a younger woman at a different point in the menstrual cycle and reassure her.

4. Refer women over the age of 35 for mammography and/or ultrasound to complement clinical examination of the 'difficult' breast.

5. By contrast, if a discrete lump is detected, it is almost always worthwhile to attempt aspiration since this will differentiate a cyst from a solid lesion. A cytological smear should be prepared from solid lesions as described below. Ideally, an ultrasound should be performed first to differentiate a solid from a cystic lump.

6. Breast cysts can occur at any age but are common in the 35–55 age range. Drainage of the cyst in most cases establishes the diagnosis, 'cures' the condition and offers immediate reassurance to the patient. It is therefore both efficient and humane. It must be emphasized, however, that if the fluid from the cyst is bloody, or if there is a residual

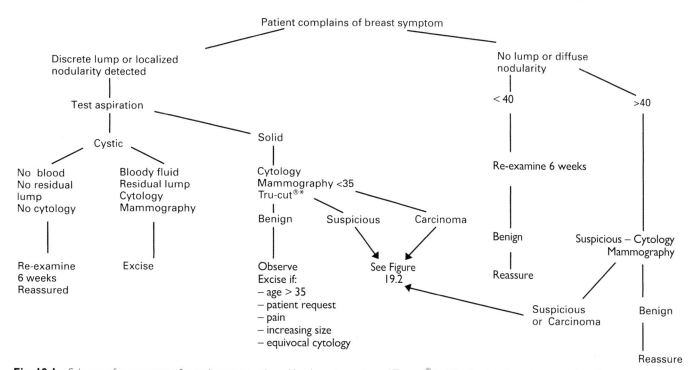

Fig. 19.1   Scheme of management for patients presenting with a breast symptom. *Tru-cut® is difficult unless lump is greater than 2 cm.

lump, then you should perform excision biopsy. Cytology of the cyst fluid is no longer considered a worthwhile procedure unless it is blood-stained or there is a residual mass after aspiration.

7. If the lump is solid with benign cytology excision is indicated if the woman is 35 or older, if the lump increases in size or is associated with pain, or if the cytology is equivocal.

8. It is often helpful to carry out core-cut or Tru-cut® biopsy of the lesion to help make a diagnosis.

9. If the diagnosis remains in doubt, carry out excision biopsy of on the first convenient operation list.

10. Frozen section should rarely be used, as it is better to await results of paraffin section from formal excision biopsy. There may still very occasionally be a place for such a stratagem when the lump is clinically suspicious of cancer, mammography and cytology are equivocal and Tru-cut® biopsy has been unhelpful.

BREAST ABSCESS

Appraise

1. Breast abscess develops most commonly during lactation. Empty the affected breast by manual pressure but permit the child to continue feeding on the opposite breast.

2. Early infection can occasionally be treated with antibiotics only but do not wait for fluctuation, as widespread destruction of the underlying breast tissue may then be found. Antibiotic therapy complicates the clinical picture, in that the abscess is walled-in and may present less acutely. Ascertain preoperatively the point of maximum tenderness and mark the point with a skin pencil. As soon as there is such a point, the time is ripe for operative intervention.

Access

Operate under general anaesthesia with the patient lying on her back and with the arm on the affected side stretched on an arm board. Do not allow traction on the brachial plexus. The arm should not be above a right angle, and the hand and forearm should be supine.

Action

1. Place the incision over the point of maximum tenderness. If this is near the nipple, where the 12–15 major ducts are lying, make a periareolar incision.

2. If pus does not at once pour out, deepen the incision or introduce a syringe with a wide-bore needle attached at varying angles until you obtain pus. Send some pus for culture and antibiotic sensitivities. If necessary, you can later give the appropriate antibiotic.

3. Introduce a gloved finger into the abscess cavity and break down all loculi in the breast tissue by moving the finger in a circular manner. This manoeuvre is necessary, since the abscess may be multiloculated.

4. If the cavity allows, introduce a retractor and examine the walls. Stop any bleeding points with diathermy.

5. Take an adequate biopsy of the cavity wall and send it for histological examination to exclude a carcinoma.

6. Ensure that the original incision is long enough to allow the wound to heal from the deepest parts upwards, otherwise there is a risk of the development of a chronic abscess.

7. A drain may be needed, although it is not strictly necessary if all pus is drained. Loose packing of the cavity is an alternative.

8. Apply a non-adhesive dressing. Advise on wearing a supportive bra. This diminishes the risk of subsequent development of a haematoma.

9. Breast feeding can recommence on both sides as soon as comfortable.

> **Key point**
>
> - Ensure all loculations are broken down so no pus remains in the breast.

MANAGEMENT OF BREAST CARCINOMA

If the diagnosis of carcinoma has been established by preoperative cytology and/or Tru-cut® or core-cut biopsy, then you should counsel the patient about treatment options of breast-conserving surgery, mastectomy or primary medical treatment, as shown in Fig. 19.2.

If the diagnosis is uncertain and the abnormality is palpable, discuss with the patient the need for excision biopsy and awaiting definitive paraffin-section report before discussing treatment options. In screen-detected lesions, if there is no palpable abnormality, proceed to stereo-tactic needle-localized cytology or core-cut biopsy by the Department of Radiology or needle localization biopsy.

Appraise

1. Selected patients with operable breast cancer can be treated with breast-conserving surgery, i.e. quadrantectomy and axillary dissection and breast irradiation, which can provide similar disease control to mastectomy with a superior cosmetic result. Axillary dissection is necessary to properly stage the patient, remove nodal disease and prevent axillary recurrence. The importance of axillary node staging has been heightened by the evidence that adjuvant cytotoxic chemotherapy in premenopausal and some postmenopausal patients can decrease the odds of death by approximately 20%. A similar benefit is seen in postmenopausal patients and premenopausal women with oestrogen-receptor-positive tumours, with the use of adjuvant tamoxifen, but this is irrespective of axillary node status.

2. Modified radical (or Patey) mastectomy provides good loco-regional control, with acceptable morbidity, for patients unsuitable for breast conservation and may be indicated for patients with a large operable primary tumour, multifocal disease or central tumours.

3. Simple mastectomy is an operation rarely indicated in patients with breast cancer. The reasons are that it has very few advantages over a well performed modified radical mastectomy and the major disadvantage of not staging or treating the axilla. The only indications for its performance in patients with breast cancer are for isolated breast recurrence after breast-conserving surgery when the axilla has been previously treated, large phyllodes tumours, multifocal duct carcinoma in situ and for those rare elderly frail women who are medically unfit for a modified radical mastectomy.

4. Mastectomy with immediate reconstruction using either an implant or a myocutaneous flap is being increasingly used by trained breast surgeons, sometimes in conjunction with plastic surgical

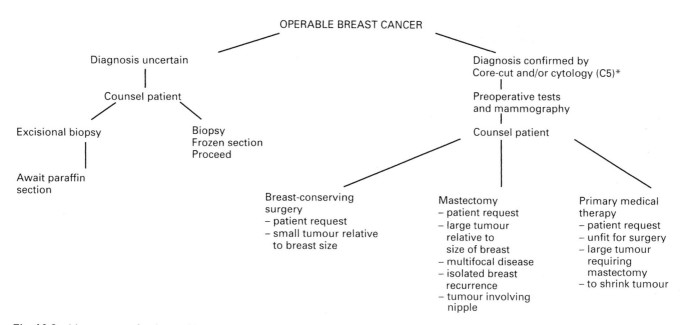

Fig. 19.2 Management of patients with operable breast cancer. *Most centres are not happy to proceed to mastectomy on a basis of cytology alone.

colleagues. This procedure is also of value in the management of extensive intraduct carcinoma and as a prophylactic procedure in patients with a very strong family history.

5. Primary medical therapy with tamoxifen may be used in frail elderly patients, and primary cytotoxic chemotherapy may be appropriate for locally advanced cases such as the 'inflammatory' carcinoma. In patients with large tumours that are operable by mastectomy, primary (or neoadjuvant) chemotherapy may be used to shrink the tumour and allow breast conservation in up to 50%.

Paget's disease

When this disease is suspected, take a biopsy of the nipple area under local anaesthetic to prove the diagnosis histologically. It may also be possible to do so with smear cytology of the area. When Paget's cells are demonstrated there is always an underlying intraduct carcinoma, which is invasive in 50% of cases. Mastectomy is usually recommended but primary radiotherapy or wide excision of the nipple and underlying breast tissue are possible alternatives.

Aspiration cytology

Aspiration cytology for outpatient diagnosis has the advantage of being applicable for the smallest of breast lumps and requiring the minimum of special equipment. It has the disadvantage of requiring the special skills of an experienced cytologist; the quality of the aspirate obtained is very much operator dependent and is associated with a definite 'learning curve'. The cytological aspirate is usually reported as containing no cells (C0), blood and debris (C1), benign epithelial cells (C2), atypical cells (C3), cells suspicious of carcinoma (C4) or carcinoma (C5), although methods of reporting vary from centre to centre. Using a combination of clinical assessment, cyto-diagnosis and mammography a preoperative diagnosis of carcinoma

can be made in most cases and enables appropriate patient counselling and planning of the operation list.

Action

1. Attach a 21G (green) or 23G (blue) needle to a 10 ml syringe and draw up 2 ml of air. Some people prefer to insert the syringe into an extractor 'gun'.

2. Fix the lump between thumb and index finger and clean the overlying skin with a swab.

3. Insert the needle into the middle of the lump and apply negative pressure on the syringe plunger. Move the needle in several different directions through the lump while maintaining negative pressure and not allowing the needle point to leave the skin. If this is done, air rushes into the needle tip and the carefully aspirated material will be drawn inside the syringe and be difficult to remove. Release the pressure and then withdraw the needle. Ask the patient or your assistant to apply pressure to the breast for 3 minutes to avoid haematoma formation.

4. Squirt a blob of aspirate on to the end of a dry microscope slide. Spread this out with another slide to make a thin smear. Avoid too much pressure and repeated smearing as this can lead to artefactual changes, making interpretation difficult.

5. Label the slide carefully, allow to dry (some centres prefer to spray with, or immerse the slide in, a fixative) and send for reporting.

6. If no aspirate is obtained the procedure can be repeated.

? Difficulty?

Obtaining good samples for cytology takes considerable practice. If the report is consistently C1 – 'inadequate' it may simply be because the area being sampled does not contain breast epithelial cells, for example a lipoma. However if any clinical doubt exists you should proceed to a core-cut biopsy or excision biopsy.

Core-cut or 'Tru-cut®' needle biopsy (Fig. 19.3)

Action

1. Infiltrate the skin over the lump with 1% lignocaine and introduce the needle into the breast, injecting the local anaesthetic deep into the breast tissue until it is judged to have entered the tumour.

2. Make a small nick in the skin with the tip of a sharp-pointed scalpel (11 blade).

3. Fix the tumour yourself or have an assistant fix the tumour within the breast between finger and thumb, to provide a static target.

4. Push the needle, in its closed position, through the skin incision until the edge of the tumour is encountered.

5. If using a Tru-cut® needle, advance the inner needle until it is judged to have entered the main tumour mass. Advance the outer sheath of the cutting needle over the inner needle, which is steadied in position, until the closed position of the assembly is re-established.

6. If using the core-cut (or Bioptycut®) needle place the needle in contact with the tumour and fire the 'gun'.

7. Remove the whole needle and open it to reveal a core of tissue measuring 2×0.1 cm

8. If no adequate core of tissue is obtained, repeat the manoeuvre. It is advisable to obtain at least two cores of tissue.

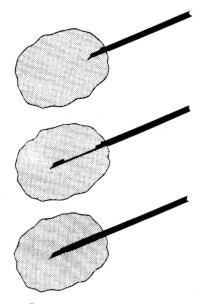

Fig. 19.3 Tru-cut® needle.

EXCISION BIOPSY

An excisional breast biopsy is an operation that should normally be reserved for patients with a solid breast lump that is clinically benign. The aim is to extract the lesion with the narrowest margin and least cosmetic defect, consistent with establishing a histological diagnosis and removing the palpable abnormality. It is not an operation that is sufficient for the removal of a breast carcinoma. Preliminary excision biopsy is occasionally necessary for that minority of patients with a breast carcinoma in whom the diagnosis cannot be established by preoperative cytology, core-cut needle biopsy and/or mammography; definitive surgery will then be required as a second procedure after paraffin-section examination, which has the advantage of allowing another opportunity for counselling prior to the definitive operation.

Prepare

1. Check that the lesion is still present on admission. Occasionally, lesions disappear. Check also that no new lesion has appeared in either breast.

2. Mark the exact site of the lesion on the breast with the patient lying in the position she will be in on the operating table. Otherwise you may be unable to find the mass once the patient has been anaesthetized.

3. Check that the appropriate preoperative investigations are available: haemoglobin, sickle test, cytology, mammography.

4. Check that you have the right patient in the anaesthetic room and are operating on the correct side.

Access (Fig. 19.4)

1. Incise over the region of the lump. Adequate excision of the lump is the first priority, but second comes the placement of the incision in the most aesthetic position. If possible, place the scar where it will be invisible under the patient's bra.

2. Periareolar incisions heal with least visible scars, but may not always be suitable.

3. Incisions in the medial half of the breast are more likely to develop keloid scars.

4. Avoid radial incisions except medially.

5. Always make your incision within the area of skin which would be removed at mastectomy if the patient required this operation subsequently, so that no unnecessary scar is added to the mastectomy scar.

Action

1. Excise the lump completely without cutting into it. Use sharp dissection with scissors or knife, and hold the specimen with Lane or Allis tissue forceps or by inserting a suture through the lesion.

2. Cut open the specimen to ensure that you have obtained the lesion. A fibroadenoma tends to be encapsulated and has a whorled appearance. Small cysts may be seen in fibrocystic disease, and the cut surface of the surrounding white fibrous tissue is convex. In

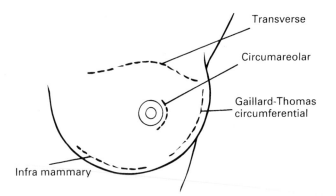

Fig. 19.4 Incisions for removal of a lump from the left breast.

contrast, drawing a scalpel across a carcinoma in two planes leaves a sharp edge and produces a 'gritty' feeling and sound, as though the knife were scratching small pieces of calcium. Cutting the specimen open does annoy many pathologists so check with them first before doing this. This procedure should always be avoided if you wish the pathologist to comment on 'margins' when cancer is suspected.

3. In mammary duct ectasia, a toothpaste-like substance may issue from transected ducts at the edge of the cavity adjacent to the nipple.

4. Introduce a finger into the cavity and place your thumb on the overlying skin. Palpate the surrounding breast tissue between finger and thumb to see if there is any more abnormal tissue that should be removed.

5. Sometimes it is impossible to remove all the abnormal tissue, particularly with fibrocystic disease, which tends not to have a well-defined edge. Under these circumstances, remove the most severely affected tissue and obtain a representative biopsy.

6. Be obsessional about haemostasis.

Closure

1. If haemostasis is absolute, then no drain is required. Otherwise a small suction or corrugated drain is a wise precaution to reduce the risk of a haematoma.

2. Use a subcuticular suture for closure, such as 3/0 synthetic material on a straight cutting needle. Circumareolar incisions always heal with an almost invisible scar, and 3/0 or 4/0 interrupted nylon can be used.

WIDE LOCAL EXCISION FOR CARCINOMA

1. The terminology used to describe breast-conserving operations for carcinoma of the breast is inexact and confusing, and includes terms such as wide local excision, lumpectomy and tumorectomy. For some surgeons these operations simply involve removing the tumour with a margin of normal tissue sufficient to obtain macroscopic clearance, while for others they involve a meticulous attempt to obtain margins clear of microscopic tumour by using intraoperative frozen-section examination.

2. The 'gold-standard' breast-conserving operation for early breast cancer is the quadrantectomy, as it is upon this operation that most of the published data comparing breast-conserving therapy with mastectomy in randomized trials have been based. Quadrantectomy is the most certain means of obtaining microscopically clear margins, and with postoperative breast irradiation gives local recurrence rates equivalent to those obtained by primary mastectomy. Wide local excision results in a significantly higher incidence of local recurrence, even when a radiotherapy boost to the primary site has been employed in the radiotherapy protocol, and for this reason quadrantectomy should be considered as the correct operation for breast cancer in those patients suitable for breast conservation.

Quadrantectomy

Prepare

1. Check that the diagnosis of breast carcinoma has been confirmed by cytology or Tru-cut® biopsy or previous excision biopsy.

2. Check that the patient is suitable for breast-conserving surgery by clinical examination. Check that the mammogram does not reveal multifocal disease.

3. Confirm that the patient has seen the Nurse Counsellor, and that she has had an opportunity to discuss her diagnosis and treatment fully.

4. Mark the side and site of the carcinoma.

Access

1. Place the patient on the table in the supine position, with the arm on the operative side extended on an arm board.

2. Prepare the skin and place the towels to allow access to the breast and axilla; the arm is wrapped separately to facilitate axillary dissection (see below).

3. With a skin marking pen, mark the position of the lump. Draw on the skin the edges of a quadrant of breast tissue that encompasses the lump at its centre; you should have drawn two radial lines extending out from the nipple at right angles to each other towards the periphery of the breast.

4. Draw on the skin your chosen line of incision. A circumferential incision is best, approximately midway between the nipple and the periphery of the breast and extending from one radial line to the other of your previously outlined quadrant. The incision should ideally lie directly over the lump, thus allowing an ellipse or crescent of skin overlying the carcinoma to be removed in continuity, but its position should allow good access to both the central and peripheral parts of the breast.

Action

1. Elevate two skin flaps centrally towards the nipple, so as to allow removal of the subareolar major duct system of the quadrant, and peripherally to the edge of the breast disc, which should thus be exposed along a quarter of its outside circumference.

2. Dissect along the edge of the breast disc down to the underlying pectoral fascia and muscle. A submammary plane of cleavage can now be raised between the breast and pectoral fascia, and the breast tissue is gradually lifted free from the chest wall. Much of the submammary dissection can be accomplished using blunt dissection, but perforating vessels should be diathermied or ligated prior to dividing with scissors.

3. Using the two radial lines marked on the skin to define the edges of the quadrant, cut vertically down through the breast tissue along these radii as far as the pectoral fascia so that the quadrant lifts free from the chest wall. Dissection continues along the two radii until they meet behind the nipple, and the major duct system is excised in continuity with the rest of the quadrant.

4. Mark the specimen with sutures to denote its three planes, i.e. superior/inferior, medial/lateral and superficial/deep.

5. Send the specimen to histology. The specimen should not be incised in theatre to look at the tumour for two reasons: first, this could theoretically contaminate the operative field with viable malignant cells; second, it could prevent adequate assessment of margins of clearance by the pathologist as the intact specimen is dipped in ink to outline the margins in histological sections.

6. Be obsessional about haemostasis.

7. Pack the cavity with a dry swab and proceed to perform the axillary dissection that usually accompanies a quadrantectomy.

Closure

1. Remove the swab, and obtain absolute haemostasis.

2. A drain is rarely needed.

3. Suture the skin edges using subcuticular sutures.

4. By closing the wound without drainage, the early cosmetic appearance is good because the large quadrantic cavity is full of air and then subsequently fills with serous fluid. The late cosmetic appearance is also good, because the seroma within the cavity gradually organizes to fill the cavity with fibrous tissue.

5. If the quadrantectomy cavity is in continuity with the axillary dissection cavity, the edges of the axillary skin should be sutured to pectoralis major so that a suction drain placed in the axilla does not suck out the air and seroma from the breast cavity.

🔑 Key point

- It is usually wise not to attempt to approximate the residual breast tissue at the edges of the cavity. However this may leave an unacceptably large defect and if this is the case mobilization of the residual breast and approximation of the edges with absorbable sutures may restore shape but tends to lead to a greater loss of breast volume.

Axillary clearance

The importance of a well-performed complete axillary dissection in the management of patients with operable breast cancer must be emphasized. The procedure provides important staging and prognostic information to allow decisions about adjuvant treatment, it removes axillary disease and prevents regional recurrence. The majority of patients with operable breast cancer should therefore undergo an axillary clearance at the time of primary breast surgery, either as part of a modified radical mastectomy or as an adjunct to quadrantectomy. While a limited 'axillary sampling' operation to biopsy a few lymph nodes in level I (lateral to pectoralis minor) may give valuable staging information, the advantage of a formal level II (up to the medial border of pectoralis minor) or level III (beyond the medial border of pectoralis minor) axillary clearance is that the operation is also therapeutic, providing local disease control without the need for axillary irradiation. Because 70–80% of breast cancer patients will have a negative axillary dissection, novel ways are being researched to avoid full axillary surgery in these patients. The technique most commonly practised is sentinel lymph node biopsy, in which the first node in the axilla draining the breast tissue around a tumour is identified perioperatively using a combination of radioisotope and blue dye. This node can then be removed and if negative is likely to indicate no further axillary node involvement. The combination of axillary surgery and irradiation is associated with the highest risk of long-term lymphoedema.

Prepare

1. Shave the axilla.

2. Warn the patient about the possibility of postoperative numbness involving the upper inner arm due to division of the intercostobrachial nerve.

Access

1. The surgeon approaching the axilla is always tempted to perform an oblique incision just behind and parallel to the lateral edge of the pectoralis major. There is no doubt that access is good via this approach but it has the disadvantage of producing an ugly scar and limitation of shoulder abduction. We tend to prefer a transverse incision with its anterior corner at the pectoral edge and the posterior angle just crossing the anterior border of latissimus dorsi. The level of the incision is judged to run 3 cm below and parallel with the axillary vein with the arm abducted at 90°. Cosmetically this produces an excellent result although two assistants are usually required to retract the skin and muscles.

2. Using a combination of sharp and blunt dissection at either end of the axillary incision, identify the lateral border of pectoralis major and the anterior border of latissimus dorsi; these landmarks will form the anterior and posterior limits of your axillary dissection.

3. Dissect up and down along the lateral border of pectoralis major and identify the underlying pectoralis minor muscle. Pass a finger under the insertion of pectoralis minor to separate it from the underlying structures and have your assistant retract the muscle forwards and medially in order to expose the axillary contents of level II.

4. If a level III clearance is desired, then both borders of pectoralis minor should be defined and its insertion into the coracoid process divided; however a level II clearance provides satisfactory disease control for the majority of cases. If axillary clearance is performed for melanoma, then a meticulous level III dissection is essential.

5. Facilitate exposure of the subpectoral area by flexing and abducting the shoulder and flexing the elbow so that the forearm lies across the patient's towelled-off face, where it may be supported by the assistant or slung from the crossbar of the anaesthetist's drape support.

6. Define the upper limit of the axillary dissection by identifying the axillary vein as it crosses behind the medial border of pectoralis minor. Blunt dissection with a Lahey 'peanut' swab is useful at this stage. Identify the inferior border of the axillary vein along its whole length. Control all vessels passing from its inferior surface into the axillary contents by surgical clips or fine ligatures. Make no attempt to clear the structures above the vein.

7. 'Stroke' the axillary contents away from the chest wall and off the subscapularis muscle using a gauze swab or 'peanut' until the nerve to serratus anterior is identified in the posterior axillary line and the nerve to latissimus dorsi is identified travelling with the subscapular vessels.

8. Identify the intercostobrachial nerve. Dissect it free from the axillary contents and preserve as many branches as feasible.

9. Now that the limits of the dissection have been defined and the nerves identified, removal of the axillary contents can be completed.

10. Achieve haemostasis.

Closure

1. Insert a vacuum drain into the axilla and suture the skin with subcuticular sutures.

2. It is your responsibility to supervise the dressing of the wound and in particular to squeeze out all blood and air from under the flaps

? Difficulty?

1. If you are unable to remove the axillary contents without severing the intercostobrachial nerve, you should not hesitate to divide this, and should inform the patient afterwards that she is likely to experience a little numbness on the medial aspect of her upper arm.

2. If you inadvertently damage the axillary vein this should wherever possible be repaired. First, obtain vascular control using small bulldog clips or other vascular clamps. The vein can then be directly repaired using a vascular suture such as 5.0 polypropylene. The patient may require postoperative anticoagulation for a time.

3. If there is heavy nodal involvement in the axilla all palpable lymph nodes should be excised, as should soft tissue disease. Only rarely is tumour found encasing the axillary vein and this is usually fairly easy to dissect off. If any tumour has to be left behind it is advisable to mark it with surgical clips to allow planning of any future radiotherapy.

into the vacuum containers in order to avoid the subsequent development of an axillary seroma.

3. Before sending the specimen to the pathology laboratory mark the apex of the flaps specimen with a stitch and the junction of level I with level II with a second stitch. This aids orientation and reporting by the pathologist.

MODIFIED RADICAL (OR PATEY) MASTECTOMY

Prepare

1. Check that the diagnosis of breast carcinoma has been confirmed by cytology or core-cut biopsy or previous excision biopsy. If the diagnosis rests on positive cytology you should ensure that you are satisfied clinically and radiologically that this is invasive carcinoma prior to undertaking an axillary dissection. In cases of genuine diagnostic doubt a preliminary biopsy for paraffin sections should be performed as it is no longer acceptable for a patient to undergo a 'Frozen section? Proceed' operation.

2. All patients undergoing mastectomy should be aware that breast reconstruction is available to them and should be offered this option either as an immediate or as a delayed procedure.

3. Confirm that the patient has seen the Nurse Counsellor and that she has had an opportunity to discuss her diagnosis and treatment fully.

4. Mark the side and site of the carcinoma.

5. If you think it advisable, have cross-matched blood available for transfusion. This is rarely required if the surgery is gentle and the bleeding points are caught as the operation proceeds.

Access

1. Place the patient on the table in the supine position, with the arm on the operative side extended on an arm board.

2. Prepare the skin and place the towels to allow access to the breast and axilla; the arm is wrapped separately to facilitate axillary dissection (see below).

3. With a skin marking pen, mark the position of the lump. Draw on the skin your chosen ellipse for the incision. This should ideally lie

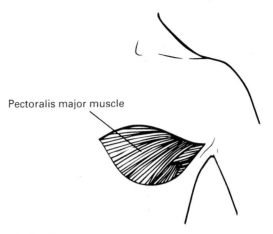

Pectoralis major muscle

Fig. 19.5 Simple mastectomy.

transversely and encompass approximately 5 cm of skin round the lesion and also the nipple (Fig. 19.5).

If the lesion is in a position that makes transverse incision impracticable, then make an oblique incision – but there is no need to take it up as far as the clavicle or across to the upper arm (this type of scar is still seen on elderly patients who had a mastectomy many years ago; it is unnecessarily ugly and may be responsible for a stiff shoulder).

4. Ensure that you will be able to approximate the wound edges at the end of the operation prior to incising along your marked lines.

Action

1. Elevate the skin flaps in the plane between subcutaneous fat and mammary fat. This can be facilitated by subcutaneous infiltration with 1:400 000 adrenaline in saline or 0.25% bupivacaine and adrenaline.

2. Have your assistant hold up the skin flaps and check after every few cuts with the scalpel or scissors that you are not in danger of making the flap too thin, resulting in 'buttonholing'. Do, however, ensure that no breast tissue is left behind in the flaps.

3. Do not allow traumatizing tissue forceps to be placed on the skin flaps but insert skin hooks into the cut edge or apply Allis forceps to the rolled back edges of the skin.

4. Raise the upper flap to the upper limit of the breast. This is usually 2–3 cm below the clavicle but varies from patient to patient. A good guide is the second intercostal space.

5. Catch any bleeding points with fine forceps and diathermy them. Take care not to burn the skin itself by contact with the diathermy needle. If this does inadvertently happen, cut away the burnt area, bevelling it off so that it will not be demonstrable later (Fig. 19.6). Burnt skin takes many weeks to heal and is painful.

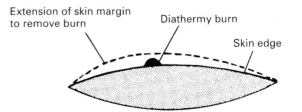

Extension of skin margin to remove burn

Diathermy burn

Skin edge

Fig. 19.6 Removal of accidental diathermy burn.

6. Raise the lower flap in a similar manner, to the lower limits of the breast.

7. Place a large tissue forceps, such as Lane's, on the breast that is to be removed, handing it to an assistant to hold, thus facilitating the subsequent dissection.

8. Return to the uppermost part of the breast and dissect down until you see the fascia of pectoralis major. Introduce a finger covered by a swab and find a submammary plane of cleavage between the fascia and the breast, as discussed under Quadrantectomy above.

9. Proceed in this plane in a downwards direction, catching and ligating the perforating vessels as they appear before cutting them; this reduces the amount of operative bleeding considerably. If the tumour appears to infiltrate into the pectoralis muscle, then excise a portion of this muscle with the specimen.

10. Continue downwards, elevating the breast alternatively laterally and medially but leaving the axillary tail of the breast in continuity with the axillary contents.

11. The medial end of the dissection proceeds to the lower limit of the breast, and the breast is elevated laterally to complete its removal from the chest wall; the breast is now only attached at the axilla. Take care to identify and ligate one or two major perforating vessels passing through the second and third intercostal spaces.

12. Place dry packs under each skin flap.

13. Identify the lateral border of pectoralis major and clear the axillary tail of the breast and the axillary contents from along this border.

14. Identify latissimus dorsi and clear the axillary contents from its anterior border.

15. Proceed as for an axillary clearance; a satisfactory result can be achieved by preserving the pectoralis minor muscle and dissecting up to level II (Fig. 19.7).

Closure

1. Insert two vacuum drains, one for the flaps and a second for the axilla.
2. Suture the skin edges with subcuticular sutures. In case of

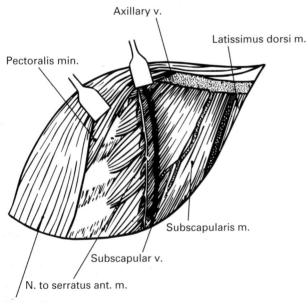

Axillary v.

Latissimus dorsi m.

Pectoralis min.

Subscapularis m.

Subscapular v.

N. to serratus ant. m.

Pectoralis maj. m.

Fig. 19.7 Left Patey's operation with preservation of pectoralis minor.

discrepancy between the lengths of the two flaps, the wound can be closed using interrupted sutures placed halfway along the incision then halfway between these lengths and so on, thus avoiding a 'dog-ear' at one end.

3. After suturing is complete, activate the vacuum drains and squeeze out all the fluid and air from beneath the skin flaps so that they adhere to the chest wall.

❓ **Difficulty?**

Rarely, you may have to apply a split skin graft to part of the wound if the skin edges cannot be opposed without tension. If so, the surgery has probably been too radical or the case selection inappropriate. A myocutaneous flap gives a better cosmetic result in these circumstances.

Aftercare

1. Supplying and arranging the fitting of a breast prosthesis for the patient is really within the operation manifesto. Artificial breasts are now available that are of a weight and consistency comparable with the removed breast. They change shape with the patient's change of posture and they take on body temperature. It is almost impossible to tell which is the side of the mastectomy when feeling through a patient's clothes, and this is of very great importance to her as a woman. She can buy clothes as anyone else does, and also wear swimsuits and evening dresses without calling attention to her deficiency. Make yourself aware of the range and variety of prostheses available. In the UK, under Health Service regulations, any women is entitled to the type and size of prosthesis of her choice. In addition, these may be replaced as frequently as necessary. If you are not willing to learn of the variety available, then at least approach the Appliance Officer at an early stage in your career to delegate this responsibility. Some centres now employ mastectomy counsellors who, as well as providing psychosocial rehabilitation of the patient, are responsible for the physical rehabilitation. This includes the prescription of a soft temporary prosthesis immediately postoperatively, which can be worn for about 6 weeks until the wound is no longer sore and then replaced by the permanent prosthesis worn within the brassiere.

2. Finally, no woman should be allowed to leave hospital with a stiff shoulder following mastectomy. Commence active physiotherapy within 24 hours of surgery and provide the patient with a list of exercises for abduction of the arm. Encourage her to brush her hair and fasten the back of her dress.

FURTHER READING

Dixon M 1995 ABC of breast disease. BMJ Publishing Group, London

Fisher B, Redmond C, Poisson R et al 1989 Eight year results of a randomized trial comparing total mastectomy and lumpectomy with or without radiation in the treatment of breast cancer. New England Journal of Medicine 320: 822–828

Hughes LE, Mansel RE, Webster DJT 1989 Benign disorders and diseases of the breast: concepts and clinical management. Baillière Tindall, London

Thyroid gland

J. R. Farndon and C. A. Fowler

Contents

General considerations
Thyroid operations

GENERAL CONSIDERATIONS

1. Thyroidectomy is the most common operation performed by endocrine surgeons for benign and malignant conditions.

2. Any patient presenting with a thyroid lump needs thorough investigation. Routinely this includes fine needle aspiration cytology (which may need to be ultrasound-guided), ultrasonography, thyroid function tests (TSH and T_4) and thyroid autoantibody measurement.

3. *Multinodular goitre* (MNG) often presents as a 'solitary nodule', which is in fact just the dominant nodule. Surgery is indicated for symptoms of dyspnoea, dysphagia, hoarseness of voice or if it is cosmetically unsightly.

4. *Retrosternal goitres* are most common in large, bulky multinodular goitres and up to 20% are recurrent goitres.

5. *Differentiated thyroid cancer*. Papillary carcinoma is usually diagnosed by cytology and, unless less than 1 cm in diameter, requires total thyroidectomy with removal of any palpable lymph nodes. Follicular carcinoma cannot be diagnosed precisely on cytology.

6. *Medullary thyroid cancer* (MTC) can be diagnosed on cytology or suspected from a family history of multiple endocrine neoplasia (MEN 2).

7. *Anaplastic carcinoma* and *lymphoma* rarely require surgery.

8. *Benign adenomas* often require surgery because cytology cannot differentiate between a follicular adenoma and follicular carcinoma.

9. *Cysts* can develop in the thyroid and are often diagnosed when FNA reveals cystic fluid with resolution of the 'lump'.

10. *Thyrotoxicosis* is most commonly due to Graves' disease.

THYROID OPERATIONS

Prepare

1. Order preoperative indirect laryngoscopy to identify compensated and unsuspected recurrent nerve palsy.

2. Render thyrotoxic patients euthyroid with antithyroid drugs (carbimazole 10–15 mg tds) and propranolol (20 mg tds) if necessary.

3. Fully discuss potential complications with the patient and record it in the notes, specifically mentioning the risk to the parathyroids and recurrent laryngeal nerve, especially if lymph node dissection is contemplated. Allow the patient the opportunity to balance potential therapeutic gains against complications. Advice sheets or pamphlets may be helpful.

Access

1. Lay the patient supine on the table; place a sandbag between the shoulders and a ring under the head so that the neck is extended, but not over-extended, particularly in the elderly. Raise the head about 15° to reduce neck vein engorgement and break the table so that the patient is semisitting and will not slide off! This also improves venous return from the legs.

2. Prepare the skin and apply a four-towel square, secured with towel clips and an adhesive drape. Stand on the patient's right to begin.

3. Incise the skin two fingerbreadths above the clavicles/suprasternal notch in, or parallel to, a skin crease (Fig. 20.1).

Extend the incision to the medial border of the sternocleidomastoid muscles. Cut through subcutaneous tissue and platysma in the line of the incision until you reach the strap muscles. Achieve haemostasis with diathermy.

> ### 🔑 Key point
>
> - Patients with thyrotoxicosis (even though medically controlled) have a hyperdynamic circulation and will bleed more from skin edges.

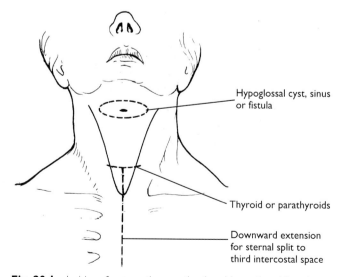

Hypoglossal cyst, sinus or fistula

Thyroid or parathyroids

Downward extension for sternal split to third intercostal space

Fig. 20.1 Incisions for operations on the thyroid, parathyroids and hypoglossal lesions.

4. Raise superior and inferior skin flaps – place two Allis forceps on the platysma superiorly and have your assistant pull vertically to demonstrate the space between the platysma and the strap muscles. Keep superficial to the deep cervical fascia and anterior jugular veins and use counter-traction to facilitate the dissection. Do not divide or injure the anterior jugular veins. Use blunt or sharp dissection and diathermize or tie any blood vessels. Dissect as far as the thyroid cartilage – recognized by its palpable notch.

Key point

● The plane you are developing to raise the flaps is essentially bloodless – if it is not you are in the wrong plane.

5. Replace the Allis forceps on to the inferior flap. Adjust your position to face towards the patient's feet. Raise the inferior flap as far as the suprasternal notch. Replace one Allis forceps on the superior flap; one remains inferiorly, both held by your assistant while you position a Joll's or similar self-retaining retractor through the platysma and subdermal tissues at the midpoint of the each flap. Fully open the retractor to give a clear view of the strap muscles.

6. Identify the midline raphe between the straps – it should be pale/white. If one lobe is very large the midline is pushed off-centre. The overlying strap muscles can be stretched very thin. Pick up the fascia on either side of the midline (your assistant holds one side) with artery forceps. Incise the deep cervical fascia using diathermy. Extend the incision superiorly and inferiorly using diathermy and scissors until you see the thyroid. Some small vessels (or the anterior jugular branches) traverse the 'bloodless' midline. Secure them as they are encountered to maintain the essential bloodless field.

7. Cut through several thin layers of fascia until you come on to the surface of the gland. Bleeding at this point can often be secured only by oversewing stitches. Take great care, therefore, as you come down on to the gland surface.

Key point

● It is very important to be in the correct tissue plane before proceeding with the next steps. The layers of fascia are often very thin and filmy – a clue as to when you are at the correct level is that the vessels coursing the surface of the gland suddenly fill up with blood as the last layer of restriction is removed. Be very careful as you dissect the last filmy slips because the thyroid veins on the surface bleed profusely if damaged.

8. Hold up the medial edge of the strap muscle with a small Langenbeck retractor and dissect between the thyroid lobe and muscle, working laterally so that the lobe can be mobilized (Fig. 20.2).

Diathermize small veins traversing this space to maintain a bloodless field. When the space is large enough, have your assistant insert a larger Langenbeck retractor. Extend the space, which should be bloodless, with your index finger or a gauze pledget around the surface of the lobe. Bleeding suggests you may be working between attenuated strap muscles.

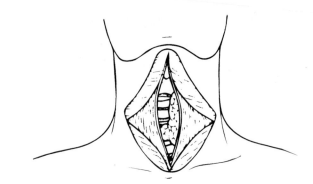

Fig. 20.2   Separation of strap muscles to expose isthmus and larynx.

10. Some surgeons routinely divide the strap muscles and others never do. Division is usually needed only for the largest goitres.

Assess

1. Adequate preoperative assessment, investigation including imaging and biopsy, exclude unexpected findings, although the true extent of some multinodular goitres or tumours is established only at operation.

2. Having uncovered the left lobe you often need to display the right lobe. Perform this from the patient's left side.

Action

1. Stand on the patient's right to deal with the left lobe and vice versa. Have the strap muscles retracted laterally and upwards and the lobe medially with two Langenbeck retractors (Fig. 20.3).

2. Develop the plane between strap muscles and thyroid by sweeping off the muscle using a pledget and identify the middle thyroid vein (Fig. 20.4). Ligate with 3/0 absorbable synthetic thread (polyglactin 910) and divide the vein to allow you to dislocate the lobe more medially and anteriorly.

Key point

● The middle vein is not as constant as the anatomy books describe! It is not always present and may consist of two or three smaller veins. Beware of the short, stubby variant, especially on the right.

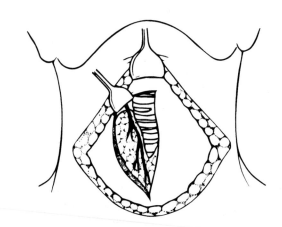

Fig. 20.3   Retraction of strap muscles to expose superior pole and blood supply.

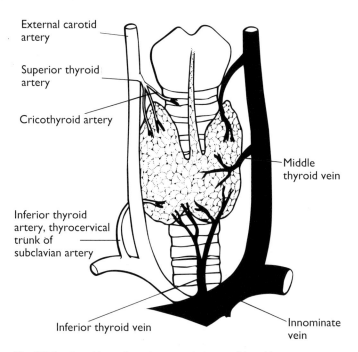

Fig. 20.4 Arterial supply and venous drainage of thyroid.

3. Apply firm traction to the lobe using a gauze swab between your index/middle fingers and the lobe so putting the tissues lateral to the lobe under tension. Your assistant continues to retract the muscles laterally.

Difficulty?

If you find difficulty in dislocating the lobe, go up to the upper pole. Secure and divide the upper pole vessels, enabling you to mobilize the lobe.

4. By blunt dissection, carefully open up the space between the gland, the oesophagus and the posterolateral tissues to seek the recurrent laryngeal nerve. Dissect parallel to the anticipated course of the nerve to minimize the risk. Identify the inferior thyroid artery as it arches forward, since this is a marker for the nerve and the superior parathyroid glands, which often lie at this junction (see below for identification of parathyroid glands).

5. Once you have identified the recurrent nerve, follow its course upwards by picking up the fascia one layer a time and dividing it. Take great care: the nerve may separate into divisions, which are easily torn or cut. Follow the nerve up to its point of entry into the larynx close to the lateral thyroid ligament (of Berry). Use a haemostatic clip with the convexity of the jaws closest to the nerve to tunnel the route parallel to the nerve and clip and tie the fascia uncovering the nerve. Do not use diathermy current within 1 cm of the nerve. Do not touch or elevate the nerve or sling it in a thread or rubber loop.

6. Move your body to face the patient's head to deal with the superior pole. Gently draw downward on the gland to aid identification of the superior pole vessels lying on the surface of the upper lobe (Fig. 20.4). Sweep the sometimes adherent sternothyroid muscle fibres off the surface of the upper pole with a pledget. Find the medial space between the larynx and medial edge of the upper lobe and make

Key point

- Identifying the recurrent laryngeal nerve. On the left the nerve runs 'north' in the tracheo-oesphageal groove or parallel to the groove, whereas on the right it nearly always takes a more oblique course. The nerve usually runs deep to the inferior thyroid artery or between its branches (Fig. 20.5).

You may be able to palpate the nerve but this may injure it. Look for the 'toothpaste' sign – the white nerve has a small red blood vessel running on its surface, giving the impression of a well-known brand of toothpaste! The nerve may be non-recurrent, especially on the right and arise high up from the vagus and pass horizontally down towards the inferior artery. Beware of alternative anatomy – do not cut/tie anything until you are sure of the structures and especially the recurrent nerve.

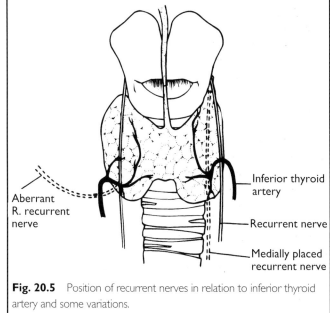

Fig. 20.5 Position of recurrent nerves in relation to inferior thyroid artery and some variations.

a small window through the fascia here with artery forceps. Pass them through the window, then laterally, tunnelling under the superior vessels to create a space. Clip the vessels individually, if you can, over the surface of the gland, well away from the external laryngeal nerve. Lahey or Pilling forceps are useful in passing a clip through this space. Place a second Lahey across, leaving enough space between them to divide the vessels. Be sure of the security of the proximal tie before cutting the thread; the vessels tend to retract, making retrieval of a bleeding branch difficult. Ease the pole downwards, sweeping off any adherent muscle fibres as you proceed. Sometimes you now see posterior branches of the superior thyroid artery and vein – secure and divide these in a similar manner. The right upper pole is higher and more difficult to isolate than the left. Take care not to damage a superior parathyroid gland, which may be lying on the surface of the upper pole or between the vessels.

7. Turn to face the patient's feet to deal with the inferior thyroid veins. Having identified the recurrent nerve, keep it in sight as you carefully isolate the inferior vessels and clip and tie them close to the gland so avoiding damage or removal of the parathyroid glands if they are sitting in the thyrothymic ligament.

8. Dissect the gland from the front of the trachea, using diathermy.

9. If you are performing a *total lobectomy*, pass artery forceps under the isthmus to free it from the trachea and divide it between forceps applied at its junction with the opposite lobe. The pyramidal lobe can arise from the isthmus or from the medial aspect of right or left upper pole. This tongue of thyroid tissue can run along the crest of the trachea (i.e. rostrally) up to the cricoid cartilage or above. For benign disease it need not be followed completely. There are often big vessels in the pyramidal lobe and an isthmic lymph node can often be identified; take it with the dissection. Ligate and divide the pyramidal lobe. This aids in dissecting the remainder of the lobe from the trachea, securing all blood vessels as you proceed. Oversew the raw surface of the residual thyroid with 2/0 synthetic absorbable thread (polyglactin 910). Stop minor oozing by suturing the anterior surface of thyroid tissue and capsule to the fascia on the side of the trachea with continuous 3/0 polyglactin 910.

10. For *total thyroidectomy* dissect the left lobe and isthmus from the trachea and continue the dissection off the right anteromedial surface of the trachea. Do not dissect too far posteriorly off the trachea otherwise you risk haemorrhage from the deep branches of the inferior thyroid artery. Move to the other side of the patient to mobilize the right lobe – identifying the recurrent nerve, securing the superior and inferior poles as described above.

11. The final point of attachment of each lobe should be at the lateral thyroid ligament (of Berry). The recurrent nerve is particularly vulnerable. Any bleeding obscures protection of the nerve. Assume that even the smallest connections to the thyroid contain a small vessel. Ligate all vessels; if they are too 'tight' and short, control them with a silver clip. Ligatures may bunch and distort tissues close to the nerve and damage it. Identify the nerve curving into the larynx and only then clip and cut safely. It is· often easier not to clip the thyroid side, controlling bleeding with pressure.

12. *Lymph node dissection* and excision is important for differentiated tumours. Although its exact role is not fully determined, for some lesions a central compartment dissection is always recommended, such as medullary and papillary thyroid cancer. This entails removal of all perithyroidal tissues, skeletonizing the trachea, oesophagus and nerve, and taking lymphatics, nodes and upper thymus. Identify and protect the parathyroids, and the nerve, which is more at risk, should be sought and protected. If lymphatic spread occurs as in papillary tumours, be prepared to take the dissection to the jugular nodes. Open the carotid sheath and carefully remove the nodes and lymphatics running vertically between jugular vein and carotid artery, identifying and protecting the vagus nerve.

13. In *subtotal thyroidectomy*, aim to leave sufficient thyroid tissue to render the patient euthyroid but with little risk of recurrent hyperthyroidism. It is better to leave smaller remnants, ensuring against hypothyroidism, and be willing to replace with thyroxine. There is no magic formula to decide on the amount of thyroid to be preserved – a strip measuring approximately 3×1×1 cm on each side. Place small artery forceps into the substance of the gland from the posterolateral aspect of the thyroid capsule, avoiding the path of the recurrent nerve. Remove each lobe by cutting through the lobe down to the trachea with a scalpel blade, leaving the forceps attached to the remnant. Oversew the oozing remnant with continuous 2/0 polyglactin 910 and then stitch it to the capsule on the surface of the trachea.

14. *Retrosternal goitres* usually lie in the anterior and superior mediastinum. Most can be removed through the standard collar incision. It may not be possible to lift the thyroid lobe anteriorly to look for the recurrent nerve until the intrathoracic extension is mobilized. Gently pull up on the lobe freeing any adhesions with your index finger.

Key point

- The secret to delivery of large retrosternal goitres is to be in the correct plane. Thinned adherent straps make the identification of this plane difficult. After division of the superior thyroid vessels it is often easiest to identify the correct plane superiorly and posteriorly and to pass the fingers downward, almost sliding in the convex surface of the gland – the so called toboggan manoeuvre.

---

15. Pressure created by the efforts to deliver the gland sometimes causes ruptures of one or more nodules and this facilitates delivery. The convexity of the lower pole can often be delivered from the inlet by using a sterile dessert spoon.

Difficulty?

Rarely, sternal split is required to deliver the gland, especially if the goitre extends into the posterior and anterior mediastinum. Be careful on delivering the gland, since the recurrent nerve may be stretched over the lateral surface of the goitre, to which it may be adherent.

---

16. *Reoperations* on the thyroid can be hazardous because adhesions often alter the anatomy such as the course of the recurrent nerve and the position of the parathyroid glands, increasing the risk of complications. Expose the thyroid in the standard manner. As in reoperative abdominal surgery, the best way to proceed is to identify 'virgin' territory and this can often, but not always, be found at the upper or lower ends of the strap muscles. Do not undertake re-operative surgery unless:

a. there is a very definite need to reintervene, such as recurrent obstructive symptoms and recurrent tumour not amenable to other therapy

b. you have had a thorough grounding in difficult primary surgery.

Checklist

1. Check for bleeding: instil physiological saline into the space once occupied by the thyroid lobe and watch – small bleeding points are more easily seen. Remove the saline with a sucker and gauze swab and secure the bleeding vessel with diathermy or, if in the vicinity of the recurrent nerve, use a silver clip. Repeat this manoeuvre until you are satisfied that the wound is completely dry. Do the same on the opposite side if total thyroidectomy has been performed.

2. Check that any parathyroids seen are vascularized – if not, slice up and reimplant.

Closure

1. Re-approximate the strap muscles and platysma with interrupted 3/0 polyglactin 910.

2. Use clips or subcuticular 2/0 polypropylene to bring the skin edges together. To aid neat closure place a skin hook at each end of the wound and ask your assistant to stretch the incision. Infiltrate the skin edges with 0.25% bupivacaine.

3. Drains are not required – they can give a false sense of security and if significant haemorrhage occurs they can block with clots.

4. Dressings are not required and similarly may hide changing contours in the neck if bleeding occurs.

5. On extubation ask the anaesthetist to look at the vocal cords and check for movement and record the findings in the operation note. Good immediate movement does not mean that a neuropraxia will not develop in the postoperative period – it does mean, however, that the nerve is in continuity.

Postoperative

1. Ensure there is a pair of clip and suture removers next to the bed of any patient who has undergone thyroid surgery.

2. Prop up the patient in a low Fowler's position with head and shoulders elevated 10–20° after recovery from the anaesthetic.

3. Thyroid surgery is well tolerated; adequate pain relief can be provided by intramuscular or oral analgesia. Sore throat often lasts for the first 24 hours.

4. Remove clips or sutures after 2 days.

Complications

1. The most immediate life-threatening complication is haemorrhage under the deep cervical fascia. This should be a rare complication.

2. Acute asphyxia can occur in the anaesthetic room or on the ward. Rarely, the patient is severely compromised and immediate removal of the skin clips and sutures is necessary to evacuate the haematoma. Call an anaesthetist in case urgent reintubation is required and arrange for the patient to return to theatre for a more controlled exploration of the wound.

3. Hoarseness in the immediate postoperative period is likely to be due to recurrent nerve injury. If cord function was documented on extubation this is likely to be a neuropraxia. Request an early examination and documentation by an independent consultant ENT surgeon. Teflon® injection of the paralysed cord may help if no recovery occurs after 3–6 months. Hoarseness may not become apparent until later and may be due to scarring or nerve infiltration (if surgery was for tumour). The patient will have an altered (huskier) voice, which will be weak. Test for shortness of breath on exercise from glottic narrowing. The stridor may be mild.

4. Damage to the external laryngeal nerve, a branch of the superior laryngeal nerve, can cause voice weakness or fatigue, mild hoarseness and loss of voice range. The upper half octave in range is lost, which can be particularly troublesome for singers and is unlikely to recover.

5. Postoperative hypocalcaemia may be permanent if the parathyroid glands are removed, or temporary if they are bruised. Replace with calcium and/or vitamin D supplements as required. Check serum calcium levels in about 2 weeks and, if they are near the upper limit of normal, reduce the dose. Hypocalcaemia beyond 6 months is likely to be permanent.

6. Hypothyroidism may develop following an over-radical subtotal thyroidectomy.

7. Tracheal collapse from tracheomalacia can follow removal of large goitres. This is exceedingly rare in western practice. Be alert to a soft, collapsing trachea moving with respiration. It may require tracheostomy.

8. Wound infection should be a rarity. Seromas usually settle following needle aspiration. Keloid scars can develop; scar excision can be tried after 1 year but a good result cannot be guaranteed.

Conclusion

A forewarned patient is less aggrieved than one experiencing unsuspected complications. Be sure you explain all these potential complications. Provide as much information as you can – perhaps accompanied by an information sheet. Record in the notes what you have told the patient.

FURTHER READING

Lazarus JH, Othman S 1991 Thyroid disease in relation to pregnancy. Clinical Endocrinology (Oxford) 34: 91–98

Reeve RS, Delbridge L, Cohen A, Crummer P 1987 Total thyroidectomy. The preferred option for multinodular goitre. Annals of Surgery 206: 782–786

Stephenson BM, Wheeler MH, Clark OH 1994 The role of total thyroidectomy in the management of differentiated thyroid cancer. In: Daly JM (ed.) Current opinion in general surgery. Current Science, Philadelphia, pp 53–59

Tunbridge WM, Evered DC, Hall R 1977 The spectrum of thyroid disease in a community: the Whickham survey. Clinical Endocrinology(Oxford) 7: 481–493

Wade JSH 1955 Vulnerability of the recurrent laryngeal nerves at thyroidectomy. British Journal of Surgery 43: 164–180

Parathyroid glands

J. R. Farndon and C. A. Fowler

PARATHYROIDECTOMY

🔑 **Key point**

● Parathyroidectomy is not an operation for the 'occasional' surgeon. It demands special training and experience. Unless you have these qualities you should not embark on surgery of the parathyroid glands.

Appraise

1. Hyperparathyroidism results from overactivity of one or more glands as primary, secondary or tertiary disease (Fig. 21.1).

2. *Symptomatic primary hyperparathyroidism* (1° HPT) is the most common indication for parathyroidectomy.

3. *Asymptomatic primary hyperparathyroidism* (1° HPT).

4. *Secondary hyperparathyroidism* (2° HPT) is most commonly seen in patients with chronic renal failure, or on peritoneal or haemodialysis.

5. Tertiary hyperparathyroidism is a rare consequence of secondary hyperparathyroidism. Autonomous hypersecretion of parathyroid hormone from one of the hyperplastic glands occurs despite correcting the underlying renal disease.

6. Familial hypocalcuric hypercalcaemia can mimic primary hyperparathyroidism biochemically except that there is a low urinary excretion of calcium (< 2 mmol/l), which should be a prompt to the diagnosis. Familial hypocalcuric hypercalcaemia is a contraindication to parathyroidectomy

Prepare

There is no adequate medical therapy that will permanently correct hypercalcaemia preoperatively. If the serum calcium is above 3.25 mmol/l, consider taking corrective measures. Ensure the patient is hydrated, with optimum renal function. Give 2-4 g/d of 1α-hydroxycholecalciferol for a few days if there is evidence of bone disease; it may help 'hungry bone syndrome' in the post-operative period.

Treat hypercalcaemic crisis by rehydrating (4–6 litres of normal saline in the first 24 hours); inhibit osteoclast action with bisphosphonates, e.g. pamidronate. Once the kidneys have responded to rehydration use a loop diuretic, e.g. frusemide, to cause forced saline diuresis.

Warn the histopathalogist to expect one or more specimens for frozen section histology.

Action

1. The incision and exposure are as for thyroidectomy.

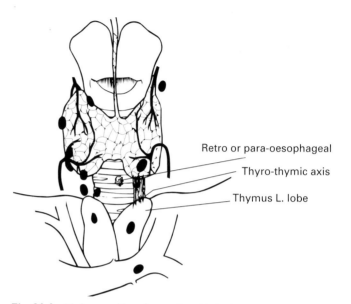

Fig. 21.1 Various positions for parathyroid glands.

Retro or para-oesophageal
Thyro-thymic axis
Thymus L. lobe

2. To assess the glands you must know their normal and unusual anatomical sites.

3. Identify all four glands before proceeding with the resection unless one gland is obviously enlarged. Remove the large gland for frozen section histology while you look for the other glands.

4. If more than one gland is enlarged and you suspect primary hyperplasia, remove the largest gland for frozen section histology; if this confirms the diagnosis remove the three most abnormal looking glands and half the fourth. Before excising half of the fourth gland or removing a biopsy specimen, identify where the blood supply enters it. Then place a silver clip across the middle and remove the specimen with a scalpel blade, from the surface of the clip away from the feeding vessels. The clip provides a useful marker for the site of the remaining gland if you have to carry out a re-exploration subsequently.

5. Ensure there is perfect haemostasis before closing.

FURTHER READING

Grant CS, Weaver A 1994 Treatment of primary parathyroid hyperplasia; representative experience at Mayo Clinic. Acta Chirurgica Australiae 26(S112): 41–44

Wong WK, Wong NA, Farndon JR 1996 Early postoperative plasma calcium concentration as a predictor of the need for calcium supplement after parathyroidectomy. British Journal of Surgery 83: 532–534

Adrenal

J. R. Farndon and C. A. Fowler

ADRENALECTOMY

Appraise

Adrenalectomy is most commonly undertaken for benign unilateral adrenal adenomas (Fig. 22.1). These are usually functional and patients present with the consequence of excessive secretion of the hormone rather than the effect of the adrenal tumour. If the anatomy of the adrenal is recalled the types of endocrine-secreting tumour can be deduced.

1. *Phaeochromocytoma* arises from the adrenal medulla and secretes adrenaline (epinephrine), noradrenaline (norepinephrine) or dopamine.

2. *Conn's syndrome* is due to an adenoma arising from the outer layer of the adrenal cortex, the zona glomerulosa, which secretes mineralocorticoids.

3. In *Cushing's syndrome*, adenomas arising in the zona fasciculata secrete excess glucocorticoids.

4. Bilateral adrenalectomy is sometimes indicated in *Cushing's disease* (pituitary-dependent adrenal hyperplasia), when a pituitary adenoma secreting ACTH has not been treated successfully.

5. Virilizing and feminizing syndromes can rarely be produced by excessive sex steroid secretion from an adenoma in the inner zona reticularis, which may be malignant.

6. 'Incidentalomas' are an increasingly common reason for adrenalectomy. They are detected coincidentally in patients undergoing investigations for a variety of conditions. Some are functioning. Others are benign, nonfunctioning adenomas and those less than 5 cm diameter may be reassessed regularly. Those over 5cm are more likely to be malignant and should be removed. Some are primary adrenocortical carcinomas or secondary metastases.

7. Neuroblastoma is a malignant tumour occurring in babies and young children. Ganglioneuroma is a benign tumour derived from sympathetic ganglion cells. It occurs in older children and adults. Both may secrete catecholamines.

8. Adrenocortical carcinomas rare tumour that is often highly malignant. Adrenalectomy is the only hope of cure, although the 5-year survival rate is only 19–35%.

9. Operative mortality should be less than 1%. Adrenalectomy for benign functioning adenomas is curative and safe if the patient has been properly investigated and treated preoperatively. There are no specific contraindications to adrenalectomy and alternative treatment is limited. Although malignant adrenal tumours may be successfully removed, metastases often develop, with no other useful treatment available.

Prepare

1. For unilateral non-functioning tumours, no special preparation is required. If excess hormone is being secreted, it is essential to optimize the patient's condition with medical therapy before surgical intervention.

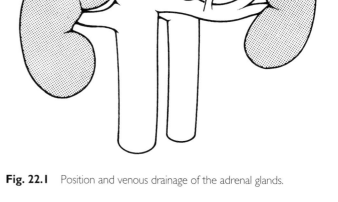

Fig. 22.1   Position and venous drainage of the adrenal glands.

2. *Phaeochromocytoma.* Noradrenaline-secreting tumours are the most common, so achieve alpha-adrenergic blockade using doxacin starting at 2–4 mg/d and increasing as appropriate.

3. *Conn's syndrome.* Spironolactone is a potassium-sparing diuretic that is an antagonist of aldosterone. Use it preoperatively for 2–3 weeks at 200–400 mg/d.

4. *Cushing's syndrome.* Metyrapone is a competitive inhibitor of 11-hydroxylation in the adrenal cortex and so inhibits production of cortisol. It can help control symptoms of the disease preoperatively.

Access

Posterolateral approach

This is the most popular open route for patients with large or potentially malignant tumours. Correctly position the patient on the side opposite the affected gland. Make the incision over the left 11th rib. Dissect out and remove the rib. Sweep the pleura superiorly and the peritoneum anteriorly to reveal the kidney. Retract it inferiorly and dissect in the fat above and medial to it; the right adrenal caps the upper pole of the kidney, the left adrenal is related to the upper medial border.

Posterior approach

This can be used for small tumours up to 5–6 cm when there is little or no risk of malignancy, or if bilateral excision is required for the treatment of Cushing's disease. Place the patient prone with the table broken to tense the lumbar fascia. Make an incision over the 11th rib and excise the rib.

Anterior transperitoneal approach

This is now rarely used. Gain access through a roof-top or chevron incision. Approach the right adrenal gland after performing Kocher's mobilization of the duodenum. On the left, gain access by incising the lienorenal ligament. Release the splenic flexure, incise the lateral colonic reflection and sweep the viscera forward.

Laparoscopic approaches

These do not offer the benefits to the patient or surgeon that other laparoscopic techniques do.

Postoperative

Glucocorticoids are required after unilateral or bilateral adrenalectomy for Cushing's disease/syndrome.

FURTHER READING

Gajraj H, Young AE 1993 Adrenal incidenaloma. British Journal of Surgery 80: 422–436

Orchard T, Grant CS, van Heerden JA, Weaver A 1993 Phaeochromocytoma – continuing evolution of surgical therapy. Surgery 114: 1153–1158; discussion 1158–1159

Arteries

P. L. Harris

Contents

INTRODUCTION

As a consequence of the high prevalence of arterial disease in western countries, and the lack of effective medical treatment, arterial operations have come to represent a considerable proportion of the total surgical workload. Accordingly, this aspect of general surgery has evolved into a speciality with a degree of complexity that is recognized in the training programmes of those who wish to make the management of vascular disease a major part of their practice. However, given the ubiquitous nature of arteries, all competent surgeons should be familiar with the basic principles of arterial repair and reconstruction.

> ### Key points
>
> There are three main reasons for operating on an artery:
> - injury
> - aneurysmal dilatation
> - occlusion.

1. *Injury*. This may result from sharp or blunt trauma. It can occur in association with fracture of long bones, especially the femur and humerus. Increasingly common are iatrogenic injuries resulting from the use of arterial access routes for various forms of investigation or treatment, and self-induced injury in main-line drug abusers.

2. *Aneurysm*. In recent years there has been a dramatic increase in the number of operations for atherosclerotic aneurysms of the abdominal aorta. The incidence of aneurysms of the popliteal artery is also rising. Dissecting aneurysms of the aorta are a distinct pathological entity for which vascular surgical intervention is sometimes required. Mycotic aneurysms are seen occasionally but those associated with syphilitic infections are now extremely rare.

3. *Occlusion and stenosis*. Most arterial occlusions result from thrombosis of a stenosed vessel, the underlying disease being atherosclerosis. In many people this is a slowly progressive condition that is part of a natural ageing process and it does not always require surgical intervention. Critical limb ischaemia is a very strong indication for operation but patients with intermittent claudication require careful assessment in order to balance the potential benefits and risks before any surgical intervention is advised for them. Occasionally an artery becomes acutely occluded by an embolus. Sudden occlusion of an otherwise normal major artery is a catastrophe that threatens both the viability of the limb and the life of the patient. Urgent treatment is required, directed towards removal or dissolution of the occluding embolus. The management of acute and chronic ischaemia is therefore quite different. Less commonly, acute limb-threatening ischaemia develops following sudden occlusion by thrombosis of a previously diseased artery or a bypass graft. The acute-on-chronic ischaemia that results poses a specially difficult problem of management since it cannot usually be treated effectively by thrombectomy alone. Because of its inherently dangerous nature, the urgency, which precludes detailed preoperative preparation, and the elderly frail condition of most of the patients, the mortality risk associated with acute arterial occlusion is high. Furthermore, the urgency of the situation may make it necessary for these patients to be treated in non-specialist units.

GENERAL PRINCIPLES

Special equipment

1. **Sutures, needle-holders and suture clamps.** Arteries are always sewn with non-absorbable stitches. There are three types. Fine monofilament material such as polypropylene has the advantage of being very smooth and slipping easily through the tissues so that a loose suture can be drawn up tight. The fact that it has a slight 'memory' can easily be compensated for with familiarity of use. Its main disadvantage is that it has a tendency to brittleness and it must never be picked up directly with metal instruments. The second type of suture is braided material coated with an outer layer of polyester to render it smooth. Examples of such sutures are Ethiflex® and Ethibond®. Sutures of this type do not slip

so easily through the arterial wall but are pleasantly floppy to handle and knot easily. Tough atraumatic needles are swaged on to each end of the suture.

Finally, PTFE (polytetrafluoroethylene) sutures are designed specifically for use with PTFE grafts. PTFE is non-compliant so that the holes in the graft made by the passage of a needle do not close around the suture, resulting in more bleeding than occurs with other types of graft. In order to overcome this problem the diameter of the needles is made smaller than that of the suture itself. This is at the expense of some loss of strength, and the fragility of these needles precludes their use in tough or calcified arteries. The suture material itself is extremely strong and has excellent handling properties. In general, use the finest suture that is strong enough for the job; as a rough guide, 3/0 for the aorta, 4/0 for the iliacs, 5/0 for the femoral, 6/0 for the popliteal and 7/0 for the tibial arteries are appropriate. For very fine work a monofilament stitch is always necessary.

In the case of double-ended sutures the end that is not being worked with should be kept out of the way by attaching to it a 'rubber-shod' clamp. This is simply a mosquito or other small clamp, the jaws of which have been cushioned with fine rubber or plastic tubing. Never apply unprotected clamps to monofilament sutures. Because arterial suturing varies from relatively crude to extremely fine, have a wide selection of needle-holders. The range must reflect the fact that some anastomoses are virtually on the surface while others may be at considerable depth so that holders varying in length from 10 cm up to 30 cm are required. They should be fine-pointed to facilitate accurate placement of sutures and have tungsten or other high-quality jaws to ensure a firm grasp of the needle.

2. **Solutions**. For local irrigation of opened vessels and instillation into vessels distal to a clamp, use heparinized saline. This is made up from 5000 units of heparin in 500 ml of physiological saline.

3. **Blood transfusion and autotransfusion**. Arterial operations, particularly emergency procedures, may be associated with significant blood loss. An autotransfusion system or cell saver reduces the requirement for banked blood and protects the patient from the risk of blood-borne infections.

4. **Grafts and stents**. The best arterial substitute is the patient's own blood vessel, usually vein. However, quite often there is no suitable vein available, because it is either absent, too small for the job required or has itself been damaged by varicosities or thrombophlebitis. Under these circumstances a prosthesis has to be chosen and three types are currently available.

a. *Dacron®*. This is an inert polymer that is spun into a thread and then either woven or knitted into the familiar cloth graft. It is available in tubes from 5–25 mm in diameter, straight or bifurcated. In general, prefer the knitted variety with a velour lining as its porosity allows tissue ingrowth and better anchoring of the internal 'neointimal' surface. The original knitted grafts needed to be carefully preclotted with blood taken from the patient prior to the administration of heparin and in an emergency such as a ruptured aneurysm it was necessary to use a woven graft, which leaks less.

However, most vascular surgeons now use knitted grafts that have been presealed with bovine collagen, gelatin or albumen. These grafts have very low porosity at the time of insertion and so do not require preclotting. Within 3 months the sealant has been absorbed and

replaced by natural fibrous tissue ingrowth, thereby providing the advantages of both woven and knitted prostheses. In the future it is likely that additional substances, for example antibiotics or anticoagulants, may be incorporated within the sealant. Dacron® grafts perform extremely well when used to bypass large arteries with a high flow rate, for example the aorta and iliac arteries, and they are the arterial substitute of choice in these situations.

b. *Expanded PTFE*. Grafts made of this material are slightly more expensive than Dacron® but their performance in terms of patency rate is superior. They are better when tubes of 6 mm diameter or less are required, for example in the reconstruction of infrapopliteal arteries. In general, therefore, Dacron® grafts are used above the groin and PTFE below the groin, although some surgeons use Dacron® in preference to PTFE for above-the-knee femoropopliteal bypass. PTFE grafts are available with an external polypropylene support to prevent compression or kinking of the graft. It is essential to use this type of graft whenever the knee or any other joint is crossed.

c. *Biological*. The first arterial substitutes tried were arterial or venous allografts or xenografts. However, these rapidly degraded and were abandoned. Modern biological grafts, of which the Dardik human umbilical vein graft is the best known, are treated to make them non-antigenic and then coated with an outer Dacron® support to prevent aneurysmal dilatation. These grafts are associated with comparatively good patency rates even in distal sites, but are subject to a risk of aneurysmal degeneration. For this reason few vascular surgeons use them.

d. *Preshaped (cuffed) grafts*. This is a recent development in graft technology. There is evidence to show that when PTFE grafts are anastomosed to small arteries below the level of the knee joint, better rates of patency may be achieved if a cuff, collar or patch of vein is interposed between the graft and the artery at the distal anastomosis. Although the mechanism involved remains uncertain, one possibility is that the configuration of a cuffed anastomosis promotes a pattern of blood flow that inhibits or redistributes the anastomotic myointimal hyperplasia that is the principal cause of graft failure. The configuration or shape of an anastomosis is not dependent upon the use of vein. Preshaped grafts have been manufactured from PTFE to reproduce an anastomosis of 'ideal' configuration without the necessity of constructing a cuff from vein. An additional benefit is that the wall of the shaped end is thinner than that of the body of the graft and this facilitates suturing.

e. *Compliant grafts*. One reason that prosthetic grafts are said to perform less well than natural vessels is that they are stiff or non-compliant. This makes them inefficient as conduits of pulsatile flow. Grafts with some degree of compliance are now available but their value in clinical practice is unproven.

f. *Stents and stent/grafts*. Metallic stents made from either stainless steel or nitinol may be used as an adjunct to balloon angioplasty in order to maintain patency of the vessel or as framework to support an endovascular graft for exclusion of an aneurysm. They are of two types: balloon expandable, e.g. Palmaz stent; and self-expanding, e.g. Wallstent. Stents for endovascular aneurysm repair are covered with Dacron®, PTFE or other fabric. They are manufactured as straight tubes or with a bifurcated construction for repair of abdominal aortic aneurysms.

Basic techniques of arterial repair and anastomosis

Arteriotomy

> ### 🔑 Key points
>
> Arteries are best opened longitudinally. This is for three reasons.
>
> - A longitudinal arteriotomy is easier to close; any thrombus that accumulates on the suture line has less tendency to narrow the lumen
> - A longitudinal arteriotomy can be rapidly extended if required
> - A transverse arteriotomy is difficult to close because the intima retracts away from the outer layers. This increases the risk of blood tracking in a subintimal plane, resulting in occlusion of the vessel.

Simple suture

Longitudinal arteriotomies in large or medium sized arteries can usually be closed by simple suture (Fig. 23.1).

Use the finest suture material compatible with the thickness and quality of the arterial wall. The aim is to produce an everted suture line that is leak-proof. This is quite different from bowel suture, where the mucosa is deliberately inverted into the lumen and the tension on the sutures is kept low to avoid necrosis of the edges. There is no need to use everting mattress sutures, which would narrow the lumen. A simple over-and-over stitch is adequate, provided that care is taken to ensure that the intima turns outwards. The needle must pass through all layers of the arterial wall with every stitch. The inner layers must be included to ensure good intimal apposition and to prevent flap dissection, and the outer layers must be included since the main strength of the arterial wall resides in its adventitia. Keep a firm, even tension on the suture at all times. Experience is required in order to judge the spacing and size of each bite, and this varies with the size and nature of the artery. Occasionally, as, for example, in aortic aneurysm repair, large, irregular stitches may be required but, in general, evenly spaced regular stitching is best.

Closure with a patch

Close vessels of less than 4 mm in diameter with a patch in order to avoid narrowing of the lumen (Fig. 23.2).

This technique may also be used to widen the lumen of a vessel that has become stenosed by disease, for example the profunda femoris artery. For small vessels use a patch of autologous vein. Never sacrifice the proximal end of the long saphenous vein for this purpose. Use either a segment taken from the ankle, a tributary or a piece of vein from another site – for example an arm vein. For larger vessels prosthetic material – either Dacron® or PTFE – may be used. When cutting the patch to shape always ensure that the ends are rounded rather than being tapered to a sharp point. This is to prevent narrowing of the lumen caused by 'clustering' of sutures at the point. After shaping the patch use just one double-ended stitch commencing close to one end and working around each side. Do not finish the stitching at the apex; carry one of the sutures around to the other margin to complete the closure and tie the knot a short distance to one side. Knots at the apex may be a cause of significant narrowing. This technique permits direct vision of the internal suture line and allows final trimming of the patch to be delayed until closure is nearly complete in order to ensure a perfect match for size.

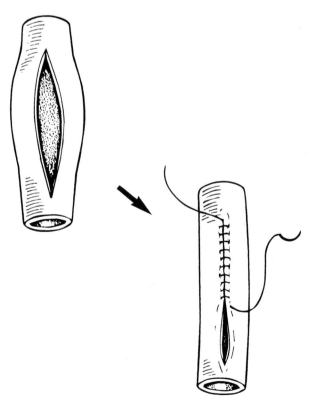

Fig. 23.1 Longitudinal arteriotomy closed by continuous everting arterial suture.

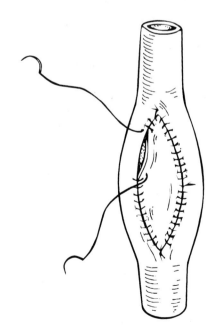

Fig. 23.2 Closure of longitudinal arteriotomy with a patch.

End-to-end anastomosis

1. For small delicate arteries this is accomplished most safely by applying the principles of the triangulation technique originally described by Carrel.[1] Join the vessels with a suture placed in the centre of the back or deepest aspect of the anastomosis (Fig. 23.3).

Be sure to tie the knot on the outside. Place two more sutures so as to divide the circumference of the vessels equally into three. Any disparity in calibre can be compensated for at this stage. Always use interrupted sutures for small vessels, in which case keep the three original stay sutures long and apply gentle traction on them to rotate the vessel and facilitate exposure of each segment of the anastomosis in turn. Complete the back or deep segments first, leaving the easiest segment at the front to be finished last.

2. For larger vessels it is permissible to use continuous sutures. Cut the ends of the vessels to be joined obliquely, then make a short incision longitudinally to create a spatulate shape. Overlapping the two spatulate ends avoids any risk of narrowing at the anastomosis.

3. A different technique of end-to-end anastomosis can be employed with great effect in operation on aneurysms. This is the inlay technique. (See below – Repair of abdominal aorta aneurysm.)

End-to-side anastomosis

1. This is the standard form of anastomosis for bypass operations. It should be oblique and its length should be approximately twice the diameter of the lumen of the graft. The end of the graft is fashioned into a spatulate shape, which will, on completion of the anastomosis, adopt a 'cobra head' appearance. The end of the anastomosis in the angle is referred to as the 'heel' and the other end as the 'toe'. The simplest way of completing it is to place a double-ended stitch at the heel and another at the toe and to run sutures along each margin, ending with a knot at the halfway point on each side. However, there is an advantage in keeping the inside of the suture line in view as much as possible. Achieve this by starting with a double-ended suture at the heel. Leave the toe free. Run the suture up each side to beyond the midpoint and then retain in a 'rubber-shod' clamp. Insert a further stitch through the toe and complete and trim the last two quadrants by tying to the previously retained threads. This is sometimes known as the 'four quadrant technique' (Fig. 23.4).

The 'toe' and 'heel' are the most crucial points of an end-to-side anastomosis. To ensure that the toe is completed as smoothly as possible, offset the starting point of the 'toe', suturing a few

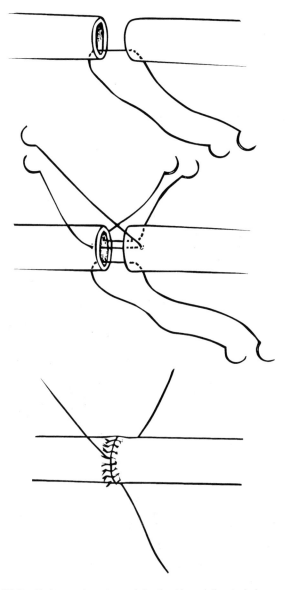

Fig. 23.3 End-to-end anastomosis by the triangulation technique.

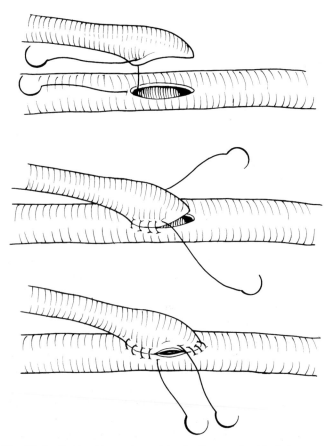

Fig. 23.4 End-to-side anastomosis by the four quadrant technique.

millimetres to one side or the other of the apex. In order to further reduce the risk of causing a stricture at this point, some surgeons prefer to place a few interrupted sutures around the toe.

2. A stricture of the heel may be avoided by stenting the vessel with an intraluminal catheter of appropriate size until this portion of the anastomosis is complete. An alternative method is the 'parachute' technique (Fig. 23.5).

This is particularly useful where access is difficult and good visualization of the anastomosis is impaired, but it is applicable to most situations. With the graft and the recipient artery separated, place a series of running sutures between them at what will become the heel of the anastomosis. These sutures are then pulled tight as the vessels are approximated.

> 🔑 **Key point**
>
> • It is essential to use a monofilament suture with this method.

EXPOSURE OF THE MAJOR PERIPHERAL ARTERIES

Common femoral artery

1. The common femoral artery needs to be exposed more frequently than any other vessel in the body and it is important to know how to do this swiftly and correctly (Fig. 23.6).

> 🔑 **Key point**
>
> • The surface marking of the artery is at the mid-inguinal point, i.e. halfway between the anterior superior iliac spine and the pubic symphysis. Remember this, since the artery is not always palpable.

2. The groin crease does not correspond in position to that of the inguinal ligament, but lies distal to it by 2–3 cm.

3. Provided that the saphenous vein will not be required during the operation, make a vertical incision directly over the artery. The midpoint of this incision should roughly correspond to the groin crease. Inexperienced surgeons tend to make the incision too low.

4. Deepen the incision through the subcutaneous fat, taking care not to cut across any lymph nodes. Expose the femoral sheath and incise it longitudinally to uncover the artery. The femoral vein lies medially and must be protected but the femoral nerve on the lateral side lies at a deeper plane and is not usually at risk.

5. Pass a Lahey clamp around the back of the artery in order to draw through a plastic sling. Gently lift the artery with the sling, which helps to identify its branches and its bifurcation into the superficial and profunda femoral arteries. Isolate these similarly with slings. Take care to avoid damage to the profunda vein, a tributary of which always passes anterior to the main stem of the profunda artery. For proper exposure of the profunda artery divide this vein between ties.

6. If exposure of the long saphenous vein is required at the same operation make a 'lazy S' incision, commencing vertically over the

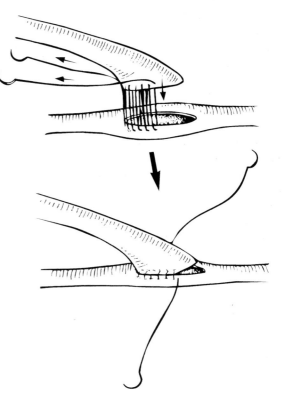

Fig. 23.5 End-to-side anastomosis by the parachute technique.

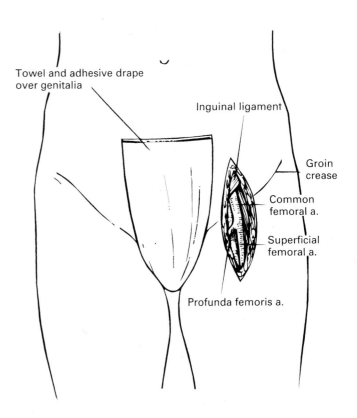

Fig. 23.6 Exposure of the common femoral artery.

Labels on figure: Towel and adhesive drape over genitalia; Inguinal ligament; Groin crease; Common femoral a.; Superficial femoral a.; Profunda femoris a.

artery at the inguinal ligament and then deviating medially over the saphenous vein in the upper thigh.

7. Transection of the many lymphatics in the femoral triangle may cause a troublesome lymphocele or lymphatic fistula after the operation. There is no sure way of avoiding this, but approach the artery from its lateral rather than its medial side and gently reflect any lymph nodes and visible lymph vessels off the femoral sheath with minimal damage.

Popliteal artery

1. The popliteal artery can be exposed above and below the knee. The most inaccessible part lies directly behind the joint line.

2. To expose the suprageniculate artery, make a longitudinal incision over the medial aspect of the lower thigh (Fig. 23.7).

If you intend to perform a bypass with a saphenous vein graft, make this incision directly over the previously marked vein. Otherwise the incision should correspond with the anterior border of the sartorius muscle. Inexperienced surgeons tend to place this incision too far anteriorly. Deepen the incision to expose the sartorius muscle, which is retracted posteriorly to reveal the neurovascular bundle enveloped by the popliteal fat pad. The artery lies on the bone. The nerve lies some distance away with the vein in between. The popliteal artery is always surrounded by a plexus of veins, which must be carefully separated and divided in order to avoid troublesome bleeding.

3. In order to expose the infrageniculate popliteal artery, make an incision on the medial aspect of the calf along the border of the gastrocnemius muscle (Fig. 23.8).

Continue the dissection between the medial head of this muscle and the tibia to reveal the neurovascular bundle. The vein is exposed first and this has to be lifted carefully away to give access to the artery. By dividing the soleus muscle along its attachment to the medial border of the tibia it is possible to expose the origin of the anterior tibial artery and the whole extent of the tibioperoneal trunk through this incision. Improve the exposure of the popliteal artery proximally by dividing the tendons of sartorius, semitendinosus and gracilis muscles. If necessary, completely divide the medial head of gastrocnemius; this leaves surprisingly little functional disability.

4. If exposure of the whole length of the popliteal artery is required

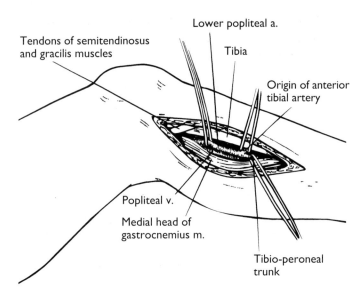

Fig. 23.8 Exposure of the infrageniculate popliteal artery.

it is better to use a posterior approach. With the patient lying prone, make a 'lazy S' incision through the popliteal fossa. Deepen the incision through the popliteal fascia and the fat pad and define the diamond between the hamstring muscles above and the two heads of gastrocnemius below; then follow the short saphenous vein into the neurovascular bundle.

Subclavian artery

1. Make a transverse incision 1 cm above the medial third of the clavicle; divide the platysma muscle in the same plane (Fig. 23.9).

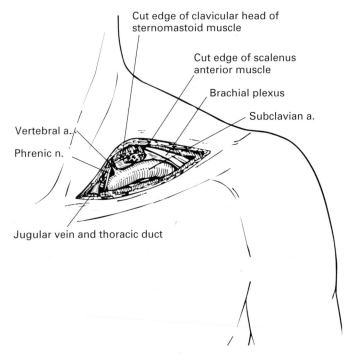

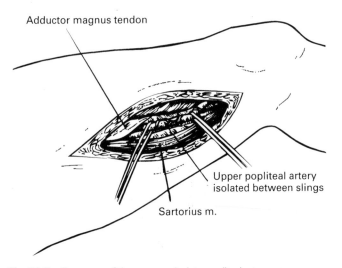

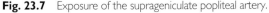

Fig. 23.7 Exposure of the suprageniculate popliteal artery.

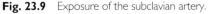

Fig. 23.9 Exposure of the subclavian artery.

This exposes the clavicular head of sternomastoid muscle, which is divided, and also a fat pad containing the scalene lymph nodes. Dissect and retract this fat pad superiorly off the surface of the scalenus anterior muscle. Identify the phrenic nerve, which passes obliquely across the front of this muscle to lie along the medial border of its tendon and usually separated from it by a few millimetres. Pass the blade of a MacDonald's dissector behind the tendon of scalenus anterior muscle, in such a way as to protect the phrenic nerve, and divide the tendon by cutting down on to the dissector with a pointed scalpel blade. Retraction of the muscle superiorly exposes the subclavian artery with its vertebral, internal mammary and thyro-cervical branches. The first thoracic nerve root and the lower trunk of the brachial plexus cross the first rib above and posterior to the artery. The subclavian vein is deep to the clavicle and is not normally seen through this approach. On the left side the thoracic duct enters the confluence of the internal jugular and subclavian veins. If it is damaged, ligate it to prevent the development of a troublesome postoperative chylous fistula.

2. Extensive exposure of the subclavian artery can be obtained by excision of the inner two-thirds of the clavicle, although this is rarely necessary. The two most common operations on the subclavian artery are carotid–subclavian anastomosis or bypass for a proximal occlusion (subclavian steal syndrome) and repair of a subclavian aneurysm. (This is usually a misnomer since most so-called subclavian aneurysms involve the first part of the axillary artery.) The former is usually completed without difficulty through the approach described above, and the latter is most conveniently accomplished with separate incisions above and below the clavicle to expose the subclavian and axillary arteries (see below).

3. Operations that involve direct exposure of the origin of the subclavian artery have been largely superseded by extrathoracic bypass procedures (carotid–subclavian and subclavian–subclavian bypass). On the rare occasions when direct exposure is considered essential this is best achieved by splitting the manubrium and upper sternum.

Make a right-angled incision with a horizontal component above the medial third of the clavicle and a vertical component in the midline over the manubrium and upper sternum. Complete the supraclavicular exposure of the artery as described above. Deepen the vertical incision through the subcutaneous tissue and periosteum. The periosteum is extremely vascular and diathermy is required to seal the small arteries. Commencing at the suprasternal notch, open a retrosternal plane by finger dissection, and then, with a sternal chisel and hammer or a properly protected reciprocating saw, divide the manubrium and sternum in the midline and spread the edges with a self-retaining retractor. Dissection of the thymus and anterior mediastinal fat is necessary to expose the arch of the aorta and the origins of the supra-aortic vessels. The innominate vein is stretched across the upper part of the incision and must be protected. It is not usually necessary to divide the sternal tendon of the sternomastoid muscle. Close with peristernal wire or strong nylon sutures, taking care to avoid damage to the internal mammary and intercostal arteries when inserting them.

The origin of the left subclavian artery, which arises far backwards from the aorta arch, can also be exposed through a posterolateral thoracotomy through the bed of the second or third ribs.

Brachial artery

It is more frequently necessary to expose the bifurcation of the brachial artery in order, for example, to remove surgically a brachial embolus. To do so, make a 'lazy S' incision in the antecubital fossa followed by division of the biceps aponeurosis (Fig. 23.10). Distal extension of this incision permits the radial, ulnar and anterior interosseous arteries to be followed into the forearm.

REFERENCE

1. Carrel A 1902 La technique operatoire des anastomoses vasculaires et de la transplantation des viscères. Lyon Medicale 99: 114–152

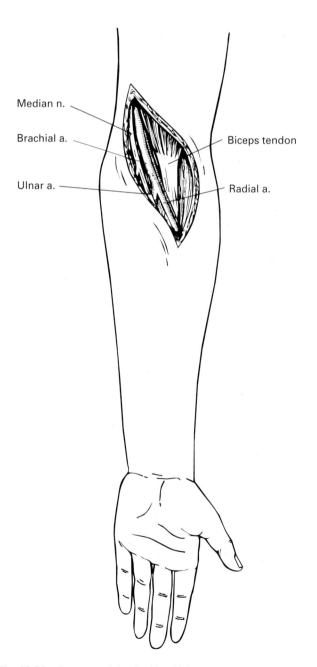

Fig. 23.10 Exposure of the distal brachial artery.

TYPES OF OPERATION

Details of the techniques used to repair or bypass damaged or diseased arteries will be included within the relevant descriptions of specific arterial operations (see below). However, it is useful at this point to summarize the range of procedures available.

1. Direct repair, interposition grafting and patch grafting for arterial trauma
2. Surgical embolectomy or thrombectomy
3. Thrombolytic therapy and percutaneous suction embolectomy
4. Endarterectomy, which, with the exception of carotid endarterectomy, has now been largely supplanted by bypass surgery as the treatment of choice for occlusive disease
5. Bypass grafting
6. Percutaneous and intraoperative (adjunctive) dilatation angioplasty. The basic technique involves the use of a guide-wire and a balloon dilatation catheter.[1] Devices exist to assist recanalization of resistant occlusions, including lasers, rotational guide-wires, high-frequency electrocoagulation ablators and various types of atherectomy catheters. None of these has yet found a major role in the routine management of vascular disease, and lasers in particular, despite increasing technological sophistication, have so far proved disappointing. The basic technique with balloon catheters has, however, made a major impact in recent years and in some centres more than half of all patients with occlusive disease are treated by this method
7. Inlay grafting for aneurysms
8. Endovascular stent/graft repair of aortic and peripheral aneurysms.

REFERENCE

1. Gruntzig A, Kumpe D A 1979 Technique of percutaneous transluminal angioplasty with the Gruntzig balloon catheter. American Journal of Roentgenology 132: 547–552

Key point

There are three basic prerequisites for success in arterial surgery. Although the relevance of each varies according to specific circumstance it is a valuable discipline to include an appraisal of all three factors when planning any arterial reconstruction:

- an unimpeded inflow tract – the run-in
- an adequate outflow tract – the run-off – and
- an efficient recanalization or bypass – the conduit.

ARTERIAL OPERATIONS

Repair of arterial injury

Appraise

1. Arterial trauma may occur as an isolated event but more often it occurs in association with other injuries, for example fracture of long bones. Under these circumstances there is a danger that the symptoms of ischaemia may be masked and therefore go unrecognized until irreversible tissue damage has occurred. Always assess the distal circulation in cases of fractured long bones or disarticulation injuries, especially those that involve the elbow or knee.

2. Arterial injury is manifest by:

a. bleeding, either externally or with the formation of a large haematoma, and
b. acute ischaemia with pallor, coldness, loss of sensation, muscle tenderness and weakness, absent pulses and absent or damped Doppler signals with reduced systolic arterial pressure in distal vessels.

3. Suspicion of arterial injury is an indication for urgent angiography, except for haemorrhage, in which case proceed directly to surgical exploration.

4. Angiographic discontinuity of a major limb vessel always requires urgent surgical exploration. Occlusion of a single tibial or forearm vessel is usually tolerated without ischaemic damage and does not as a rule require reconstruction.

5. Beware the concept of 'arterial spasm'. It is true that the smooth muscle of arteries contracts protectively in response to injury so that an important vessel may appear quite small both angiographically and on direct inspection. However, luminal discontinuity is always due to a mechanical fault and demands surgical repair. Never attempt to treat such lesions with vasodilator drugs.

6. In the case of multiple injuries co-operate closely with colleagues of other specialities in planning surgical treatment. Repair of damaged major arteries always takes precedence over orthopaedic fixation of fractures. However, there is a danger that vascular anastomoses may become disrupted during the manipulation of fractures. In these circumstances it may be advisable to restore vascular continuity initially by inserting a temporary intraluminal plastic shunt, and completing the repair once the fractures have been stabilized, when the length of the arterial defect can be accurately measured.

7. Run-in. This is not usually relevant in arterial trauma.

8. Run-off. There is a risk that blood clot may form and occlude vessels distal to the site of injury. The procedure must include measures to deal with this problem (see below), otherwise the run-off vessels are usually normal.

9. Conduit. In the case of limb injuries this is either the original artery repaired directly or an interposition graft of autogenous vein. Since only short segments are required, problems are rarely encountered in finding a vein of suitable quality and calibre.

10. For closed injuries to major arteries (e.g. iliac, subclavian) with tearing or rupture of the vessel consider endovascular repair with a covered stent in hospitals with facilities for this type of procedure.

Prepare

Once the presence of major arterial injury has been established, undertake surgical exploration without delay. Have cross-matched blood available and correct serious hypovolaemia.

Access

1. In the case of limb injury, prepare and drape the limb so as to permit direct inspection of skin perfusion and palpation of pulses distal to the site of injury.

2. Consider also the possibility that a segment of healthy undamaged vein of suitable size may need to be harvested for construction of a graft.

3. First, gain proximal control of the artery and then gain distal control. This requires a skin incision that extends well beyond the confines of the injury. Make this incision along the axis of the injured vessel and directly over it.

4. Do not enter the haematoma until the vessel has been dissected and controlled by passing rubber slings around it proximally and distally.

Assess

1. On entering the haematoma there may be brisk fresh bleeding, in which case apply clamps at the proximal and distal control points already prepared.

2. If there is complete disruption of the artery find the ends and apply soft clamps. It is unlikely that they will be actively bleeding at the time of exploration.

3. It is always the case that the vessel is traumatized for some distance proximally and distally from the principal site of injury. Therefore trim each end back a few millimetres at a time until undamaged intima is reached.

4. Assess the length of the defect. Attempt direct end-to-end anastomosis only if there will be no tension. In most cases it is more prudent to insert an interposition graft of autologous vein, even if this is only a centimetre in length.

5. If the artery is in continuity there may be bruising of the adventitia at the site of injury and absence of downstream pulsation. These are sure signs of internal disruption. The intima and inner layers of the media split transversely and the edges roll back to form a flap, which obstructs flow, causing secondary thrombosis. It is never sufficient, therefore, to simply inspect the outer surface of such a vessel and it is totally unacceptable to treat such lesions by topical application of vasodilator substances. Excise the damaged segment completely, cutting back each end of the artery as before to find healthy intima.

6. Active arterial bleeding usually signifies incomplete disruption or a lateral wall defect that inhibits protective retraction and constriction of the vessel.

Action

1. Before commencing repair of the artery pass a Fogarty catheter distally and proximally to withdraw any propagated clot and then instil heparinized saline.

2. If there are associated orthopaedic injuries consider inserting a temporary intraluminal shunt (see above).

3. The adventitia tends to prolapse over the end of a normal artery that has been cut across. Trim this back to prevent it intruding inside the anastomosis.

4. If direct end-to-end anastomosis is possible, accomplish it by the triangulation technique (see Basic techniques) and in most cases employ interrupted sutures in preference to continuous.

5. If the defect is too great to permit direct repair, harvest a segment of vein of appropriate size. Complete the proximal anastomosis first, in end-to-end fashion, using the triangulation technique with interrupted sutures for small or inaccessible vessels or the oblique overlap technique for larger vessels. Remember to reverse the vein to avoid obstruction to blood flow by competent valves. Apply a clamp to the distal end of the graft and allow arterial pressure to distend it in order to determine the optimum length to avoid both excessive tension and kinking. Finally, complete the distal anastomosis.

6. A small puncture or lateral wall defect, as may result from iatrogenic injury following arterial access for investigation or treatment, may be repaired by direct suture or by closing the arteriotomy with a patch.

? Difficulty?

1. Technical difficulty may be encountered in effecting satisfactory end-to-end anastomoses, usually because of awkward access. Under these circumstances the ends of the artery may be ligated and the area of trauma bypassed with end-to-side anastomoses at remote, more accessible sites.

2. Magnification is advisable for small-vessel anastomoses.

3. If there is any doubt about the effectiveness of the repair, obtain an on-table angiogram.

4. Recurrent thrombosis despite a technically satisfactory repair warrants immediate systemic heparinization.

5. It may be difficult to decide whether or not to repair associated damage to veins. As a rule, repair major axial veins such as the femoral vein and, in the case of near-amputation of a limb, restore continuity to two veins for each artery repaired. Construct venous anastomoses obliquely and with interrupted sutures.

Closure

1. Where possible, effect primary closure of the incision with suction drainage.

2. In the case of blast injuries and other causes of extensive skin and soft tissue damage, observe the general principles of wound management. Where primary closure is either not possible or inadvisable, always cover the arterial repair with healthy viable tissue, which in practice usually means a muscle flap.

Aftercare

1. Except in cases where continued bleeding is a serious problem, maintain anticoagulation with heparin for several days.

2. Arrange regular half-hourly observation of the distal circulation during the immediate postoperative period and be prepared to re-explore immediately in the event of recurrent occlusion.

Complications

1. Early thrombosis or bleeding at the site of the repair demands immediate re-exploration and re-assessment.

2. A false aneurysm may result from a contained anastomotic leak and this also requires early re-exploration and repair.

3. The risk of associated deep venous thrombosis is high, so take appropriate preventative measures.

4. Repair of arterial injuries in young, healthy people is usually very successful and long-term disability associated with ischaemia is rare.

Surgical embolectomy

Appraise

1. Embolic occlusion of a major artery results in acute ischaemia, which, if not relieved quickly, may progress to irreversible tissue damage and limb loss.

2. The differential diagnosis is from acute thrombosis occurring within an already diseased artery. Differentiation between these two conditions may be impossible on clinical grounds alone, especially since embolization is nowadays more commonly associated with ischaemic heart disease than valvular stenosis, and most patients therefore have generalized arteriosclerosis.

3. If there is an immediate threat to the viability of the limb, evidenced by muscle tenderness and paralysis and loss of sensation, then immediate surgical exploration is required irrespective of the cause.

4. Revascularization of a limb that is already totally non-viable invariably has fatal consequences and is absolutely contraindicated. Urgent amputation may be life-saving.

5. Under other circumstances urgent angiography is indicated to establish the diagnosis and to permit proper appraisal of the various options for treatment.

6. Surgical embolectomy is indicated for embolic occlusion of:

a. the common femoral artery and vessels proximal to the groin, e.g. saddle embolus, and
b. the brachial and axillary arteries.

8. For patients in whom there is no immediate threat to the viability of the limb, more distal emboli, such as those in the popliteal artery, are more appropriately treated by thrombolytic therapy.

9. Preoperative appraisal includes an assessment of the underlying cardiac disease. Surgical embolectomy can be performed under local anaesthesia but general anaesthesia is preferable in the absence of serious anaesthetic risk.

10. Run-in, run-off and conduit usually are not relevant to surgical embolectomy in the absence of associated arterial disease.

Prepare

1. The urgency of the situation dictates that preoperative preparation must be limited. Treatment may be required for heart failure or dysrhythmia.

2. Commence systemic anticoagulation with heparin.

Access

1. For lower limb emboli, expose the common femoral artery (see above, Exposure of the major peripheral arteries).

2. For upper limb emboli, expose the brachial artery in the antecubital fossa (see above).

Action

1. Make a short longitudinal arteriotomy. In the case of the femoral artery make this directly over the origin of the profunda artery.

2. Select an embolectomy catheter of a size that is appropriate to vessel: 3F for axillary and brachial arteries, 4F for the superficial and profunda femoral arteries and 5F for the aortic bifurcation.

3. A number of different makes of embolectomy catheter are available. Choose one with a central irrigating lumen that permits injection of heparinized saline or X-ray contrast medium into the vessels beyond the balloon.

4. Pass the uninflated catheter proximally through the vessel beyond the clot. Inflate the balloon and withdraw the catheter slowly while adjusting the pressure within the balloon to accommodate changes in the diameter of the vessel. Avoid severe friction between the balloon and the arterial wall since this can cause serious damage to the vessel.

5. Instruct an assistant to control bleeding from the vessel during this process by applying gentle traction to the rubber sling previously placed around it.

6. Repeat the procedure until no more thrombus is retrieved and forceful bleeding is obtained from the vessel. Avoid all unnecessary passages of the catheter.

7. Instil heparinized saline into the artery and gently apply a clamp.

8. Repeat the same procedure distally.

9. Fill the vessels with heparinized saline and close the arteriotomy. Directly suture the common femoral artery but use a small vein patch for the brachial artery always.

? Difficulty?

1. *The catheter will not pass proximally or forceful forward bleeding is not obtained.* This can be due to pre-existing arterial disease or to the catheter having been introduced in a subintimal plane. Avoid direct aortoiliac reconstruction under these circumstances if at all possible and perform either a femorofemoral crossover or an axillofemoral bypass (see below).

2. *The catheter will not pass distally.* Obtain an on-table angiogram. This may show embolus impacted at the popliteal bifurcation and in the tibial arteries or evidence of atherosclerotic occlusion. Instil a small amount of a thrombolytic agent (streptokinase, urokinase or tissue plasminogen activator) locally through a small catheter advanced to the site of occlusion. Then pass a small Fogarty catheter 15 minutes later; more embolus may be retrieved. Alternatively, expose the infrageniculate popliteal artery to enable Fogarty catheters to be introduced directly into the tibial vessels. This requires the administration of a general anaesthetic. If there is a long-standing atherosclerotic occlusion of the superficial femoral artery, restoration of blood flow to the profunda system alone is likely to be sufficient to save the limb. However, if distal perfusion remains poor, then proceed to femoropopliteal bypass.

Closure

Close the wound in layers with interrupted skin sutures or clips after instituting suction drainage.

Aftercare

1. Arrange long-term anticoagulation therapy to prevent recurrent embolization for younger patients. But, in the case of the very elderly, weigh the risks of this strategy against the benefits.

2. Evaluate and treat the underlying cardiac disease.

Percutaneous thrombolytic embolectomy/thrombectomy

Appraise

See Surgical embolectomy, above.

Prepare

1. Thrombolytic therapy is contraindicated in patients who have suffered a stroke and in those with intracardiac thrombus. Obtain an echocardiogram to eliminate the latter.

2. Streptokinase is antigenic and may induce severe anaphylactic shock if administered more than once. Therefore ascertain that the patient has never received streptokinase previously. Note that urokinase and tissue plasminogen activator (TPA) may be given repeatedly without risk of this specific complication, but they are considerably more expensive.

3. Administer systemic anticoagulation with heparin.

Action

1. Puncture the common femoral artery with a Potts–Cournand needle and pass a short guide-wire into the superficial femoral artery.

2. Remove the needle and insert a 6F introducer sheath over the wire.

3. Under X-ray control advance a long guide-wire through the vessel beyond the embolus.

4. Pass a small-bore (4F) catheter over the guide-wire so that the tip enters the clot.

5. Withdraw the guide-wire and infuse the thrombolytic agent according to the manufacturer's instructions. Appreciate that, by infusing the agent locally into the thrombus, relatively small amounts are required. The high incidence of serious bleeding complications associated with systemic administration is thereby reduced.

6. After 30–60 minutes ascertain by X-ray the progress of clot lysis and advance the catheter again over a guide-wire into the embolus. Repeat this process until all blood clot has been dissolved.

7. More rapid and efficient lysis of thrombus can be achieved by the 'pulse-spray' technique. This involves pulsed high-pressure injection of the thrombolytic agent through a catheter with multiple side holes. Special equipment is required that is not available in all hospitals.

8. Finally, withdraw the catheter and apply pressure to the puncture site in the groin for a minimum period of 10 minutes to ensure haemostasis.

Difficulty?

The embolus may fragment and impact in more distal vessels. Further administration of the thrombolytic agent may be effective but it must be infused directly into the clot. Alternatively, small fragments may be removed by suction applied to a larger catheter (suction embolectomy). Provided that the viability of the limb has been secured, small residual fragments of this type may be of no consequence and they may lyse spontaneously in time if left.

Complications

1. In order to minimize haemorrhagic complications, monitor coagulation tests repeatedly and adjust the dose of thrombolytic agent accordingly.

2. There is a risk of blood clot forming around the catheter itself. Therefore maintain heparin anticoagulation throughout the procedure.

3. Groin haematomas will usually resolve spontaneously but expanding haematomas and false aneurysms require surgical repair.

PRINCIPLES OF REPAIR OF ABDOMINAL AORTIC ANEURYSM

Appraise

1. The abdominal aorta is the commonest site for aneurysms. These are dangerous lesions, death being the likely outcome in the event of rupture. The rate of growth and the risk of rupture increase exponentially with the diameter of the aneurysm, with a watershed level for serious risk at about 5.5 cm. Therefore, unless the patient is gravely ill from other causes, any aneurysm wider than 5.5 cm should be operated upon electively.

2. With improvements in anaesthetic management and progressive modification of surgical technique the mortality rate associated with elective aneurysm surgery is less than 5% in the best centres. In the UK small aneurysm trial the in-hospital mortality rate was 5.8%. The important surgical principles are:

a. minimal dissection
b. inlay technique of anastomosis
c use of straight rather than bifurcated grafts whenever possible.

3. Emergency operation is indicated for a patient with an aneurysm who develops severe abdominal or back pain with or without circulatory collapse, unless he is already moribund. The mortality risk associated with emergency aneurysm surgery is between 30% and 60%. The overall risk of death from a ruptured aneurysm is, however, more than 90%, since many patients die without reaching hospital.

Access

1. Make a midline incision extending from the xiphisternum to the pubis, skirting the umbilicus.

2. Displace the omentum and large bowel superiorly and the small bowel with its mesentery to the right.

3. The duodenum lies across the upper part of the aneurysm and must be displaced.

4. Once the neck of the aneurysm has been identified, carefully make a space on each side to accommodate the jaws of a straight clamp and apply this immediately from the front.

Assess

1. Confirm the position of the neck of the aneurysm relative to the renal arteries. 95% of aneurysms are infrarenal.

2. Assess the aortic bifurcation and the iliac arteries. A minor degree of ectasia of the iliac arteries can be accepted and it should be possible to use a straight graft in 60–70% of patients. A bifurcated graft is required if the common iliac ostia have been separated by the aneurysm or if one or both of the iliac arteries are grossly aneurysmal.

3. Assess the inferior mesenteric artery. Usually it is totally occluded. However, if it is widely patent it is advisable to observe the effect of temporary clamping of this vessel on the bowel circulation before it is finally sacrificed.

Action

1. No attempt should be made to encircle either the aorta or the iliac arteries. To do so risks trauma to veins with serious venous bleeding.

2. Carefully dissect a narrow space on each side of the aorta and of both common iliac arteries to permit access for the jaws of straight or slightly angled clamps applied from the front.

3. In elective cases only give heparin intravenously and allow 3 minutes for it to circulate before closing the clamps. Apply only sufficient pressure to occlude blood flow and no more.

4. Open the aneurysm longitudinally and scoop out the laminated thrombus, degenerate atheromatous material and liquid blood it contains. Always send a specimen to the laboratory for microbiological analysis.

5. Using 3/0 polypropylene sutures, construct an end-to-end anastomosis to the proximal aorta. This is done from within the sac by the inlay technique (Fig. 23.11).

6. Apply a soft clamp to the graft and gently release the aortic clamp to test the anastomosis. Place additional sutures as required.

7. If a straight tube is to be used, construct a similar anastomosis at the aortic bifurcation.

8. If a bifurcated graft is necessary it may be possible to construct an end-to-end anastomosis by the inlay technique to the iliac bifurcation on both sides.

9. Before completion of the distal anastomosis flush the graft to eliminate any blood clots and also to ensure that the recipient vessels bleed back satisfactorily. If this is not the case pass embolectomy catheters to retrieve any distal blood clots.

10. Give the anaesthetist several minutes warning before releasing the clamps and re-perfuse one leg at a time in order to minimize the risk of declamping shock. In the case of a bifurcation graft the anastomosis on one side may be completed and this limb perfused before the second anastomosis is constructed. A slight fall in blood pressure on release of a clamp is reassuring evidence that the limb is in fact being adequately perfused.

11. Having made quite certain that all anastomoses are blood-tight and that there is no bleeding from any other source, fold the redundant aneurysm sac over the graft and fix it with a number of catgut sutures. Make sure that the graft is covered completely.

Complications

There are six important potential complications to remember.

1. Haemorrhage
2. Occlusion

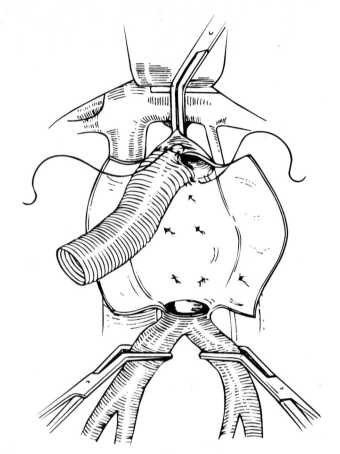

Fig. 23.11 The inlay technique of anastomosis.

3. Renal tubular necrosis
4. Adult respiratory distress syndrome (ARDS)
5. Myocardial infarction
6. Graft infection.

FURTHER READING

Fahal AH, McDonald AM, Marston A 1989 Femorofemoral bypass in unilateral iliac artery occlusion. British Journal of Surgery 76: 22–25

Kunlin J 1949 Le traitement de l'arterite obliterante par la greffe veineuse. Archives Chirurgie Mal Coeur 42: 371–372

Moody P, Gould DA, Harris PL 1990 Vein graft surveillance improves patency in femoro-popliteal bypass. European Journal of Vascular Surgery 4: 117–121

Veins

K. G. Burnand and M. Waltham

Contents

VARICOSE VEIN SURGERY

Appraise

1. Most patients seek treatment for their varicose veins because they dislike the appearance of the large, tortuous veins on their exposed legs. The greater number of varicose vein operations performed in women may reflect the greater importance they attach to attractive legs.

2. Many patients complain that the veins ache – a symptom that is often worse at the end of the day or after prolonged standing.

3. Minor varicose veins can often be made symptom-free by elastic support stockings.

4. Recurrent attacks of superficial thrombophlebitis or extensive bleeding from a ruptured varix are clear-cut indications for surgical treatment.

5. In patients with normal deep veins the severe pre-ulcerative changes of lipodermatosclerosis may be reversed and venous ulcers prevented by appropriate surgery to sites of superficial and communicating vein incompetence.

6. Surgical ligation and stripping remains the treatment of choice for major incompetence of the long and short saphenous veins, as injection sclerotherapy provides only short-term benefit. Varicose branch veins may be avulsed through local incisions at the time of saphenous surgery, but in the absence of saphenous incompetence are treated equally well by injection sclerotherapy.

7. Persistent or recurrent varicosities after saphenous surgery can also be treated by injection sclerotherapy if there are no residual connections with the femoral or popliteal veins.

8. Coincidental varicose veins are often erroneously diagnosed as

---

Key point

- Exclude arterial ischaemia, lymphoedema, arthritis of the hips and knees, and referred pain from the back as a cause of the patient's symptoms.

---

the cause of painful or swollen legs.

9. Most patients with uncomplicated and clear-cut varicose veins require little in the way of investigation beyond a careful history and an examination of the legs to determine the competence or incompetence of the major sites of communication between the superficial and deep venous systems. Inspection, palpation and the cough, percussion and tourniquet tests provide this information.

10. Patients who have lipodermatosclerosis, past ulceration or a history of limb fracture or deep vein thrombosis should undergo bipedal ascending phlebography or Duplex scanning to enable an accurate assessment of the deep and calf communicating veins to be made.

11. Patients with complicated or recurrent varicose veins are more accurately assessed by varicography, in which low-osmolality contrast medium is injected directly into the surface veins to display their course and deep connections. Duplex examination of reflux in the long and short saphenous trunks provides useful additional information.

12. An examination of calf pump function provided by ambulatory foot vein pressure measurements, plethysmography or foot volumetry is useful in a patient with healed venous ulcers. Duplex scanning is also used to quantify reflux in the deep veins and to evaluate reflux in the calf communicating veins.

13. Carefully re-examine patients admitted for varicose vein surgery. Incompetence in the long and short saphenous veins, and in the calf perforating veins, must be confirmed or excluded. Large branch varicosities and the sites of major communicating vein incompetence should be marked with an indelible pen. Suspect incompetence of the calf communicating veins in patients with lipodermatosclerosis. Preoperative marking with Duplex may be useful.

High saphenous ligation (Trendelenburg's operation) and stripping of the long saphenous vein

Appraise

1. Perform the operation on patients with varicose veins who have evidence of long saphenous reflux at the groin on clinical, Doppler or Duplex examination.

2. Avoid the operation if the long saphenous vein is a collateral for obstructed deep veins.

Prepare

1. Place the patient supine in Trendelenburg's position with approximately 30° of head-down tilt.

2. Abduct both legs about 15° from the midline and place the ankles on a padded board held under the cushions of the operating table. This position facilitates access and reduces bleeding.

Access

1. Make a short oblique incision parallel to and below the inguinal ligament in the groin crease, over the saphenofemoral junction. This is approximately 2 cm lateral and 2 cm below the pubic tubercle.

2. Deepen the incision through the subcutaneous fat, which is spread by digital retraction or by the insertion of a self-retaining retractor such as Traver's, West's or Cockett's.

Assess

The long saphenous vein normally appears as a dark-blue longitudinal trunk in the centre of the dissection as the subcutaneous fat is spread. If it is difficult to find, trace a small tributary back to the main trunk.

🔑 Key point

- Do not divide the long saphenous vein until the saphenofemoral junction has been identified.

Action

1. Dissect the long saphenous vein out of the surrounding fat and follow it up towards the saphenofemoral junction.

2. All the tributaries that join the long saphenous vein near its termination must be dissected out, ligated with 2/0 polyglactin 910 and divided. The superficial inferior epigastric vein, the superficial circumflex iliac vein, and the superficial and deep external pudendal veins all join the saphenous trunk near its termination. In addition the posteromedial and anterolateral thigh veins terminate close to the saphenofemoral junction (Fig. 24.1). One or more of these veins may join before emptying into the saphenous trunk.

3. After these tributaries have been divided, approach the saphenofemoral junction. The long saphenous vein dips down through the cribriform fascia over the foramen ovale to the femoral vein; carefully separate the subcutaneous fat off the vein by blunt dissection to trace its path. Display the femoral vein for approximately 1 cm above and below the saphenofemoral junction, and clear any small branches entering from either side.

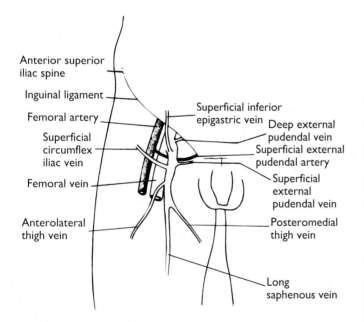

Fig. 24.1   The termination and tributaries of the long saphenous vein in the groin.

Anterior superior iliac spine
Inguinal ligament
Femoral artery
Superficial circumflex iliac vein
Femoral vein
Anterolateral thigh vein
Superficial inferior epigastric vein
Deep external pudendal vein
Superficial external pudendal artery
Superficial external pudendal vein
Posteromedial thigh vein
Long saphenous vein

4. Ligate the long saphenous vein in continuity with 0 polyglactin 910 flush with the saphenofemoral junction and divide it. For greater safety doubly ligate or transfix the saphenous stump. Alternatively, overview the termination with a 3/0 polypropylene continous suture.

5. Place a ligature around the long saphenous trunk and hold it up to occlude the flow of blood from below. Make a small side-hole in the vein above the ligature through which the tip of the stripper can be introduced. Use either a flexible steel stripper or a disposable plastic stripper with a suitably sized head. Gently manipulate the tip of the stripper into and down the vein until it is approximately a hand's breadth below the knee, where it may remain in the saphenous vein or pass into a tributary. Tie the ligature at the top end to prevent bleeding from the long saphenous trunk. Alternatively, a pin stripper with a small hole at the top can be used to invert and extract the vein. This technique has not been shown to have any benefit.

6. Make an oblique incision in one of Langer's lines, 1–2 cm in length, over the tip of the stripper. The incision must be large enough to allow the head of the stripper to pass. Palpate the vein containing the stripper and dissect it out, freeing any branches of the saphenous nerve. Make a small side-hole in the vein through which the tip of the stripper can be delivered and attach the T-shaped handle to the stripper.

7. Strip the long saphenous vein from the groin to the knee with steady downward traction. Ease the stripper and the bunched up vein through the lower incision. Clamp the attached long saphenous vein and any tributaries, divide and ligate it with 2/0 polyglactin 910.

8. Prevent excessive bleeding from the stripper track, either by tightly applying a sterile elasticated bandage while withdrawing the stripper, or by gently rolling a swab along the course of the vein before applying bandages. Some surgeons apply a tourniquet to the leg to prevent excessive haemorrhage.

❓ Difficulty?

1. The retrograde passage of the stripper may be impeded by competent valves, varicosity of the saphenous vein or false passage into small tortuous tributaries. Attempts to forcibly pass the stripper often result in perforation of the vein wall; if difficulty is encountered, withdraw the stripper and repass it. Twisting the free end to rotate the tip may help to negotiate irregularities in the vein. If hold-up occurs around the knee, the passage of the stripper may be aided by flexing and extending the joint, with gentle external compression over the tip of the stripper to prevent passage into superficial tributaries.

2. If these measures fail, leave the stripper in situ and pass a second stripper into the long saphenous vein from below the knee. If the second stripper passes without difficulty, gradually withdraw the first ahead of the advancing stripper passed from below.

3. If neither stripper will bypass the obstruction, cut down over the tips of both strippers. One stripper may be redirected through the cut-down incision and passed on down the vein, but if this fails, strip out the two halves of the vein leaving a short residual portion between the two incisions. Alternatively, forcibly avulse this segment of residual vein.

4. Control sudden massive haemorrhage by applying direct pressure to the bleeding point with a finger or swab. Summon experienced vascular help. Never attempt to blindly apply artery forceps.

Closure

1. Insert interrupted 2/0 polyglactin 910 into the subcutaneous tissue and fascia.

2. Close the skin with a 3/0 subcuticular suture and adhesive tapes, or with interrupted 4/0 nylon.

Postoperative

1. Keep the legs elevated 15° above the horizontal in bed.

2. Encourage early mobilization after applying additional compression bandages over the bandages put on in theatre. This reduces haematoma formation and provides better support when the patient stands. Patients should walk when up, and not stand still or sit with their feet down.

3. Discharge fit patients between 24 hours postoperatively, to reattend for removal of any non-absorbable sutures a week later.

4. The bandages should be worn for at least a week, and are usually re-applied in the daytime for 2–3 weeks.

Complications

1. Complications are uncommon. They include haematoma formation, oedema, wound infection and nerve damage. Accidental stripping of the femoral vein and artery have also been described.

2. Expect varicosities to recur in up to 15% of patients.

Short saphenous ligation and stripping

Appraise

1. This operation is indicated if there is gross dilatation and reflux in the short saphenous trunk or its tributaries.

> **Key point**
>
> - The termination of the short saphenous vein in the popliteal or femoral vein is extremely variable and must be accurately identified and marked.

2. Preoperative varicography, on-table saphenography and duplex scanning all provide accurate information about the termination of the short saphenous vein and its proximal tributaries.

Prepare

1. Place the anaesthetized, intubated patient prone with pillows under the chest, midriff and pelvis, and 30° of head-down tilt.

2. Slightly abduct the legs to ease access.

Access

1. Make a short transverse incision behind the lateral malleolus.

2. Make a longer incision in the popliteal fossa over the saphenopopliteal junction at the marked site.

Assess

1. Identify the short saphenous vein and carefully dissect it from the sural nerve behind the ankle.

2. A stripper passed up the vein may 'flick' as it enters the popliteal vein, indicating the position of the saphenopopliteal junction. More accurate information is obtained from the imaging techniques described and careful preoperative marking.

Action

1. Find the short saphenous vein posterior to the lateral malleolus at the ankle by dissecting it from the fat and its accompanying sural nerve.

2. Ligate the vein distally with 2/0 polyglactin. Pass a second ligature under the vein, elevate it with an artery forceps and make a small incision in the vein to insert the stripper.

3. Having inserted the stripper, pass it up the vein in an identical manner to that described for the long saphenous vein. Tie the ligature at the ankle to prevent blood loss.

4. Make a transverse incision 3–5 cm in length in the popliteal fossa over the saphenopopliteal junction, which has been identified by one of the methods described. Divide the deep fascia vertically or in the line of the incision and define the short saphenous vein beneath containing the easily palpable stripper. Pull the stripper back slightly.

5. Gently expose the termination of the vein using blunt dissection to separate it from the surrounding fat until the T-junction with the popliteal vein is identified. Deep retraction by Langenbeck's by an experienced assistant is helpful. Doubly ligate the stump of the short saphenous vein with 2/0 polyglactin, extract the head of the stripper from the lumen and tie the vein to the stripper.

6. Strip out the vein, and firmly wrap the leg in an elasticated bandage.

Closure

1. Insert interrupted 2/0 polyglactin into the subcutaneous tissue and fascia.

2. Close the skin with a 3/0 subcuticular suture and adhesive tapes, or with interrupted 4/0 nylon.

Postoperative

Manage the patient in the same manner as described for long saphenous ligation and stripping.

Complications

The sural nerve is easily damaged if it is not dissected free from the vein at the ankle. For this reason some surgeons never strip the short saphenous vein.

Avulsions or local ties

Appraise

1. Large branch veins that are not in close proximity to the saphenous or perforator systems must be occluded or excised to prevent unsightly local recurrences and provide a satisfactory cosmetic result.

2. A number of alternative techniques have been used to achieve this, including surgical avulsion, transcutaneous suturing and transcutaneous diathermy.

> **Key point**
>
> - Carefully mark branch veins on either side preoperatively to ensure that they are easily found through the small stab incisions.

Action

1. Make minute stab incision in Langer's lines directly over the course of the tributaries. Draw out a loop of vein by gentle blunt dissection with a mosquito artery forceps.

2. Divide the loop between mosquito forceps and tease out the vein in either direction by steady traction and gentle blunt dissection under the skin flaps with fine mosquito forceps or specially designed venous hooks.

3. Ease out the vein by gentle rotary movements during maintained traction.

4. Stop traction when the vein starts to stretch, and at this point tie off both ends with polyglactin . Alternatively, continue the traction until the vein breaks. Control bleeding by local pressure until traumatic venospasm develops.

5. Place incisions about 5 cm apart along the course of each tributary. The whole vein may be satisfactorily avulsed using the technique described above.

Difficulty?

Thin-walled 'blue' veins avulse poorly compared with thick 'white' veins and, if the veins tear easily with extensive blood loss, use local ligations in preference to avulsion.

Closure

Use interrupted 4/0 monofilament nylon mattress sutures or 2/0 polyglactin 910 in the subcutaneous tissues and adhesive tapes for the skin.

FURTHER READING

Cockett FB 1955 The pathology and treatment of venous ulcers of the leg. British Journal of Surgery 43: 260–278

Doran FSA, Barkat S 1981 The management of recurrent varicose veins. Annals of the Royal College of Surgeons of England 63: 432–436

Scott A, Dormandy J 1976 Outpatient percutaneous ligation of varicose veins. Proceedings of the Royal Society of Medicine 69: 852–853

Transplantation

K. Rolles

Contents
Introduction
Kidney transplantation
Liver transplantation

INTRODUCTION

1. Solid whole-organ transplantation has been one of the main events in the evolution of 20th-century patient care. Within the field of general surgery a kidney transplant offers a quality of life unattainable by long-term dialysis and the lack of long-term artificial support for end-stage disease of the liver, heart and lungs makes it likely that there will be a demand for organ transplantation into the foreseeable future.

2. Immunosuppressive agents that reduce or abolish graft rejection are vital to the success of organ transplantation.

3. The donor pool comprises:

a. *brain-stem dead*: heart-beating 'cadavers' – over 90% of solid organ donors, usually providing multiple organs
b. *non-heart-beating cadavers*, providing suitable organs for kidney transplantation but not transplantable livers or hearts
c. *living related donors*, such as identical twins, siblings, parents, children, first-order cousins, providing excellent sources for kidney transplants; with development of appropriate techniques, segments of livers, pancreas and lung can be grafted
d. *living unrelated donors*: spouses, partners, friends, altruists and paid donors (illegal in the UK).

KIDNEY TRANSPLANTATION

1. Donor kidneys for transplantation may be obtained from:

a. Living related donors
b. Living unrelated donors
c. Unrelated brain-stem-dead heart-beating cadaver donors
d. Unrelated non-heart-beating cadaver donors.

2. Kidney transplantation currently offers the best chance of long-term survival combined with near normal quality of life for those suffering from end-stage chronic renal disease.

3. End-stage renal disease of all types comprise the indications for renal transplantation.

Action

1. Mobilize both the external iliac artery and vein and control them with nylon tapes. Carefully ligate and seal with diathermy the perivascular lymphatic vessels.

2. Remove the prepared donor kidney from ice.

3. Perform an end-to-side anastomosis between the renal vein and the external iliac vein using continuous 5/0 polypropylene or PDS.

4. Perform an end-to-side anastomosis between the donor renal artery and the external iliac artery using similar suture materials.

5. Remove the clamps from the iliac vessels, thus perfusing the graft, and secure haemostasis.

6. Fill the bladder with physiological saline from the previously attached infusion line to distend it and help identify the bladder in the pelvis.

7. Spatulate the end of the ureter, pass below the spermatic cord and perform an anastomosis to the dome of the bladder using continuous 4/0 catgut or PDS. Fashion a submucosal tunnel by incising the bladder muscle down to the mucosa over a 2 cm distance in line with the ureter. Lay the distal ureter in the groove created and close the bladder muscle loosely over the top of the ureter using interrupted absorbable sutures. Test the anastomosis by refilling the bladder with saline (Fig. 25.1).

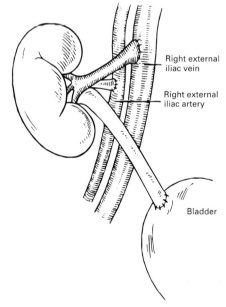

Right external
iliac vein

Right external
iliac artery

Bladder

Fig. 25.1 Renal transplantation. The renal vessels have been united end-to-side to the external iliac vessels. The ureter is joined to the dome of the bladder.

8. Take a renal biopsy before closing the wound in layers over a large silicone tube drain.

LIVER TRANSPLANTATION

Appraise

1. More than 72 000 liver transplants have been performed in over 200 liver transplant centres worldwide since Starzl reported the first liver graft in 1963.

2. In 70% of cases transplantation is for end-stage chronic liver disease due to cirrhosis arising from a variety of different causes such as primary biliary cirrhosis, primary sclerosing cholangitis, post-hepatitic cirrhosis, autoimmune chronic active hepatitis and alcohol-related liver disease. In approximately 12% it is for primary hepatic malignancy and in another 12% for acute liver failure resulting from fulminant hepatitis acute (drug) poisoning or idiosyncratic drug reactions.

Metabolic disease account for 6% of cases, including:

a. where the liver is itself a target organ of the metabolic abnormality (e.g. Wilson's disease and α_1-antitrypsin deficiency and tyrosinosis)
b. where a hepatic enzyme defect leads to damage and failure to other organs (e.g. primary hyperoxaluria, familial hypercholesterolaemia and some forms of familial amyloidosis).

Access

Make a bilateral subcostal incision with upward extension to the xiphoid. Pin back the abdominal wall flaps so created to the lower chest wall.

Excise

Excise the failed liver, retaining the common bile duct, hepatic artery, portal vein, and the cut ends of the inferior vena cava.

Replace (Fig. 25.2)

1. Remove the new liver from ice.

2. Begin the reimplantation with the suprahepatic vena caval anastomosis using a continuous 2/0 polypropylene, polydioxanone (PDS) or polyester suture. Follow this with the infrahepatic vena caval anastomosis using a continuous 3/0 polypropylene suture.

3. Anastomose the donor and recipient portal veins with an end-to-end reconstruction using 5/0 polypropylene.

4. Reconstruct the hepatic arterial supply as an end-to-end anastomosis between the donor and recipient common hepatic arteries using interrupted 6/0 polypropylene.

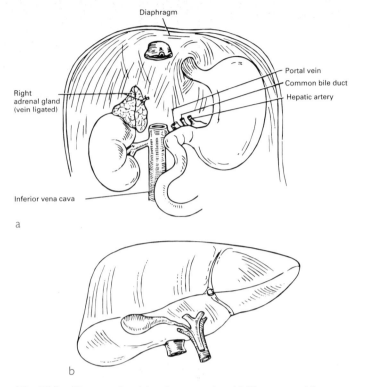
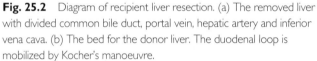

Fig. 25.2 Diagram of recipient liver resection. (a) The removed liver with divided common bile duct, portal vein, hepatic artery and inferior vena cava. (b) The bed for the donor liver. The duodenal loop is mobilized by Kocher's manoeuvre.

5. Reconstruct the biliary tract as an end-to-end, duct-to-duct anastomosis using interrupted 5/0 PDS.

6. Perform a donor cholecystectomy and a liver biopsy.

7. Check thoroughly for haemostasis, inspecting all anastomoses and placing extra sutures when necessary, and then close the abdomen in layers over two large silicone tube drains.

FURTHER READING

Advisory Group on the Ethics of Xenotransplantation 1996 Animal tissues into humans: recommendations and report. Department of Health, London

Lancet 1976 Diagnosis of brain death (editorial). Lancet ii: 1069–1070

Medawar PB 1944 The behaviour and fate of skin autografts and skin homografts in rabbits. Journal of Anatomy, London 78: 176–199

Thorax

T. Treasure, R. R. Kanagasabay and A. R. Makey

Contents

INTRODUCTION

1. Cardiothoracic surgery demands a precise knowledge of the topographical anatomy of the thorax when viewed from the lateral, anterior or posterior aspect; this knowledge is necessary for the accurate dissection that is required. It is essential that no vessel is sacrificed other than those of the diseased area because of the consequent increased loss of lung function and the risk of lung infarction. The safety margin during intrathoracic dissection is small.

2. The accurate placing of good-calibre drainage tubes is essential to secure rapid and full re-expansion of the lung, by removing fluid and air in the postoperative period. Meticulous and accurate technique, coupled with prophylactic antibiotic therapy, minimizes the incidence of infection, which can cause secondary haemorrhage and interfere with bronchial and chest wall healing.

In cardiovascular surgery, similar techniques are employed, coupled with the ability to perform accurate, leak-free anastomoses and blood-tight closure of openings in the cardiac chambers.

CHEST DRAINS

Appraise

The insertion of chest drains is a frequent cause of morbidity, and attention to a few key points can help to avoid most problems.

1. In general, drains are inserted to drain air or fluid (blood, effusion, pus, chyle). It is customary to place drains for air in the apex and the others basally, but provided that the pleural space is not loculated then the actual position is probably not important. To avoid injury to underlying structures drains should be inserted into the 'triangle of safety'. This is bounded by the anterior axillary line, the mid-axillary line and the level of the nipple. It is important to be above the nipple to avoid any risk of diaphragmatic injury.

2. Place the patient in the lateral position having checked the chest X-ray. Clean the skin and infiltrate with the maximum quantity of local anaesthetic permitted according to the patient's weight. Leave this for at least 10 minutes to work before continuing. In anxious patients, further analgesia with a non-steroidal anti-inflammatory given 1 hour previously can be helpful

3. Make a short skin incision sufficient to admit a finger. Using a blunt artery clip, dissect down to the pleura immediately above a rib and enter the chest by blunt dissection. The pleura will be felt to 'give' as a distinct 'pop'. Insert a finger to confirm that you are safely in the chest and sweep away any adhesions. Place a simple suture across the midpoint of the incision to close the wound when the drain is removed and tie a knot in the end. Place another suture at the corner of the incision to secure the drain. The drain may now be safely inserted, with the aid of a Roberts clamp if necessary.

UNDERWATER SEAL DRAINAGE

1. Connect the drainage tube from the patient to the long tube, which passes well below the level of a measured amount of water in the bottle so that the fluid provides a seal preventing entry of air into the chest. If necessary, connect the short tube, which allows escape of air, to a source of suction; this is usually increased up to a negative pressure of 20 cmH$_2$O or 20 mmHg (3–5 kPa; Fig. 26.1).

2. Check free drainage by noting a free swing of fluid in the long tube on inspiration, if no suction is connected.

3. When suction is used, the apparatus must not be turned off and left connected to the bottle or the drain is effectively blocked. Any suction device used must be a low-pressure, high-volume device to prevent obstruction. (Wall suction with a regulated adapter is ideal.)

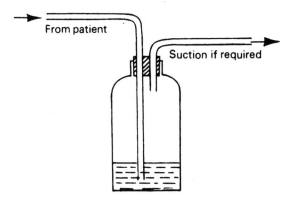

Fig. 26.1 Underwater seal drainage.

Drains inserted after a pneumonectomy must never be placed on suction as massive mediastinal shift may occur.

4. The drainage tube arrangement must not be reversed (i.e. the short tube connected to the patient) as, again, obstruction results.

5. Clamping a chest drain is almost never indicated and is potentially dangerous. Clamping drains while patients are being transferred is not appropriate; however the drainage bottle must not be lifted above the patient or fluid may enter the chest.

6. Connect the drain up to an underwater seal bottle. Suction may be used if desired. It may be helpful in the following situations:

a. where there is a pneumothorax and the lung does not inflate with simple drainage
b. after performing a pleurodesis
c. when draining a haemothorax or empyema, to help avoid the drains blocking.

(SUCTION SHOULD NEVER BE USED AFTER A PNEU-MONECTOMY.)

Note. If suction is not used the resistance to drainage will increase as the bottle fills with fluid. Change the bottle once it is more than half full to ensure good continued drainage

POSTEROLATERAL THORACOTOMY

Appraise
This is the usual route of access for:

1. pulmonary operations
2. some oesophageal operations
3. posterior, middle mediastinal and mainly unilateral anterior mediastinal lesions
4. repair of coarctation, division of patent ductus arteriosus, and thoracic aneurysms.

Access
1. Place the patient in either the lateral or the prone position (Fig. 26.2).
2. Approach all standard lobectomies through the fifth interspace.
3. Cut the skin in a smooth curve, running from midway between the midline and medial border of the scapula posteriorly, skirting the

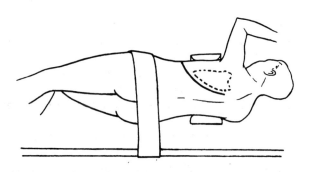
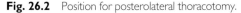
Fig. 26.2 Position for posterolateral thoracotomy.

angle of the scapula by 2.5 cm, and passing forward to the anterior axillary line.

Action
1. Divide the muscles, using the diathermy point with coagulation of the vessels as required. The muscles are arranged in two layers: the superficial layer consists of the trapezius and latissimus dorsi muscles; the deeper layer is composed of the rhomboid and serratus anterior muscles. Preserve the serratus anterior muscle almost intact by dividing this layer through the aponeurosis below the muscle fibres right to the anterior extent of the wound (Figs 26.3, 26.4). It is often possible to avoid dividing it at all.
2. Count the ribs from the apex by passing a hand up under the scapula. It is hard to feel the first rib and so the uppermost rib you can feel is usually the second. The second rib has a characteristically flatter, broader shape than the third, and has superior muscle attachments. The space below the second rib is wider than that below the third rib. The most common mistake is to make the incision through the sixth space.
3. Divide with the diathermy point the periosteum of the rib selected.
4. Strip the periosteum from its upper border, using a curved rougine, working posteroanteriorly. Some surgeons prefer to divide

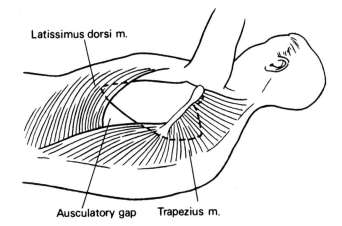
Fig. 26.3 Arrangement of superficial muscle layers.

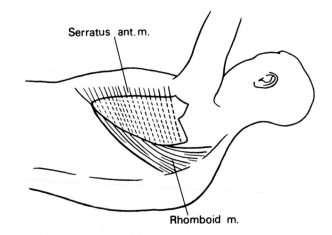
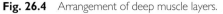
Fig. 26.4 Arrangement of deep muscle layers.

the intercostal muscle above the rib using diathermy without stripping the periosteum.

5. Resection or division of a rib is rarely necessary, provided that the costotransverse ligament is freed posteriorly using a notched chisel and the retractor is opened very gradually and gently.

6. Open the pleura along the length of the wound after warning the anaesthetist to allow the lung to fall away. The periosteal separation may be extended anteriorly deep to the wound.

7. Insert the customary rib spreader (Finochietto) after pads have been placed over the wound edges.

8. Intercostal nerve blocks may be performed now or delayed until the time of closure.

9. If light or filmy adhesions are present, divide them with scissors or diathermy.

10. When widespread and marked adhesions are present, use a mounted gauze swab and blunt dissection to strip the lung in the extrapleural plane. Use a hot pack to control the diffuse oozing; later, bleeding points may require coagulation with diathermy. Sometimes the extrapleural strip need only be over an area of dense localized adherence, the rest of the lung being free.

Closure

1. Insert apical and basal drains posterolaterally through the second intercostal space below the wound after muscle layers have been put on stretch with Lane's forceps. Pass the apical tube up the apex of the chest. It may be tethered to the chest wall with a light catgut suture looped around it. This tube is usually sited anterior to the basal drain, the lowest side-hole of which is level with the dome of the diaphragm (Fig. 26.5). Be sure that the exit sites of the drains are sufficiently anterior so that the patient will not lie on the drains in his bed, as this may cause considerable postoperative discomfort.

2. Insert two or three pericostal sutures of no. 1 nylon or polyglactin (doubled) when healing is likely to be poor. Pass the pericostal sutures around the upper rib and, to avoid the intercostal nerve, through an awl hole in the lower rib, or around the rib hugging the bony groove (Fig. 26.6).

3. Using a Holmes Sellors approximator or by crossing the pericostal sutures to bring the ribs together, close the intercostal layer with a continuous suture of no. 1 catgut, approximating the edge of the stripped intercostal layer above to the intercostal muscle below the rib that has been stripped. In the majority of cases, this intercostal closure is sufficient and the use of pericostal sutures can be avoided. This may help to prevent chronic post-thoracotomy pain due to nerve entrapment.

4. Unite each muscle layer with a continuous suture (no. 1 catgut), which must pass through the whole thickness of the muscle to ensure haemostasis. Suture the superficial fascia with a fine (00) catgut suture.

Polyglycolic acid or polyglactin is commonly used instead of catgut.

MEDIAN STERNOTOMY

Appraise

1. This is commonly performed for cardiac operations using cardiopulmonary bypass, as it provides the best overall access. Postoperative pain is less and least respiratory upset is caused.

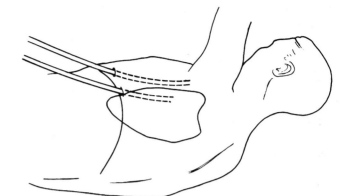

Fig. 26.5 Siting of drainage tubes.

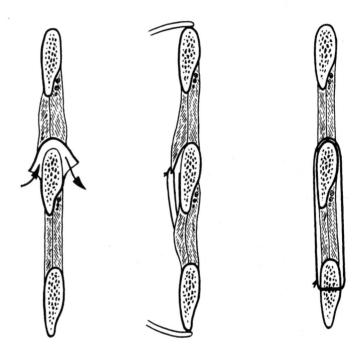

Fig. 26.6 Technique of opening and closing modified intercostal incision and insertion of pericostal suture.

2. The incision is used for removal of anterior mediastinal tumours such as thymomata, germ cell tumours, and rarely for retrosternal goitre.

3. This incision can be performed very quickly with the appropriate equipment but, in the emergency situation without access to a sternal saw, an anterior thoracotomy may be more judicious.

Prepare

1. Place the patient supine with the arms by the side on a soft mattress or water blanket.

2. Attach ECG electrodes to shoulders and chest wall.

3. Insert percutaneously a radial artery catheter for arterial pressure monitoring. Insert a central venous pressure line via the internal jugular vein.

4. Insert a urinary catheter, rectal and nasopharyngeal temperature probes.

5. Prepare the skin to allow access to groins and also to leg in coronary artery bypass operations.

6. In patients with very stocky necks, placing a sandbag under the shoulder blades and extending the neck can make exposure a little easier.

7. If internal defibrillator paddles are not available, place external paddles in case of arrhythmias.

Action

1. Make an incision from the lower margin of the suprasternal notch to 2 inches below the xiphoid process.

2. Divide the subcutaneous tissue with the diathermy point down to the periosteum of the sternum to obtain haemostasis. Keep in the gap between the pectoralis major muscles and precisely mark the midline of the sternum with the diathermy point. The sternum is least wide at the second space.

3. Divide the linea alba for a short distance below the xiphoid process. Be careful of veins that lie in the immediate suprasternal region. Avoid them by keeping very close to the upper border of the bone. Likewise there is often a large vein crossing the xiphisternal junction, which requires control with diathermy.

4. Free tissues from the deep surface of the manubrium by passing a finger up from beneath. This avoids the danger of catching a fold of pericardium in the saw and risking injury to the heart.

5. Divide the sternum longitudinally with an electric or pneumatic Stryker saw, hugging the posterior surface to avoid damage to the heart, ascending aorta or left innominate vein. If this is not available, a Gigli saw may be used, which is withdrawn from above after an extra-long Roberts forceps has been passed upwards behind the sternum hugging its posterior surface. With the latter method it is possible to open the pleura, especially on the right, which often lies well across the front of the mediastinum. In emergency, and for the shorter divisions, a Lebsche chisel may be used from above.

6. Secure haemostasis on both aspects of the sternum by diathermizing the periosteal vessels and using bone wax to control the bleeding from the exposed marrow.

7. Insert a self-retaining retractor and incise the pericardium in the midline. The heart should be visible moving freely behind the pericardium; if it is not, suspect that there are pericardial adhesions and take great care in opening the pericardium. Avoid the use of diathermy near to the heart if defibrillator paddles are not available. Extend the incision up to the reflection on the aorta, avoiding the left innominate vein, and down to the diaphragm. Sew the pericardial edges to the skin to form a well and improve the exposure of the heart.

Closure

1. If the pericardium has been opened, introduce pericardial and anterior mediastinal drains (24–28F catheter) through separate skin incisions below the xiphoid process and through separate openings in the rectus sheath.

2. Using an awl or heavy trocar-pointed needle, pass stainless-steel wire sutures through each side of the sternum; make a firm closure by twisting the wire to obtain close approximation. Alternatively, pass the needle close to the edge of the sternum, from the second space caudally, avoiding the internal mammary vessels.

3. Approximate the muscle and the subcutaneous layers with polyglactin sutures, 1 and 00 respectively. Suture the linea alba accurately to avoid an incisional hernia.

COMPLICATIONS OF CHEST TRAUMA

Patients with chest injuries frequently have multiple injuries that all require treatment. The key to successful management of such patients is prompt and appropriate prioritization of injuries. The acute trauma life support (ATLS) protocol is one such system that can be recommended.

Rib fracture

1. Rib fractures of themselves are of only limited significance and rarely require special treatment other than adequate analgesia.

2. Simple analgesia is generally all that is required. Fixation of fractured ribs is not helpful.

Flail segment

1. Multiple fractures may result in a flail or paradoxical segment, where a portion of chest wall becomes completely mobile, embarrassing respiration. This is often associated with underlying pulmonary contusion.

2. Treatment of the flail segment and the underlying contusion are supportive, and ventilation is often required. Strapping the chest or wiring the fractures is not considered beneficial.

Sucking chest wounds and pneumothorax

1. A special category of chest injury is where there is a breach in the integrity of the chest wall leading to a sucking wound. This will lead to a pneumothorax. Pneumothorax may also occur in the absence of a sucking wound, due to damage to the lung from sharp fragments of fractured rib. The diagnosis of a tension pneumothorax is a clinical one, with absence of air entry, shift of the mediastinum to the contralateral side, raised jugular venous pressure (although note that in the hypovolaemic trauma patient this feature may not be apparent) and incipient circulatory collapse.

2. Immediate insertion of an intercostal chest drain. In extremis, a needle thoracocentesis may be a quicker life-saving manoeuvre. Any sucking chest wound should be covered with an air-tight dressing once adequate intercostal cheat drainage has been established.

Lung injury

Lung lacerations may be caused by fractured ribs protruding into the chest cavity. The resulting pneumothorax will often respond to simple drainage, but large air leaks may require open repair, particularly if the lung remains collapsed. Simple repair with a running 4/0 polypropylene suture is usually sufficient. Stapling devices may also be usefully employed. The severely injured or 'burst' lung may require more major formal resection. In cases of large air leak, a tracheal or proximal bronchial injury should be specifically excluded by means of bronchoscopy.

Diaphragmatic injury

1. These injuries are often overlooked in the immediate resuscitation period, but any patient presenting with major chest trauma and with evidence of a poorly defined hemidiaphragm, or basal chest shadowing, particularly on the left side, should raise suspicion of a diaphragmatic injury. Plain chest X-ray and CT scanning may be

helpful, but diaphragmatic ultrasound and/or barium studies of the small bowel are probably the investigations of choice.

2. Repair either by direct suture or with the aid of a polypropylene mesh is usually straightforward in the acute setting. Delayed surgery is often complicated by adhesions.

Penetrating stab wounds or perforating wounds

These usually seal quickly and do not result in suction pneumothorax.

Action

1. Such wounds may not necessarily demand a thoracotomy. Treat the patient conservatively and deal with the wounds locally if there is no clinical evidence of serious internal damage, absence of bleeding and a satisfactory chest X-ray. Note the direction of the wound.

2. Remember that stab wounds in the lower half of the chest may be associated with diaphragmatic puncture and intra-abdominal injury to the spleen, liver or hollow viscera.

3. Undertake thoracolaparotomy if in doubt after very careful assessment. Fatal results have followed strangulation of an incisional hernia resulting from an overlooked penetration of the diaphragm sustained a long time before.

4. Transthoracic echocardiogram may show the presence of a pericardial effusion. This is highly suggestive of a cardiac injury and should be followed by surgical exploration provided that adequate facilities are available.

WOUNDS OF THE HEART AND PERICARDIUM

Appraise

1. Many gunshot wounds are rapidly fatal but some patients, especially those who sustain stab or knife wounds, reach the surgeon with a haemopericardium and evidence of cardiac tamponade.

2. Diagnose by the clinical picture of falling cardiac output – peripheral vasoconstriction, tachycardia, low blood pressure associated with rising venous pressure. Intravenous resuscitation increases the venous pressure further.

The site of the wound is likely to be atrial or a minor ventricular injury for the patient to survive.

3. Confirm the clinical diagnosis with X-ray and ultrasonography.

Prepare

Establish a good intravenous infusion and order adequate blood replacement. This is mandatory because on opening the pericardium rapid and profuse bleeding may occur.

Action

1. Aspirate the pericardium to confirm the diagnosis. This may be adequate to relieve the condition.

2. Expose the heart through a left anterolateral thoracotomy via the fifth space if bleeding persists, recurs or is obviously severe and requires emergency operation. Median sternotomy may be preferable for central or right-sided penetrating wounds, especially if bypass is available and indicated. If there are wounds on both sides, a bithoraco-

sternotomy ('clamshell incision') may be fashioned by performing bilateral anterior thoracotomies through the fourth space and joining them by dividing the sternum transversely.

3. Control atrial wounds by finger pressure or an appropriate atraumatic clamp, such as a Brock's mitral clamp or, occasionally, a Duval forceps. Suture with 3/0 or 4/0 vascular sutures. Restore adequate blood volume once bleeding is under control.

4. Control ventricular wounds by finger pressure and then suture with 2/0 sutures. Use a pad of Dacron®, Teflon® or pericardium to reinforce the closure if the muscle is friable.

5. *Injured coronary vessels*. Under-running a transected coronary artery may allow control of ventricular bleeding and subsequent more meticulous repair of the coronary injury. Bypass with a segment of vein may be possible but is demanding without the availability of cardiopulmonary bypass. Small arterial branches and cardiac veins may be safely ligated.

6. Some penetrating wounds may be associated with valvular damage, which requires investigation and may need treatment later.

7. Drain the pericardium adequately and close the chest in routine fashion.

ASPIRATION OF THE PERICARDIUM

This is performed to treat cardiac tamponade due to the accumulation of blood following trauma or fluid due to inflammation of the pericardium.

Prepare

Sit the patient up at 45° (Fig. 26.7). Confirm the clinical diagnosis with echocardiography.

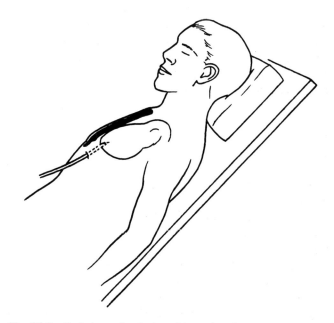

Fig. 26.7 Technique of aspiration of the pericardium.

Action

1. Infiltrate the skin below the xiphisternum and to the left of the midline with local anaesthesia.

2. Advance the needle obliquely upwards to just touch the back of the sternum and then guide it more deeply (approximately at an angle of 45°) until the inferior aspect of the pericardium is felt as a definite resistance.

3. Push the needle through the pericardium and aspirate the fluid.

4. It is possible to introduce a plastic catheter of the intracath variety through a larger-bore needle or a small cannula if aspiration needs to be maintained.

5. An ECG electrode attached to a metal aspiration needle will warn when contact with the ventricle is made (the trace will suddenly show a high-voltage waveform), but this technique is cumbersome and is rarely needed.

6. A pericardial drain should be left in situ for at least 24 hours to encourage obliteration of the space and limit reaccumulation of the effusion.

FURTHER READING

Sabiston DC, Spencer FC 1990 Surgery of the chest, 5th edn. WB Saunders, Philadelphia

Seremetis MG 1970 The management of spontaneous pneumothorax. Chest 57: 65–68

Shields TW 1989 General thoracic surgery, 3rd edn. Lea & Febiger, Malvern

Trinkle JK, Marcos J, Grover FL, Cuello LM 1974 Management of the wounded heart. Annals of Thoracic Surgery 17: 230–236

Head and neck

M. P. Stearns, R. Farrell and M. Hobsley

Contents

GENERAL PRINCIPLES

1. Details of anatomy tend to be more important in the head and neck than in other regions. Numerous structures are crowded into a small volume and many of them, such as the facial nerve, perform important functions – some are vital to life itself, such as the recurrent laryngeal nerve and the internal carotid artery.

2. The airway may be threatened by the accumulation of blood, by laryngospasm, etc., so insist on endotracheal intubation for all but the simplest procedures.

Minimize blood loss

1. Venous bleeding is more difficult to control than arterial. Venous pressure, and therefore venous bleeding, can be minimized by paying careful attention to posture.

2. Diathermy is a valuable aid to haemostasis, but use it carefully.

3. After the operation, use suction drainage to obliterate the dead space under the skin flaps, thereby reducing the risk of reactionary haemorrhage and haematomas.

EXCISION BIOPSY OF A RODENT ULCER OF THE FACE

Appraise

1. A rodent ulcer (basal cell carcinoma, BCC) may be treated by surgery or by radiotherapy. If surgery is chosen, the ulcer must be excised with a wide margin of normal tissue, both around the lesion and deep to it. A 'wide margin' means preferably 1 cm, but in regions where skin is precious, for example near the eye, 0.5 cm is acceptable.

Sometimes the ulcer is small and occurs in a region where there is plenty of redundant skin. In these circumstances, primary closure of the elliptical wound may be possible. Often, however, a skin graft is needed. A full-thickness graft is desirable; the cosmetic result of a split skin graft on the face is unacceptable. The description below includes two sites for obtaining a free full-thickness skin graft. Plastic surgeons can rotate flaps to cover large defects, but do not attempt these unless you have experience with the techniques.

Assess

1. The extent of the lesion, and of the area of excision required, is carefully assessed by inspection and palpation. The depth of excision required may be difficult to assess at this stage.

2. In planning the incision, remember to take into account the direction of Lange's lines of skin tension. After the excision, you may find it is possible to close the defect by primary suture, and the scar then lies in the skin crease.

Action

1. Mark out the oval of skin that you have decided to excise.

2. Cut vertically through the skin along the oval line, until the superficial fat is clearly visible everywhere in the wound. It is not possible to make a curved incision with a straight knife-blade, but a series of short linear incisions will permit your incision to approximate closely to the oval you have marked.

3. Deepen the incision at one end of the longer diameter of the oval. Raise the skin at the end of the diameter with a pair of toothed dissecting forceps and, using either a clean scalpel or a pair of scissors, start raising the oval of skin and some subcutaneous tissue towards the region of the lesion.

4. At this stage you will find it easier to decide by palpation how deeply the lesion extends. Make sure that your plane of cutting is sufficiently deep to give a wide margin of normal tissue below, as well as all round, the tumour.

5. Complete the excision. You may find it more convenient to do this by starting again at the opposite pole of the ellipse, the two planes of section meeting deep to the lesion.

6. Inspect the wound for bleeding and stop it with diathermy.

7. Take a single sheet of petroleum jelly (Vaseline) gauze, lay it on the wound and cut out a piece the shape and size of the wound. This piece of gauze will serve as a pattern for cutting a full-thickness (Wolfe) graft of skin.

8. Lay the piece of Vaseline gauze on the skin at the site you have chosen for supplying the skin graft. Suitable areas, where even a large oval defect can be closed by primary suture without tension, are the loose skin immediately below the clavicle, or the groove between the side of the head and the medial aspect of the posterior part of the pinna. Cut out an area of skin corresponding in size and shape to the pattern; take the full thickness of the skin, but as little as possible subcutaneous fat. Clean off any subcutaneous fat adhering to the deep surface of the skin, using a sharp scalpel for this purpose. Sew up the defect in the donor area.

9. Lay the full-thickness skin graft on the defect produced by the excision of the rodent ulcer, having first made certain that there is no bleeding. Stitch the edges of the graft to the margins of the defect with a series of interrupted non-absorbable sutures, tying the knots so that they lie on the surrounding intact skin rather than on the skin graft. Arrange these sutures to achieve sufficient tension in the graft to discourage the formation of a haematoma beneath it, but less tension than will produce a strangulation effect on the graft and cause its death.

10. Spray the grafted area with an artificial skin preparation such as Nobecutane. Use the spray sparingly and allow the liquid film to harden, then repeat the procedure several times to produce a firm dressing. Protect the patient's eyes, nostrils, mouth and hair during the spraying.

Checklist

1. Do not forget to dress the donor site.

2. Check that the specimen, properly labelled and accompanied by the appropriate request forms, is sent to the histopathologist.

LOCAL EXCISION OR BIOPSY OF AN INTRAORAL LESION

Appraise

1. Small lesions in the surface of the oral mucosa, whether on cheek, tongue, palate, floor of mouth or inner surface of the lips, are best dealt with by excision biopsy, i.e. excision with a sufficiently wide margin of normal tissue to ensure that excision is complete.

2. Make sure, however, by careful palpation beforehand, how deeply the lesion penetrates beneath the mucosa. Remember that you must achieve an adequate margin of normal tissue on the *deep* aspect of the lesion as well as around it.

3. The oral tissues are very vascular, so take special precautions to minimize haemorrhage and so prevent aspiration of blood into the lungs.

Access

1. Ask the anaesthetist to pass a pernasal endotracheal cuffed tube and to distend the cuff. As a further precaution against aspiration of blood, have him pack the pharynx with 2.5 cm ribbon gauze.

2. Fix the patient's mouth in the open position by means of a dental prop or Ferguson's forceps inserted between the teeth or gums of the molar region on the side opposite to the lesion.

3. Position the patient with a head-up tilt of about 15°, sufficient to cause the external jugular vein to collapse. Use a head-ring to stabilize the position of the head.

Assess

1. Palpate the lesion carefully again to assess its depth. Tissues often feel different when the patient is anaesthetized, and you may occasionally change your decision about the depth of penetration of the lesion.

2. If you are still sure that you can remove the lesion with a wide margin of normal tissue on all aspects, and without producing deformity or serious loss of function, proceed to excision biopsy (see below). If you are not sure, however, change your plan of action to biopsy of the lesion (see below).

Excision biopsy

Action

1. Form a mental picture of the exact position and shape of your incision.

2. Using a 3/0 absorbable suture on a half-circle 30 mm or 50 mm cutting needle (according to the depth of bite required), insert a stitch through the tissues near each end of your proposed incision. The stitches must traverse the tissues far enough from the incision that they will not be cut when you make the incision. Bear in mind particularly the *depth* of stitch you will require if you are to get the depth of excision that you need. Leave the two ends of each untied but held in four artery forceps.

3. Excise the lesion with at least a 5 mm margin in all directions. Make the wound roughly oval, the direction of the long axis of the oval being dictated by the need to minimize damage to neighbouring structures. Do this as speedily as possible, as you cannot control bleeding until the excision is complete.

4. Pull each stitch end across the wound towards the opposite end of the other stitch, i.e. the stitch ends form a cross. This should control the worst of the bleeding. Get your assistant to maintain traction on the stitch ends.

5. Inspect the excised specimen to make sure that, at least to the naked eye, the excision is complete. If it does not seem to be complete, you must consider taking more tissue from the appropriate region of the wound.

6. Assuming that the excision does appear complete, tie the stitches in the form of the cross, as your assistant has been holding them.

7. Complete haemostasis with diathermy and/or further sutures while maintaining the field clear of blood with the sucker.

Biopsy

Appraise

Decide where you will take your biopsy. Plan to get from the rim of the lesion a piece of tissue that includes a generous portion of the lesion in continuity with a generous portion of the neighbouring normal tissue. In general, the piece of tissue removed will be an oval with its long axis at right angles to the margin of the lesion.

Action

1. Insert one or two deep sutures of 3/0 absorbable material through normal tissues on either side of your proposed excision, and leave the ends united. Do not put sutures into the lesion itself, since such a procedure may spread neoplasm.

2. Excise the specimen, taking care not to cut your sutures.

3. Tie the suture or sutures. Usually this stops all bleeding, but if it fails to do so, use diathermy or more sutures.

Checklist

1. Was there any blood on the deeper parts of the pharyngeal pack? If there was, monitor the possibility of chest complications later.

2. Are you sure that the specimen has been correctly bottled and labelled, that the request form for the pathology department has been accurately filled out and that you are satisfied with the arrangements for conveying the specimen to the laboratory?

3. Should you send part of the specimen for bacteriological examination (e.g. if the lesion may be tuberculous)? Remember that any such sample must be sent in a sterile container without formalin.

WEDGE EXCISION OF THE LIP

Appraise

Early tumours of the lip can be removed with a wide margin by this operation. Particularly in elderly people, up to one-third of the length of the lip can be removed in this way with an acceptable functional and cosmetic result. If the patient is young, or if a length of lip greater than one-third must be sacrificed, various plastic operations are available (see Ch. 32). These plastic operations are more difficult than they look, so attempt them only if you are expert.

Assess

1. Inspect and palpate the lesion and its surroundings with care.
2. Decide on the width and length of wedge necessary to excise the lesion with a clear margin, 0.5–1.0 cm, of normal tissue.

Action

1. Cut out the wedge, taking the full thickness of the lip, using bipolar diathermy to control the bleeding, if it is available. Alternatively control bleeding with finger pressure or use non-crushing intestinal clamps.
2. Close the defect with three layers of interrupted sutures: 3/0 absorbable sutures for the muscle, the same for the mucosa and very fine non-absorbable sutures for the skin and the vermilion border. Pay special attention to the accuracy with which you make the two edges of the vermilion border, and of the mucocutaneous junction, meet. It is useful to 'tack' these first.

EXCISION BIOPSY OF CERVICAL LYMPH NODE

Appraise

1. Never attempt this operation under local anaesthesia if general anaesthesia is available. Cervical lymph nodes may feel superficial yet lie deeply in the neck, and the dissection to remove them may be much more difficult than you expect.
2. Depending on the position of the lymph node, neighbouring structures may be at risk during the operation. An example commonly encountered is the accessory nerve, either in the anterior triangle of the neck at the junction of upper and middle thirds of the anterior border of the sternomastoid muscle, or in the posterior triangle at the junction of the middle and lower thirds of the sternomastoid.
3. Handle lymph glands very gently during dissection. Rough handling is likely to distort the internal structure of the node and make histological interpretation difficult.
4. The operation described here is for a lymph node lying under cover of the anterior border of the sternomastoid muscle near the junction of its upper and middle thirds. The principles illustrated can be applied to an operation on a lymph node anywhere else in the neck.

Access

1. Position the patient supine with the upper half of the operating table tilted upwards sufficiently to cause the external jugular vein to collapse. Turn the patient's head to the opposite side.
2. Clean the skin from the level of the mouth to the clavicle and from the anterior midline of the neck to as far posteriorly as can be reached. Tuck a pad of sterile wool beneath the neck and scapular regions.
3. Towel up to leave exposed a circular area of radius about 5 cm around the palpable lymph node.
4. Make an incision across the palpable lump and extended for 1 cm beyond its margins in both directions, in the direction of the lines of skin tension (in this case roughly horizontally, with a slight convex curve downwards). Deepen this incision through skin and platysma.
5. Achieve haemostasis with diathermy.

Assess

1. Feel the lump carefully again. Is it covered only with fascia or is any other structure between your fingers and the swelling?
2. If the intervening tissues are fascia only, deepen your incision through these tissues with a clean scalpel until you can see the surface of the lymph node itself.
3. If there is some structure other than fascia in the way, you must move it out of the way, excise it or cut through it so as to reach the surface of the lymph node. Exactly what you do depends upon the nature of the structure. The commonest in this particular site is the anterior border of the sternomastoid muscle. Usually it is easy to spread apart the edges of the wound in the skin and platysma with retractors, to divide the fascia where it joins the anterior border of the muscle over a distance of about 3 cm and to retract laterally the anterior border of the muscle. The fascia overlying the lymph node can now be incised.

Action

1. Dissect the lymph node free from its surroundings. A good way to do this is to lay a small, curved artery forceps along the surface of the node, with the curve of the forceps corresponding with the curvature of the surface. Insert the tips of the blades of the forceps between the gland and the free edge of investing fascia where you have cut the fascia in order to reach the swelling. Gently push the forceps further along this plane and then separate the blades, thereby stripping the fascia off the lymph node. Cut the fascia with scissors between the separated blades of the forceps, so as to increase the exposure.
2. Repeat this process of combined blunt and sharp dissection all over the superficial aspect of the lymph node. Minimize bleeding by the use of diathermy on vessels before you cut them, if that is possible. A really dry field facilitates the dissection.
3. During this superficial clearance, there is no need to handle the lymph node at all. As you approach the deep aspect, it becomes necessary to push the gland in one direction so that you can free it in that area of its bed from which you are displacing it. This manipulation is likely to damage the gland; be very gentle, and use a finger rather than a metal instrument.
4. Somewhere in this deep aspect you will nearly always find a fairly large feeding artery to the gland. In this region also it is easy to damage neighbouring important structures such as the accessory

nerve, because the exposure is limited by the overhanging gland. The safe rule is to cut only tissues that you can see perfectly.

5. When you have completed the dissection deep to the lymph node, it will be lying free. Remove the node, cut it into two equal parts, put one into a container that will later be filled with formol-saline and sent for histological examination, and put the other into a sterile empty container so that it can be sent for culture (including for tuberculosis).

Closure

1. Ensure complete haemostasis. Ask the anaesthetist to flatten the operating table; this change of posture raises venous pressure and sometimes starts bleeding, and it is better that this should happen while you have the wound still open rather than after you have sewn up.

2. Sew up any deep muscle that you have had to divide and platysma, using 2/0 absorbable sutures.

3. Close the skin wound using a subcuticular polypropylene or a blanket stitch using nylon.

Postoperative

1. Is there any sign of a haematoma forming?

2. Are the two portions of the specimen being properly dealt with?

FURTHER READING

Freidberg J 1989 Pharyngeal cleft sinuses and cysts and other benign neck lesions. Paediatric Clinics of North America 36: 1451–1469

Jesse RH, Ballantyne AJ, Larson D 1978 Radical or modified radical neck dissection: a therapeutic dilemma. American Journal of Surgery 136: 516–519

Radkowski D, Arnold J, Healy GB 1991 Thyroglossal duct remnants: pre-operative evaluation and management. Archives of Otolaryngology Head and Neck Surgery 117, 1378–1381

Razack M 1977 Influence of initial neck node biopsy on the incidence of recurrence in the neck and survival in patients who subsequently undergo curative resectional surgery. Journal of Surgery and Oncology 9: 347–352

Orthopaedics and trauma: amputations

N. Goddard and G. Harper

Contents

GENERAL PRINCIPLES

1. Approximately 5500 amputations are performed each year in England, the number steadily increasing as the population ages. 75% of the patients are over 60 years of age, and 65% are men.

> **Key point**
>
> • The aims of amputation surgery are to fully excise all abnormal pathology and to reconstruct for maximal limb function.

2. The main indications for amputation are:

a. vascular disease, arterial or venous
b. diabetes (these two categories accounting for about 85% of amputations)
c. trauma (10%)
d. tumours (3%)
e. infection (now only responsible for 1.5% of amputations)
f. neurological causes such as nerve injury and its secondary effects
g. congenital problems.

3. Major upper limb amputations are rarely required (only 3% of the total).

4. Explain the proposed surgery carefully to the patient and obtain consent to amputate, if necessary, more proximally than you intend.

5. If in any doubt about the necessity for amputation obtain a second opinion from a senior colleague.

> **Key point**
>
> • In elective cases contact the regional limb fitting centre, if available, for advice prior to amputation to discuss the best level and type of procedure for your patient. Remember, the best results occur with informed involvement of a trained team including nursing staff, physiotherapists, occupational therapists, prosthetists and social workers.

6. Proceed under general anaesthesia whenever possible.

7. The level of amputation (and the type of prosthesis) is influenced by:

a. viability of soft tissues
b. underlying pathology
c. functional requirement
d. comfort
e. cosmetic appearance.

Conservation of energy expenditure is also an important consideration with lower limb surgery. The level of amputation can make a vast difference. Energy expenditure with a bilateral below-knee amputation is still less than that of a unilateral above-knee amputation.

As a rule, preserve every possible dynamic structure, preserve the knee joint and preserve the epiphysis in children.

8. Vascular appraisal
Assess the blood supply of the limb clinically by looking at the skin for colour changes, shiny atrophic appearance and lack of hair growth. Feel the skin for temperature changes, check the peripheral pulses and perform Buerger's test. Further studies that may help include:

a. transcutaneous Doppler recordings and measurement of the ankle-brachial index, etc.
b. thermography
c. radioactive xenon clearance
d. transcutaneous P_{O_2} measurement.

9. Bony appraisal
Assess the bone by taking plain radiographs in two planes, tomograms or a radioisotope bone scan.

For bone or soft tissue malignancy, ensure that the lesion has a confirmed diagnosis with a biopsy. Computerized tomography and magnetic resonance imaging are essential in fully staging the lesion and assessing the necessity for amputation. Limb-sparing surgery has recently become more feasible for the right indications and in the hands of expert tumour surgeons.

Prepare
1. Obtain consent and explain possible complications.
2. Give prophylactic antibiotics: penicillin (or erythromycin) plus one other broad-spectrum antibiotic. Swab and culture any wounds preoperatively.
3. Clean the limb and seal off the infected or necrotic areas.

4. Arrange for the disposal of the limb after amputation to the pathology department or straight to the incinerator.

5. Clearly mark the limb with indelible marker.

Action

General techniques

1. Use a tourniquet except in peripheral vascular disease. Exsanguinate the limb by elevation for 2–4 minutes rather than an Esmarch bandage.

2. Prepare the skin and apply the drapes.

🔑 **Key point**

- Mark the proposed skin flaps preoperatively. The flaps should be roughly the same length with their base at the level of bone section. Leave the flaps too long rather than too short. In traumatic cases preserve all viable skin to create an adequate stump. Handle the flaps gently. In vascular cases do not undermine the edges.

---

3. Wherever possible include underlying muscles in the flap (myoplastic flap) as this greatly improves the blood supply and covers and protects the stump. Muscles provide power, stabilization and proprioception to the stump. In emergency cases remove all dead muscle (this avoids gas gangrene), and leave viable muscle (red, bleeding and contracting). In elective cases cut the muscle with a raked incision angled towards the level of bone section.

4. Double ligate major vessels with strong silk or linen thread. Ligate other vessels with chromic catgut or polyglycolic acid.

5. Gently pull down nerves, divide them cleanly and allow them to retract into soft tissue envelopes. Ligate major nerves with a fine suture prior to and just above the site of division. This stops bleeding from accompanying vessels and decreases neuroma formation.

6. Prepare to cut the bone at the appropriate level. Remember that the stump must be long enough to gain secure attachment to the prosthesis and to act as a useful lever but short enough to accommodate the prosthesis and its hinge or joint mechanism. Divide the periosteum and cut the bone with a Gigli or power saw. During bone section, cover the soft tissues with a moist pack and irrigate afterwards to remove bone dust and particles from the soft tissues. Round off sharp bone edges with a rasp.

7. Check that the flaps will approximate easily.

8. Release the tourniquet and secure haemostasis.

9. Insert a suction drain.

10. Suture the flaps together without tension, starting with the muscle. Handle the skin carefully and close with staples, if available, or interrupted nylon sutures.

11. If infection is present, or if there is doubt about the viability of the flaps, approximate the muscles loosely (to avoid them contracting) over gauze soaked in saline or proflavine. Do not close the skin. Arrange delayed primary closure at 5–7 days.

Aftercare

1. Apply a well-padded compressible but not crushing dressing, using either cotton wool or latex foam. Hold this in place with crepe bandage taking care to avoid fixed flexion or other deformity of neighbouring joints.

2. Wherever possible apply a *light* shell of plaster of Paris (maximum four layers) over the dressing, except in cases with infection or doubtful flap viability. This will make the patient more comfortable and more mobile in bed. In specialist centres a prosthetist will apply a rigid dressing to which a temporary pylon can be attached for early ambulation.

3. Leave the dressing undisturbed if possible for 10 days. Increasing pain, seepage of blood or pus through the dressing, rising temperature and pulse are indications for earlier inspection of the wound.

4. Order regular physiotherapy to prevent joint contractures.

5. Encourage mobilization and use of the stump as soon as the patient is comfortable.

6. When the wound has healed and sutures have been removed, apply regular stump bandaging to maintain the shape of the stump.

7. Refer as soon as possible to the local limb fitting centre if you had not already done so before operation.

Special situations

Amputations in children

Children's amputations can present their own special problems. Growing bones at the site of amputation will overgrow by apposition (not related to growth at the proximal growth plate) and revision is often needed to prevent skin problems. Epiphyseal growth plates should always be preserved if possible.

Children suffer less from the complications of amputation such as phantom pain, neuroma, etc. Children can adapt amazingly well to prostheses if fitted correctly at an early age.

Decision-making for amputations in major trauma

Objective criteria can help predict amputation after lower extremity trauma. The Mangled Extremity Score (MESS) is one such system. It uses four significant criteria of skeletal/soft tissue injury, limb ischaemia, shock and patient age. Such systems can accurately discriminate between salvageable limbs and those better managed by primary amputation.

Complications

Haematoma

🔑 **Key point**

- Avoid this complication by meticulous haemostasis at the time of amputation. Double-ligate major vessels and try to prevent infection, which may cause secondary haemorrhage. Never close the stump before releasing the tourniquet.

Infection

1. Amputation stumps are more at risk of infection than most other surgical wounds because of the frequency of poorly vascularized tissues in the stump, infected lesions in the distal extremity and frail, elderly patients with poor resistance to infection.

2. Give prophylactic antibiotics to all lower limb amputees. The antibiotics should be active against gas gangrene organisms, *Escherichia coli* and staphylococci.

3. Handle all soft tissues with care and avoid leaving dead muscle and long sections of denuded cortical bone in the stump.

4. Treat wound infections promptly with antibiotics. Incise and drain any collection of pus.

5. If a chronic sinus fails to dry up with a course of antibiotics lasting up to 6 weeks, explore the stump under general anaesthesia. A focus of infection such as a small bony sequestrum or a lump of infected suture material will usually be found.

Flap necrosis

1. Prevent this complication by carefully assessing skin viability prior to amputation and by handling all skin edges and flaps with the utmost care. Use a myoplastic flap wherever possible as this always has a better blood supply.

2. Treat small areas of wound necrosis conservatively. The wound will granulate beneath the patch of blackened, sloughing skin, which will eventually separate spontaneously.

3. Major flap necrosis will require either a wedge resection down to and including bone or a re-amputation to a higher level.

Joint contractures

> **🔑 Key point**
>
> • Particularly important at the hip and knee, contractures are common in the elderly and immobile, in patients with serious head injuries, prolonged coma or chronic pain.

1. Treat or prevent mild contractures by early active and passive exercises, corrective posturing and prosthetic fitting and mobilization. Hip contractures may be avoided by regular prone lying, for example.

2. Severe contractures may require serial plasters or surgical release; otherwise the use of a prosthesis is likely to be impossible.

Neuroma

1. All cut ends of nerves form neuromata but they are painful only if trapped in scar tissue or exposed to repeated trauma. It is important that the transected nerves lie deep within the normal tissues of the limb proximal to the end of the stump.

2. Treat painful neuromata by resecting the neuroma and a length of the affected nerve well away from the area of scar tissue.

Phantom limb sensation

1. Always warn the patient before amputation that after the operation he will have a feeling that the missing part of his limb is still present. Do not introduce the concept of phantom pain, however.

2. After amputation, reassure the patient that this feeling will gradually fade away. Meanwhile warn him of the danger of attempting to use a limb that is not present.

Phantom pain

1. This difficult complication is most common with proximal rather than distal amputations, in patients who had severe pain before amputation and in those who have been in contact with other patients with phantom pain.

2. The cause is unknown and the pain is untreatable even by nerve section or cordotomy. Be continually optimistic and supportive and remember that this distressing symptom occasionally leads to suicide. Management requires a team approach.

Failure to use prosthesis

> **🔑 Key point**
>
> • The earlier a prosthesis is applied, the more likely it is that it will be used. In specialist centres, rigid casts are applied to the stump to which a prosthesis can be attached. Patients are mobilized within 48 hours of operation. The advantages are: reduced postoperative oedema, considerable reduction in pain, profound psychological benefits, fewer complications of immobility (e.g. joint contracture and osteoporosis), reduced hospital stay, earlier maturation of the stump and earlier return to full social activities.

BELOW-KNEE AMPUTATION

Appraise

1. Assess carefully the viability of the soft tissues of the lower leg when amputation at this level is being considered for peripheral vascular disease, diabetic gangrene or trauma.

> **🔑 Key point**
>
> • Use a long posterior flap, or a skew flap, in peripheral vascular disease, diabetes and trauma. Equal flaps are suitable for amputation for tumours and severe acute infection.

2. Do not consider this amputation in the non-ambulant patient. But otherwise always try to preserve the knee.

3. A third of its length is the optimal level for tibial section. Do not make it longer than this as the resulting flaps will not contain enough muscle to maintain its viability. The minimum length is 6 cm. If there is a fixed flexion deformity of the knee then the required tibial lengths are as indicated in Table 28.1.

Action

1. Seal off any infected, gangrenous areas by enclosing in a polythene bag.

2. Use general or epidural anaesthesia.

3. Apply a tourniquet to the thigh unless the amputation is for peripheral vascular disease.

4. Place the patient supine on the operating table with a padded, inverted bowl underneath the proximal tibia.

5. Mark the skin flaps (Fig. 28.1).

Table 28.1

Fixed flexion deformity	Tibial length
35°	6–10 cm
15°	10–15 cm
5°	>20 cm

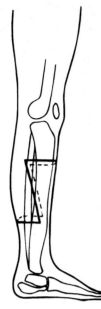

Fig. 28.1   Incision for below-knee amputation.

Start the anterior incision at the base of proposed bone section and pass transversely round each side of the leg to a point two-thirds of the way down each side. Then take the incisions distally on each side passing slightly anteriorly to a point well below the length that is likely to be required. Join the two incisions posteriorly.

6. Dissect the longitudinal incisions down to deep fascia. Anteriorly incise straight down to bone and then on to the interosseous membrane. Ligate the anterior tibial vessels at this point. Elevate the periosteum of the tibia for 1 cm proximal to the level of section. Divide the tibia using a Gigli or amputation saw. Bevel the anterior half of the tibial stump with the saw and a rasp. Divide the fibula 1 cm proximally and bevel the bone laterally.

7. Use a bone hook to distract the distal part of the tibia. Divide the deep posterior muscles of the calf at the same level as the tibia. At this stage identify and ligate the posterior tibial and peroneal vessels and divide the posterior tibial nerve cleanly and allow it to retract.

8. Use a raking cut through the soleus and gastrocnemius muscles down to the end of the posterior flap. Remove the limb.

9. Complete the smoothing and bevelling of the tibia and fibula using bone nibblers and a rasp.

10. Bevel gastrocnemius and soleus medially and laterally, and trim the excess skin to fashion a rounded, slightly bulbous stump.

11. Release the tourniquet and secure haemostasis.

12. Insert a suction drain brought out medially through the wound.

13. Bring the posterior flap forwards over the bone and suture it anteriorly to the deep fascia of the anterolateral group of muscles, using a strong absorbable suture.

14. Close the skin, preferably with closely placed staples, or with interrupted nylon sutures and adhesive tapes. Do not leave any 'dog ears' laterally.

15. Apply a dressing of gauze and sterile plaster wool and apply gentle compression over the stump with a crepe bandage. Apply a further layer of plaster wool and then a light plaster cast to mid-thigh level. Mould the plaster over the femoral condyles to prevent it slipping down. Do not use plaster in infected cases.

Aftercare

1. Elevate the leg.

2. Remove the drain at 48 hours by pulling it gently out of the top of the plaster cast.

3. Mobilize early and retain the plaster cast undisturbed for at least 10 days.

4. Remove the sutures at 14 days.

5. Apply a daily stump bandage.

6. Arrange for daily hip and knee physiotherapy.

7. As soon as the wound has fully healed arrange for the fitting of a temporary pylon, either patellar-tendon-bearing or ischial-bearing, depending on the quality of the stump. Arrangements for definitive limb fitting may then proceed.

AMPUTATION OF THE TOES

1. Use a tourniquet with exsanguination.

2. Mark out a racquet incision for amputation of individual toes. For amputation of all the toes the incision should be transverse, passing across the root of the toes on the plantar aspect (i.e. overlying the proximal phalanx) and across the metatarsophalangeal joints on the dorsum. The eventual scar should lie dorsally.

3. Take the flaps straight down to bone and dissect off the proximal phalanx.

4. Preserve the base of the proximal phalanx where possible, dividing the bone just distal to the insertion of the capsule. A small wound cavity is thereby created, which heals quickly, and the amputation does not damage the transverse metatarsal ligaments. Otherwise, perform a careful disarticulation.

5. Secure haemostasis.

6. Close the skin with interrupted nylon sutures.

7. Apply a bulky compression dressing, passing a few turns of crepe bandage round the ankle to hold the dressing in position.

Aftercare

1. Elevate the leg.

2. Remove the sutures at 10 days and mobilize the patient.

3. Where individual toes have been amputated, ask the chiropodist to supply a toe spacer.

4. Where all the toes have been amputated, order from the surgical appliances department a special insole that incorporates a combined metatarsal and cavus support plus a cork toe-block faced with sponge rubber.

FURTHER READING

Angel JC, Weaver PC 1979 Amputation surgery. In: Rob and Smith's Orthopaedics, Part 1. Butterworths, London

Limb salvage versus amputation. Preliminary results of the Mangled Extremity Severity Score. Clinical Orthopedics 1990 256: 80–86

Symposium on Amputations 1991 Annals of the Royal College of Surgeons of England 73(3): 133–176

Tooms RE 1987 Amputations. In: Crenshaw AH (ed) Campbell's Operative orthopedics. CV Mosby, St Louis, pp 597–646

Orthopaedics and trauma: general principles

N. Goddard

Contents

PREOPERATIVE PREPARATION

Appraise

1. Most elective orthopaedic operations are carried out on otherwise healthy patients but always assess the patient's fitness for operation beforehand. When operating for trauma ensure that the patient is adequately resuscitated.

2. Postpone elective operations until any concomitant illness such as a chest or urinary infection or hypertension has been corrected. This is especially so if one is contemplating implanting a prosthetic device, e.g. a total joint replacement.

3. Correct blood loss and dehydration before emergency operations.

4. *Antibiotics*. It is recommended practice usually to administer an antibiotic intravenously at the time of induction of anaesthesia, followed up by two further doses at 8-hourly intervals, making three doses in all. The choice of antibiotic depends upon the nature of the operation, the likely infecting organism and the patient's potential sensitivity. It is usual to use a broad-spectrum antibiotic (cephradine: 500 mg tds) or alternatively an agent that has a potent antistaphylococcal activity.

> **Key point**
>
> ● Infection of bone and non-living implants is a potentially catastrophic complication. Give prophylactic antibiotics for all but the most minor operations on bone, when an implant is used and if there is an open wound.

5. *Anticoagulation*. The routine use of prophylactic anticoagulants for major orthopaedic operations, particularly on the hip joint, is controversial.

Tourniquets

Appraise

1. Most orthopaedic operations on the limbs, especially the hand, are facilitated if performed in a bloodless field using a pneumatic tourniquet.

It has been said that attempting to operate on a hand without a tourniquet is akin to trying to repair a watch at the bottom of an inkwell!

2. Use a tourniquet with caution if the patient suffers from peripheral vascular disease or if the blood supply to damaged tissues is poor. Peripheral vascular disease, however, is not an absolute contraindication to the use of a tourniquet.

> **Key point**
>
> ● Do not exsanguinate the limb in the presence of distal infection, suspected calf vein thrombosis or foreign bodies, so as to avoid propagating the infection, dislodging any blood clot or shifting the foreign body. Take care when exsanguinating an injured limb or a limb that is fractured.

Action

1. Apply a pneumatic tourniquet of appropriate size over a few turns of orthopaedic wool around the proximal part of the upper arm or thigh.

2. Exsanguinate the limb either by elevation (Bier's method), or with a soft exsanguinator (Rhys-Davies). Use an Esmarch bandage where the latter is not available, but take particular care if the skin is friable, as in a patient with rheumatoid disease. A stockinette applied over the skin prior to exsanguination reduces the likelihood of shear stresses and potential skin damage.

3. Secure the cuff and inflate until the pressure just exceeds the systolic blood pressure for tourniquets on the upper limb, and to twice the systolic blood pressure for tourniquets on the lower limb. In practice, 200 mmHg is appropriate for the upper limb and 350 mmHg for the leg. Higher pressures are unnecessary and may cause soft tissue damage by direct compression, especially in thin patients. Never allow the pressure to exceed 250 mmHg in the arm or 450 mmHg in the leg.

4. If the tourniquet is accidentally deflated or slips during the operation, allowing partial or complete return of the circulation, deflate the cuff completely, reposition and re-fasten it and elevate the limb before reinflating the cuff.

> **Key point**
>
> ● Record the time of inflation of the tourniquet and the duration of its application, which must be kept to a minimum by careful planning of the operation. Exsanguination after preparing the skin can save 5 minutes or more of ischaemia time. 60–90 minutes is usually regarded as a safe period for an arm. Up to 3 hours is acceptable, but not desirable, for the leg. If necessary, temporarily release and then reinflate the tourniquet, but be prepared for a poorer operative field.

5. I prefer to release the tourniquet and achieve satisfactory haemostasis before closing the wound. Some surgeons, however, prefer to close and dress the wound prior to tourniquet release. Under these circumstances a drain is usually necessary and any plaster must be split.

Aftercare

1. On completion of the operation always ensure that the circulation has returned to the limb. Locate and mark the position of the peripheral pulses to facilitate subsequent postoperative observations.

2. Reduce the likelihood of swelling by applying a bulky cotton wool and crepe bandage dressing for at least 24 hours after the operation. Encourage and supervise active exercises A good orthopaedic maxim is: 'Don't just lie there – do something!'

Skin preparation

Elective surgery

1. There should be no break or superficial infection in the skin of a limb or the area of the trunk that is to be operated on. If necessary, postpone the operation until any wound has healed or infection eradicated.

2. Instruct the patient to bathe or shower within 12 hours of the operation using an antiseptic soap. Preoperative shaving is a matter of personal preference, but should be performed as late as possible and by an expert. Poor preoperative shaving may result in multiple skin nicks, which in turn become colonized with bacteria, increasing the risk of postoperative infection.

3. Mark the limb or digit to be operated on with an indelible marker. Give instructions to re-mark it if the mark is accidentally erased before the operation.

4. Prepare the skin with either iodine or chlorhexidine in spirit or aqueous solution. Iodine solutions are more effective skin antiseptics but are also the most irritant. Avoid pooling of alcohol-based solutions beneath a tourniquet or diathermy pad, with an attendant risk of explosions!

Emergency surgery

1. Prepare the skin in the anaesthetic room after induction of anaesthesia.

2. Cover open wounds with a sterile dressing held in place by an assistant.

3. Clean the surrounding skin with a soft nail brush and warm cetrimide solution, removing ingrained dirt and debris.

4. Remove the dressing and clean the wound itself in similar fashion to remove all dirt and debris, controlling bleeding by local digital pressure.

5. Irrigate the wound with copious volumes of physiological saline. A pulsed lavage system may be extremely helpful in this regard.

6. Complete the cleansing and irrigation of the wound in the theatre as part of the definitive surgical treatment.

OPEN WOUNDS

1. Resuscitate the patient, if necessary, according to ATLS principles and guidelines before dealing with an open wound.

2. Take a culture swab from the wound and send it for culture and sensitivities. This may be useful in the management of later infection.

> ### Key point
>
> - Clean open wounds in the accident and emergency department and cover them with an iodine-soaked dressing. Leave this dressing undisturbed and do not repeatedly uncover the wound to inspect it until the patient is in theatre. This will significantly reduce the rate of wound infection.

3. If possible take a Polaroid® picture prior to the dressing being applied to give you (or the treating surgeons) an idea of the extent and configuration of the underlying wound.

4. Stop the bleeding by applying local pressure. Elevate the limb if necessary. Do not attempt blind clamping of a bleeding vessels, to avoid damaging adjacent structures.

Appraise

1. Determine how the wound was sustained and whether it is recent and clean or long-standing and dirty, and superficial or deep. The longer the period since the injury, the deeper and dirtier the wound, the greater the need for antibiotics and tetanus prophylaxis.

2. Consider what structures may have been damaged and test for the integrity of arteries, nerves, tendons and bones.

3. Make an initial assessment of skin loss or damage and look for exit wounds following penetrating injuries.

4. An X-ray will show the extent of bone damage and the presence of radio-opaque foreign bodies (remember that not all foreign bodies are radio-opaque).

5. Always request X-rays of the skull, lateral cervical spine, chest and anterioposterior views of the pelvis in multiply injured patients, but do not let this delay treatment.

6. Depending on the extent of the wound, carry out further assessment and treatment without anaesthesia or with regional or general anaesthetic. Avoid local infiltration anaesthesia.

Prepare

1. Give a broad-spectrum antibiotic, unless the wound is clean, superficial and recent in origin.

2. If the wound is dirty, deep and more than 6 hours old give 1 g of benzyl penicillin and 0.5 ml of tetanus toxoid intramuscularly if the patient has been actively immunized in the past 10 years.

3. If the patient has not been actively immunized, give 1 vial (250 units) of human tetanus immunoglobulin in addition to the toxoid. Ensure that further toxoid is given 6 weeks and 6 months later.

4. Clean the wound and prepare the skin, as described above.

5. Apply a proximal tourniquet when appropriate.

Assess

1. Gently explore the wound, examining the skin, subcutaneous tissues and deeper structures. Follow the track of a penetrating wound with a finger or a probe to determine its direction and to judge the possibility of damage to vessels, nerves, tendons, bone and muscle. If you suspect muscle damage, slit open the investing fascia and take

swabs for an anaerobic bacterial culture. Decide into which category the wound falls, since this determines the subsequent management.

2. Simple clean wounds have no tissue loss, although all wounds are contaminated with microorganisms, which may already be dividing. In clean wounds seen within 8 hours of injury, the bacteria have not yet invaded the tissues.

3. Simple contaminated wounds have no tissue loss. However, they may be heavily contaminated and if you see them more than 8 hours after the injury, they can be assumed to be infected. Late wounds show signs of bacterial invasion, with pus and slough covering the raw surfaces, and redness and swelling of the surrounding skin. Although there is no loss of tissue from the injury, the infection will result in later soft tissue destruction.

4. Complicated contaminated wounds result when tissue destruction (e.g. loss of skin, muscle or damage to blood vessels, nerves or bone) has occurred, or foreign bodies are present in the wound. Recently acquired low-velocity missile wounds fall into this category since there is insufficient kinetic energy to carry particles of clothing and dirt into the wound.

5. Complicated dirty wounds are seen after heavy contamination in the presence of tissue destruction or implantation of foreign material, especially if the wound is not seen until more than 12 hours have elapsed.

6. High-velocity missile wounds deserve to be placed in a category of their own. For instance, when a bullet from a high-powered rifle strikes the body it is likely to lose its high kinetic energy to the soft tissues as it passes through, resulting in extensive cavitation. Although the entry and exit wounds may be small, structures within the wound are often severely damaged. Muscle is particularly susceptible to the passage of high-velocity missiles and becomes devitalized. It takes on a 'mushy' appearance and consistency and fails to contract when pinched or to bleed when cut. If the bullet breaks into fragments or hits bone, breaking it into fragments, the spreading particles of bullet and bone also behave as high-energy particles. The whole effect is of an internal explosion. In addition, the high-velocity missile carries foreign material (bacteria and clothing) deeply into the tissues, causing heavy contamination.

The risk of tetanus and gas gangrene is increased when the wound is sustained over heavily cultivated ground in which the organisms abound. Devitalized ischaemic muscle makes an excellent culture medium. As haematoma and oedema formation develop within the investing fascia, tissue tension rises, further embarrassing the circulation and causing progressive tissue death. Although handgun bullets, shotgun pellets, shrapnel from shells and fragments from mine, grenade and bomb explosions have a relatively low velocity, they behave as high-velocity missiles when projected into the tissues from nearby. When a shotgun is fired from close to the body, the wad and the pellets are carried in as a single missile.

7. *Open fractures* can be classified in a variety of ways.

Action

1. Stop all bleeding. Pick up small vessels with fine artery forceps and cauterize or ligate or them with fine absorbable sutures. Control damage of major arteries and veins with pressure, tapes or non-crushing clamps, so as to permit later repair.

2. Irrigate clean simple wounds with copious volumes of sterile saline solution without drainage. Do not attempt to repair cleanly divided muscle with stitches but simply suture the investing fascia. Close the skin accurately.

> ### 🔑 Key point
>
> - Never close simple infected wounds immediately. Take a swab for culture. Remove any retained foreign material, radically excise and debride any dead or devitalized tissue and drain any potential pockets of infection. Systemic antibiotic or local instillations may be started but will not make up for poor technique. Pack the wound with gauze soaked in sterile isotonic saline solution and cover with an occlusive dressing. Plan to renew the packing daily until the wound is clean and produces no further discharge. Provided there is no redness or oedema of the surrounding skin, close the wound by delayed primary suture, usually after 3–7 days.

3. Complicated contaminated wounds can be partially repaired after excising the devitalized tissue. Damaged segments of major arteries and veins should be repaired by an experienced surgeon using grafts where appropriate. Loosely appose the ends of divided nerves with one or two stitches in the perineurium, so that they can be readily identified and repaired later when the wound is healed and all signs of inflammation have disappeared. Similarly, identify and appose the ends of divided tendons in preparation for definitive repair at a later date. Do not remove small fragments of bone that retain a periosteal attachment, or large fragments whether they are attached or unattached. Excise devitalized muscle, especially the major muscle masses of the thigh and buttock. Remove foreign material when possible. Some penetrating low-velocity missiles are better left if they lie deeply, provided damage to important structures has been excluded. Remove superficial shotgun pellets. Low-velocity missile tracks do not normally require to be laid open or excised, but do not close the wound. Excise damaged skin when the deep flap can be easily closed, if necessary by making a relaxing incision or applying a skin graft. Do not lightly excise specialized skin from the hands; instead leave doubtful skin and excise it later, if necessary, on expert advice.

4. Stabilize any associated fracture. It may be possible merely to immobilize the limb in a plaster cast, cutting a window into it so that the wound can be dressed. An open fracture, however, is not an absolute contra-indication to surgical stabilization using the appropriate device (plates and screws, intramedullary nails), but such should be undertaken only by an experienced trauma or orthopaedic surgeon. In an emergency situation it is preferable to use temporary skeletal traction and external fixator.

5. Complicated dirty wounds require similar treatment of damaged tissues such as nerves and tendons, but do not attempt to repair damaged structures other than major blood vessels. Pack the wound and change the dressings daily until there is no sign of infection, then close the skin by suture or by skin grafting.

6. Lay open high-velocity missile wounds extensively. Foreign matter, including missile fragments, dirt and clothing, is carried deeply into the wound, so contamination is inevitable. Explore and excise the track, since the tissue along the track is devitalized, lay open the investing fascia over disrupted muscle to evacuate the muscle

haematoma and excise the pulped muscle, leaving healthy contractile muscle that bleeds when cut. This leaves a cavity in the track of the missile.

7. Mark divided nerves and tendons for definitive treatment later. Excise the skin edges and pack the wound with saline-soaked gauze. Treat any associated fracture as described above. Change the packs daily until infection is controlled and all dead tissue has been excised. Only then can skin closure be completed and the repair of damaged structures be planned.

External fixation

There are many types of external fixator, ranging from the simple unilateral frame (Denham, Orthofix) through to the more complicated circular frames (Ilizarov) and hybrid devices. The essential feature of the external fixator is that it provides a stable reduction of any fracture by using percutaneously introduced wires or pins into the bone, which are then attached to an external frame.

The Ilizarov and similar circular frames are beyond the scope of this chapter but in an emergency you should be familiar with the principles involved, and the techniques of applying a simple unilateral frame. Such a frame is constructed from one or more rigid bars, which are aligned parallel to the limb, to which the threaded pins that are drilled into the fragments of bone are attached. In the more sophisticated devices (Orthofix, AO, Monotube, Hoffman) this is done by clamping the pins to universal joints, which allow the position of the fragments to be adjusted before the clamps are finally tightened. In the simplest form, here described, the pins are held to the bar with acrylic cement (Denham type; Fig. 29.1).

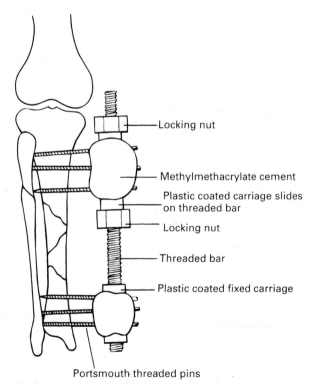

Locking nut

Methylmethacrylate cement

Plastic coated carriage slides on threaded bar

Locking nut

Threaded bar

Plastic coated fixed carriage

Portsmouth threaded pins

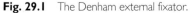

Fig. 29.1 The Denham external fixator.

Prepare
1. Treat the wound as outlined above.
2. Reduce the fracture, either open under direct vision, or closed using an image intensifier
3. Maintain the reduction using bone clamps, traction or temporary wires.

Action
1. Make a stab wound through healthy skin proximal to the fracture site, bearing in mind the possible need for subsequent skin flaps.
2. Drill a hole through both cortices of the bone approximately at right angles to the bone with a sharp 3.6 mm drill. Take care in drilling the bone that the drill bit does not overheat, which may in turn cause local bone necrosis leading to the formation of ring sequestra with subsequent loosening and infection of the pins. Measure the depth of the distal cortex from the skin surface.
3. Insert a threaded Schantz pin into the drill hole so that both cortices are penetrated.
4. If possible insert two more pins approximately 3–4 cm apart into the proximal fragment and three pins into the distal fragment in similar fashion. Biomechanically the stability of the fixator is enhanced if there are three pins in each of the major fragments with the nearest pin being close to the fracture line.
5. Loosen the locking nuts that hold the carriages on to the rigid bar and hold the bar parallel to the limb and 4–5 cm away from the skin.
6. Place one carriage opposite the protruding ends of each set of three pins and adjust the locking nuts to hold the carriages in position.
7. Fix the pins to the carriages with two mixes of acrylic cement for each carriage, moulding the cement around the pins and the carriage, maintaining the position until it is set.
8. Remove any temporary reduction device and carry out the final adjustment on the locking nuts to compress the bone ends together.
9. Dress the wound.

Aftercare
1. Keep the pin tracks clean and free of scabs and incrustations by daily cleaning with sterile saline or a mild antiseptic solution. A rigorous regime will minimize the risk of pin-tract infection and premature pin loosening.
2. An external fixator is essentially only a temporary measure before definitive treatment can be carried out. It is seldom used as the sole method of fracture management and should therefore be removed at a time when the wound is healthy at which time it may be possible to definitively stabilize the fracture.
3. Fixator removal is simple. Cut the pins with a hacksaw or bolt cutters and then unscrew them. The acrylic cement can be removed from the carriages, which may be used again.

OPEN (COMPOUND) FRACTURES

Appraise
1. Assess the patient according to ATLS principles and resuscitate as necessary.
2. Manage the wound as outlined above.

3. X-ray the bone to determine the pattern of the fracture and to decide on the appropriate method of reduction and fixation.

Prepare
1. Anaesthetize the patient.
2. Prepare the skin.
3. Clean the wound.

Action
1. Explore and reassess the wound.
2. Expose and assess the fracture. Remove only small and completely unattached fragments of bone. Retain any bone that has a remaining periosteal attachment, as this bone is potentially still viable.
3. Free the bone ends from any adjacent fascia and muscle through which they may have buttonholed.
4. Wash away any blood clot and other debris.
5. Strip the periosteum for 1–2 mm only from the bone ends to allow accurate reduction without the interposition of soft tissues.
6. Using a combination of traction, bone clamps, levers and hooks, reduce the major fragments into an anatomical position. If necessary, extend the original wound to improve access.
7. If the fracture is stable, immobilize in a plaster cast after definitive treatment of the wound. Leave a window in the cast to permit wound inspection and changes of dressings.
8. Apply an external fixator when the wound is contaminated or there is extensive skin loss.

> **Key point**
>
> - If the fracture is unstable and there is a simple, clean wound, then it may be appropriate to internally fix the fracture. If there are multiple injuries or if the wound is contaminated an external fixator may be more appropriate. Do not forget the possibility of immediate amputation if the limb is severely mutilated with associated neurovascular injuries (Gustillo grade IIIB or C).

SKELETAL TRACTION

Appraise
1. Temporary skeletal traction can be applied using skin traction, and indeed this is the method of choice when using a Thomas splint for immobilization of a femoral fracture as a first aid measure.
2. Skeletal traction is a simple and safe method of immobilizing a limb after injury or operation. It may be seen as a temporary measure, as definitive treatment, or as a supplement to treatment.
3. There are two types of pin in common usage (Fig. 29.2). Each has a triangular or square butt, which inserts into a chuck, and a trocar point. The Steinmann pin is uniform throughout but the Denham pin has a short length of screw thread wider than the main shaft near its centre, which screws into one cortex of the bone and minimizes sideways slip during traction.

Prepare
1. Clean the skin and drape the limb, leaving about 10 cm exposed on either side of the site of entry.

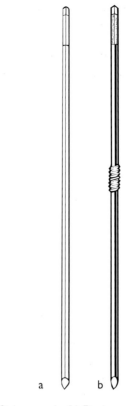

Fig. 29.2 (a) Steinmann pin; (b) Denham pin.

2. Anaesthetize the skin, subcutaneous tissue and periosteum on both sides of the bone at site of entry and exit of the pin with 1% lignocaine.
3. Make sure that the pin selected fits the sockets in the stirrup.

Action
1. To insert the pin through the upper tibia, make a 5 mm stab incision in the skin on the lateral side of the bone 2.5 cm posterior to the summit of the tibial tuberosity; this avoids damage to the common peroneal nerve when a medial approach is used. If the tibial plateau is fractured, make the nick and insert the pin 2.5–5.0 cm distally.
2. To insert the pin through the calcaneus, make a 5 mm stab incision in the skin on the lateral side of the heel 2.5 cm distal to the tip of the lateral malleolus.
3. Introduce the point of the pin through the nick at right angles to the long axis of the limb and parallel to the floor with the limb in the anatomical position. Avoid obliquity in either plane.

> **Key point**
>
> - Drill the pin through both cortices of the bone with a hand drill until the point just bulges under the skin on the opposite side of the limb. Take care that the pin does not suddenly penetrate the skin to impale your hand or the opposite limb. This is particularly likely if the bone is thin and porotic.

4. Incise the skin over the exit point and gently push the pin through until equal lengths are protruding on either side. When using the

Denham pin the threaded section should be screwed into the cortex a further 6–8 mm so that the thread engages the bone.

5. Make sure that the skin is not distorted where the pin passes through. Make tiny relieving incisions if necessary.

6. Dress the punctures with small squares of gauze soaked in tincture of benzoin.

7. Attach traction cords or a traction stirrup to the pin. Three types of stirrup are available (Fig. 29.3):

a. the Bohler stirrup, for general use
b. the Nissen stirrup, for more accurate control of rotation
c. the Tulloch-Brown 'U' loop for Hamilton Russell traction.

8. Put guards on the ends of the pin.

9. Attach a length of cord to the centre of the stirrup through which the traction will be applied.

Aftercare

1. Keep the pin tracks clean and free of scabbing and incrustation as described above.

2. Continually monitor the position of the fracture and adjust the traction as necessary so as to maintain an accurate reduction.

3. Monitor the condition of the patient as the enforced prolonged period of recumbence predisposes them to chest infection and pressure sores.

Simple skeletal traction

Simple skeletal traction over a pulley fixed to the end of the bed usually suffices for relatively stable fractures, for example, of the tibial

plateau. Unstable fractures need the support of a splint. Support the calf on two or three pillows with the point of the heel clear of the bed. Have the traction string horizontal and apply sufficient traction weights so as to reduce the fracture and restore alignment and length of the bone. Usually 4–5 kg is sufficient depending upon the weight of the patient.

Hamilton Russell traction

This is a convenient method for fractures and other conditions around the hip, e.g. dislocation or acetabular fractures. It controls the natural tendency of the leg to roll into external rotation and avoids the use of a Thomas splint, the ring of which causes discomfort if the hip is tender.

Action

1. Set up the apparatus as in Figure 29.4, passing the cord through the pulleys as indicated.

The sections of string x and y must be parallel to the horizontal and the section z must lead in a cephalic direction. Support the calf either on two ordinary pillows or on slings of Domette bandage attached to the 'U' loop with safety pins.

2. Attach between 2 and 5 kg of weight (w) to the end of the cord and make sure that it is clear of the floor. Remember that the effective traction is doubled as a result of the pulley arrangement.

3. Keep the point of the heel clear of the bed to avoid pressure sores.

4. Place a foot rest between the bars of the loop to maintain the foot at a right angle to the leg.

5. A separate cord running from the Nissen stirrup through the more proximal pulley can be attached to a handle so facilitating knee flexion exercises.

Calcaneal traction

Use calcaneal traction with the leg supported on a Bohler–Braun frame in the conservative treatment of unstable fractures of the tibia. It may be combined with a padded plaster cast to provide more lateral stability.

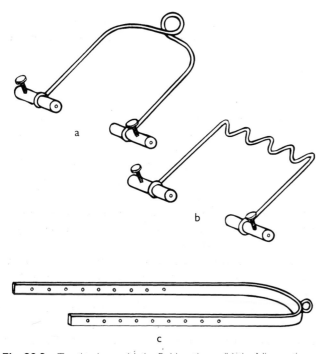

Fig. 29.3 Traction loops: (a) the Bohler stirrup; (b) the Nissen stirrup; (c) the Tulloch-Brown 'U' loop.

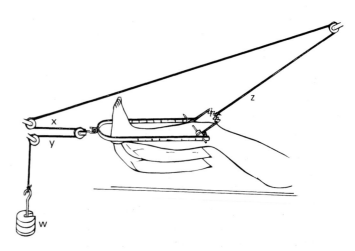
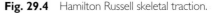

Fig. 29.4 Hamilton Russell skeletal traction.

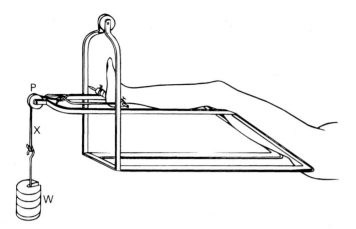

Fig. 29.5 Calcaneal skeletal traction with a Bohler-Braun frame.

Set up the apparatus as shown in the diagram (Fig. 29.5).

Apply 2–4 kg of weight (w). Support the calf and thigh from the side-bars of the frame with slings of Domette bandage. Pad under the limb with cotton wool.

PERIPHERAL NERVE REPAIR

Complete disruption of a peripheral nerve may be associated with both open and closed injuries and recovery will not take place unless continuity is re-established surgically. Peripheral nerve repair (Fig. 29.6) is a specialist technique but faced with it in the field, you should be aware of the principles. If you feel unable to attempt a primary repair then mark the nerve ends with a non-absorbable suture to assist their location at the time of the definitive operation.

Appraise

1. Always assume that a peripheral nerve injury in the presence of an open wound is the result of a complete division of the nerve fibres (neurotmesis). You must therefore identify the nerve when the wound is treated and satisfy yourself as to its integrity. If it is divided, either mark or appose the ends in their correct orientation for secondary repair later.

2. Some form of magnification is essential in repairing a peripheral nerve. While an operating microscope may not be available, simple magnifying loupes will usually suffice.

> **Key point**
>
> - Primary repair undoubtedly gives the best results and may sometimes be undertaken in specialist centres. If the patient is stable and fit for transfer, then do so. Secondary repair is safer and sometimes easier when the wound is soundly healed and the danger of infection has passed.

3. It is entirely acceptable to treat a peripheral nerve injury conservatively in the absence of an open wound. A neurapraxia (block to conduction of nerve impulses without disruption of the axon or its supporting cells) will usually recover spontaneously in days or weeks,

and an axonotmesis (the axon undergoes Wallerian degeneration) in the time it takes for the axons to regenerate. This is calculated by measuring the distance from the site of injury (e.g. a fracture) to the point at which the motor nerve enters the first muscle innervated distal to the lesion. Axons regenerate at a rate of 1 mm per day and so it will take approximately 90 days, for example, for reinnervation of the brachioradialis to occur following an injury to the radial nerve at the distal end of the spiral groove of the humerus. Electrophysiological studies (EMG, nerve conduction) may give some pointers as to the likely nerve lesion and will help in documenting recovery.

4. If recovery fails to occur in the predicted time and if the nerve conduction studies show no improvement then explore the course of nerve and treat any lesion appropriately.

Primary apposition of a divided nerve

1. Prepare the skin.
2. Apply a tourniquet.
3. Clean and explore the wound.
4. Identify the ends of the nerve and place them in their correct rotational orientation.
5. If you are sufficiently experienced it may be appropriate to proceed to immediate primary repair at this point (see below). If there is any doubt it is safer to mark or appose the nerve ends for later exploration and repair.
6. Appose the ends with two or three fine non-absorbable sutures (4/0 nylon or equivalent) for ease of later identification. Pass the needle through the epineurium 2–3 mm from the cut ends.
7. If the ends cannot be apposed without tension, tack them to the underlying soft tissues to prevent retraction until definitive repair is undertaken.
8. Release the tourniquet and secure haemostasis.
9. Close the wound when appropriate.
10. Carry out secondary suture when the wound is healed and free from induration, ideally 6 weeks later or as soon as possible thereafter.

Secondary nerve repair

1. Prepare the skin.
2. Apply the tourniquet.
3. Excise the previous scar if necessary, and extend the wound proximally and distally along the course of the nerve.
4. If there was no wound, make an incision 15 cm long along the course of the nerve centred at the site of injury. Use a 'lazy S' incision if the incision crosses the flexor crease of a joint.
5. Always begin by exposing the nerve in normal tissue on either side of the site of injury and then work towards the site of the injury.
6. Carefully dissect along the course of the nerve towards the point of injury. In the case of an open wound there may be extensive scar tissue and adhesions. The previously placed marker sutures will help to identify the nerve ends.
7. Free the ends of the nerve from the surrounding soft tissues and place a marker suture through the perineurium 2–3 cm proximally and distally from the site of injury to facilitate later alignment of the ends.
8. Cut transversely across fibrous scar tissue that may be joining the ends together.

9. Hold one end of the nerve firmly using a special nerve-holding clamp (a finger and thumb will suffice in extremis), and carefully cut thin slices of tissue from the exposed end with a sharp razor blade at right angles to the long axis of the nerve until all the scar tissue has been excised and the nerve bundles can be seen pouting from the cut surface (Fig. 29.6a).

10. Repeat the procedure on the other end of the nerve. It may be necessary to resect a centimetre or more from each end of the nerve because of the intraneural fibrosis (neuroma) caused by the initial injury.

11. Mobilize the nerve from the surrounding soft tissues proximally and distally as far as is necessary to bring the ends together without tension, carefully preserving and dissecting out the main branches. A

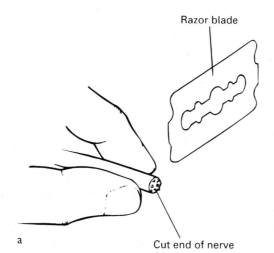

Razor blade

Cut end of nerve

a

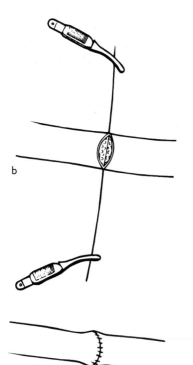

b

c

Fig. 29.6 Nerve suture: (a) cutting back to pouting fibres with a razor blade; (b) first and second sutures in place; (c) sutures completed.

neighbouring joint may be flexed if necessary. If it proves impossible to appose the nerve ends then an interposition graft may be necessary.

12. Release the tourniquet and secure haemostasis.

13. Ensure that the ends of the nerve are correctly orientated by aligning the marker sutures.

14. Place an 8/0 nylon stitch through the perineurium on one side of the nerve. Cut the suture 3 cm from the knot and hold the ends in a small bulldog clip (Fig. 29.6b).

15. Place a second suture directly opposite the first and place another bulldog clip on the ends. These act as stay sutures and facilitate rotation of the nerve while placing further sutures.

16. Place further sutures through the perineurium, 1.5 mm or so apart, around the circumference of the nerve.

17. After completing the repair of the superficial surface, turn the nerve over by passing one bulldog clip suture under and the other over the nerve.

18. Complete the repair. Cut the first pair of sutures and turn the nerve back to the correct position (Fig. 29.6c).

19. Close the soft tissues and skin without altering the position of the limb if there is any danger of putting tension on the suture line.

20. Apply a padded plaster without increasing the tension on the repair.

21. Remove plaster and skin sutures after 3 weeks and gently mobilize the limb. If joints were flexed to avoid tension they must only be extended gradually over the next 3 weeks, if necessary by applying serial plasters at weekly intervals, or by incorporating a hinge with a locking device to allow flexion but no more than the set amount of joint extension.

TENDON SUTURE

Appraise

1. Tendons are relatively avascular structures and heal by the ingrowth of connective tissue from the epitenon. When the tendon is divided within a fibrous sheath on the flexor surface of the hand, for example, the sheath is also damaged and the connective tissue from the healing sheath grows into the healing tendon, causing adhesions. For this reason injuries to the digital flexor tendons within the sheath should preferably be treated by experienced hand surgeons.

> **Key point**
>
> • It is entirely safe to perform a delayed primary repair of a divided flexor tendon up to 7 days postinjury without adversely affecting the final outcome.

2. Tendons may also require suturing as part of another procedure such as tendon transfer.

Assess

1. Examine the wound. As with nerve injuries, if it is in the vicinity of a tendon and there is no distal action, assume that the tendon is divided until it is shown to be intact on clinical examination.

2. If no action is demonstrated or if there is doubt, explore the wound.

Action

1. Prepare the skin.

2. Apply the tourniquet.

3. Explore the wound and extend it if necessary in order to identify any divided tendons.

4. If the wound is suitable for primary closure then proceed to repair the tendons. If not, delay the repair until the wound is healed and is no longer indurated, maintaining full mobility of the joints in the meantime by physiotherapy.

5. When several tendons are divided (for example at the wrist), make sure that the cut ends are correctly paired. It is not unheard of to suture the proximal end of one tendon to the distal end of another or even to the cut end of a nerve!

6. Draw the cut ends together after picking up the paratenon round each end of the tendon with fine mosquito forceps, flexing neighbouring joints if necessary.

7. Secure the cut ends of the tendon by passing one needle into an exposed tendon end and bring it out of the side of the tendon about 1.5 cm from the cut end. Now pass this needle transversely through the tendon 3–4 mm nearer to the cut end. Reinsert this needle on the other side of the tendon to create a mirror image and bring it out through the cut end (Fig. 29.7a).

8. Freshen the ends of the tendon by cutting them with a no. 15 blade.

9. Use a 3/0 braided non-absorbable suture with a 15 mm straight needle at both ends using a modified Kessler core stitch (Fig. 29.7a). Repeat this process using the second needle on the other tendon end.

10. Make a half hitch and approximate the tendon ends till they just meet. Complete the knot with at least six throws. Cut the knot flush; this should now have been buried within the tendon (Fig. 29.7b).

11. Complete the repair with a simple running suture of 6/0 monofilament nylon with a small curved needle. The final repair must be smooth, with no bunching at the repair site.

12. Release the tourniquet and secure haemostasis.

13. Close the wound with suction drainage if necessary.

14. Apply a padded plaster so that the suture line is not under tension and remove after 3 weeks in the upper limb and 6 weeks in the lower limb.

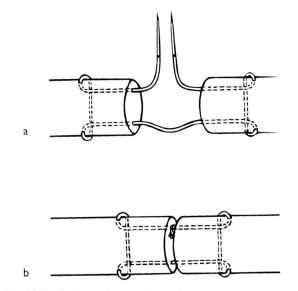

Fig. 29.7 End-to-end suture of a tendon.

FURTHER READING

Dixon RA 1978 Nerve repair. British Journal of Hospital Medicine 20: 295–305

Klenerman L, Miswas M, Hughland GH, Rhodes AM 1980 Systemic and local effects of the application of a tourniquet. Journal of Bone and Joint Surgery 62B: 385–388

Lowbury EJL, Lillie HA, Bull JP 1960 Disinfection of the skin of operative sites. British Medical Journal ii: 1039–1044

Nade S 1979 Clinical implications of cell function in osteogenesis. Annals of the Royal College of Surgeons of England 61: 189–194

Patzakis MK, Gustilo RV, Chapman MW 1982 Management of open fractures and complications. In: Frankel VH (ed) Instructional course lectures. American Academy of Orthopaedic Surgeons vol 31. CV Mosby, St Louis, pp 62–88

Seddon H 1975 Surgical disorders of the peripheral nerves, 2nd edn. Churchill Livingstone, Edinburgh

Stewart JDM, Hallet JP 1983 Traction and orthopaedic appliances. Churchill Livingstone, Edinburgh

Orthopaedics and trauma: upper limb

CHAPTER

30

N. Goddard

Contents

Approaches to the wrist
Ganglion of the dorsum of the wrist
Median nerve decompression in the carpal tunnel
Approaches to the hand and fingers
Pyogenic infections of the hand
Operations on the nails

APPROACHES TO THE WRIST

Anterior (volar) approach (Fig. 30.1)

Prepare

1. Position the anaesthetized patient with the affected limb on a large arm table.
2. Use a pneumatic tourniquet on the upper arm.
3. Clean the forearm and fingers and drape the limb as described for the upper arm, but leave the fingers and hand exposed.

Access

1. Incise the skin in line with the radial border of the ring finger as far

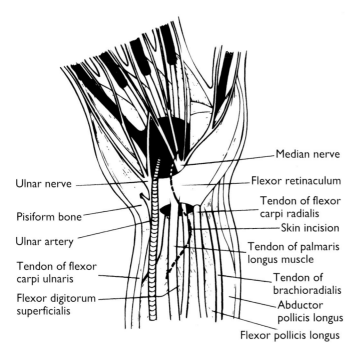

Fig. 30.1 Anterior approach to the wrist.

Ulnar nerve

Pisiform bone

Ulnar artery

Tendon of flexor carpi ulnaris

Flexor digitorum superficialis

Median nerve

Flexor retinaculum

Tendon of flexor carpi radialis

Skin incision

Tendon of palmaris longus muscle

Tendon of brachioradialis

Abductor pollicis longus

Flexor pollicis longus

as the midpoint of the transverse palmar crease. Cross the wrist crease either transversely in the skin crease for 1 cm or with a small zigzag incision, and then extend the incision proximally along the radial side of the flexor carpi radialis tendon for 3–4 cm.

2. Retract the skin edges with skin hooks exposing the palmar aponeurosis. The transverse carpal ligament will be exposed in the distal part of the wound and is continuous proximally with the deep fascia of the forearm.

3. Carefully incise the palmar fascia further exposing the transverse carpal ligament (flexor retinaculum) between palmaris longus and flexor carpi radialis. Incision of the transverse carpal ligament will then expose the median nerve and its recurrent branch, which is motor to the muscles of the thenar eminence.

4. Retract the median nerve and palmaris longus towards the ulnar side to expose the tendon of flexor pollicis longus, which should also be retracted medially.

5. The pronator quadratus lies in the floor of the wound. Carefully elevate this from its radial border to expose the lower end of the radius and the radiocarpal joint.

GANGLION OF THE DORSUM OF THE WRIST

Appraise

A simple ganglion is the result of cystic degeneration of fibrous tissue. They commonly arise from a synovial joint or less frequently from a tendon sheath. The commonest site is on the dorsal aspect of the wrist where they nearly always originate from the scapholunate joint. Recurrence is common unless care is taken in removing the ganglion.

Prepare

As for anterior approach. There may be advocates for performing this operation under purely local anaesthetic, but this does not really permit the use of a tourniquet. My preference therefore is to perform the operation under either a regional block or general anaesthetic, which allows a tourniquet to be used and permits a better exposure of the neck of the ganglion, so theoretically reducing the risk of recurrence.

Action

1. Make a transverse incision in a skin crease over the apex of the swelling.
2. Deepen it carefully until the bluish-grey surface of the ganglion is seen.
3. Carefully dissect around the ganglion with small curved scissors.
4. Do not grasp it with toothed forceps, to avoid puncturing it.
5. The swelling is often multilocular and passes between the

223

tendons. With care its attachment to the capsule of the joint can be identified.

6. Trace the ganglion down to its origin and remove the small portion of the capsule (or tendon sheath) to which the ganglion is attached, as well as the ganglion itself.

7. Remove the tourniquet and close the skin.

Aftercare

1. Apply a compression dressing for 24 hours and then replace this with a small adhesive dressing.

2. Remove the stitches at 10 days.

MEDIAN NERVE DECOMPRESSION IN THE CARPAL TUNNEL

Appraise

1. Decompress the median nerve if conservative treatment (night splints, steroid injections, diuretics) fails to relieve the symptoms of carpal tunnel syndrome, or if abnormal neurological signs are present. Look in particular for wasting and weakness of the thenar muscles and dryness of the skin over the radial two-thirds of the hand.

2. I always advise preoperative nerve conduction studies prior to surgical decompression.

3. Combine decompression with flexor tendon synovectomy in rheumatoid arthritis when the proliferating synovium is the cause of compression of the nerve.

Prepare

As for anterior approach.

Action

> **Key point**
>
> - Incise the skin in line with the radial border of the ring finger as far as the midpoint of the transverse palmar crease. This avoids potential damage to the palmar cutaneous branch of the median nerve.

1. Deepen the incision down through the longitudinal fibres of the palmar aponeurosis to expose the transverse fibres of the flexor retinaculum.

2. Insert a small self-retaining retractor.

3. Incise the flexor retinaculum longitudinally with a scalpel to expose the median nerve. Pass a McDonald's dissector deep to the retinaculum to protect the nerve while the remaining transverse fibres are divided.

4. Ensure that the proximal part of the retinaculum has been adequately released where it disappears under the skin at the proximal end of the wound, by passing a dissector along the surface of the median nerve. This is a common site of inadequate decompression, which can result in persistent symptoms.

5. Take care not to damage the transverse palmar arch at the distal end of the incision.

6. If there is an associated hypertrophic synovitis affecting the flexor tendons (as in rheumatoid disease), perform a flexor synovectomy by stripping the synovium with a fine pair of bone nibblers.

Closure

1. Release the tourniquet; the nerve will 'blush' at the site of compression.

2. Stop any bleeding.

3. Close the skin.

Aftercare

1. Apply a firm compression dressing and then replace it with an adhesive dressing after 24 hours.

2. Instruct the patient to exercise the fingers immediately after the operation.

3. Remove the stitches at 10 days.

APPROACHES TO THE HAND AND FINGERS

The unique sensibility and mobility of the hand and fingers call for special care whenever surgical treatment is contemplated.

Palmar approach (Fig. 30.2)

Appraise

> **Key point**
>
> - Incisions may be made anywhere in the palm of the hand provided that they do not cross the skin creases at right angles. Skin creases should be crossed obliquely (Brunner incisions) or, as far as possible, parallel to but not within the creases (Fig. 30.2). They may have to take into account any pre-existing lacerations or injuries.

Prepare

1. Use a general anaesthetic or regional block.

2. Attach the arm table to the operating table.

3. Apply a pneumatic tourniquet to the upper arm.

4. An unscrubbed assistant grasps the forearm immediately below the elbow while the skin is cleaned from the assistant's forearm to the patient's fingertips.

5. Place the towels as if the operation were to be on the wrist.

6. Place the hand on the hand table in a supinated position and secure the fingers and thumb with a 'lead hand'.

Action

1. Incise the skin and subcutaneous tissue obliquely crossing the skin creases at their apices. Extend the incision proximally and distally over the structure to be exposed.

2. Carefully dissect the skin and subcutaneous tissue from the underlying fascia and retract the edges with skin hooks.

3. Expose the deeper structures with incisions made according to anatomical considerations and not necessarily following the skin incisions.

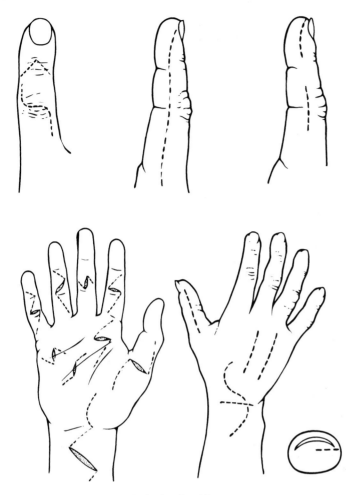

Fig. 30.2 Skin incisions in the hand and fingers.

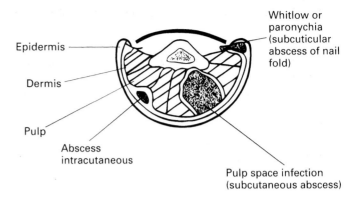

Fig. 30.3 Superficial and deep infections of the digits.

2. Incise and drain as soon as an abscess develops or you detected the presence of pus, either visually or because of increasing pain and tenderness.

3. Open subcuticular, intracutaneous and subcutaneous infections where they are most superficial and take a swab for bacteriological analysis. Local anaesthetic is not always necessary and many abscesses can be incised using a freezing spray (ethyl chloride) or no anaesthetic at all.

4. Web and palmar space infections are rare. Very little swelling is obvious in the palm, but the back of the hand is oedematous and pain is severe.

5. Tendon sheath infections cause swelling and tenderness along the line of the sheath, and the finger cannot be extended passively because of excruciating pain.

Action

Superficial infections

1. Accurately localize the most tender point with the tip of an orange stick before induction of anaesthesia.

2. Prepare the hand for a palmar approach but do not exsanguinate the limb.

3. When the infection is superficial, make a cruciate incision over the most tender point and cut away the corners of the skin to saucerize the lesion. Take a swab for bacteriological analysis.

4. If pus extends under the nail, remove only that portion of the nail that has been raised from the nail bed.

5. Incise in the line of the skin crease over the most tender part when a web or palmar space is infected. Do not incise the web itself.

6. Carefully explore between the deeper structures (Fig. 30.4) by blunt dissection and follow the track to the abscess cavity.

7. Insert a small latex drain.

8. Cut back the skin edges to ensure adequate drainage but do not insert a drain.

9. Leave the incision open to ensure drainage.

Tendon sheath infections

1. Drain tendon sheath infections through transverse incisions at either end of the sheath (Fig. 30.5).

2. Irrigate the sheath with antibiotic solution through a fine ureteric catheter until the effluent is clear.

3. Leave the catheter in place for subsequent irrigation if

Closure

1. Release the tourniquet and control bleeding.
2. Close the skin.
3. Apply a non-adherent dressing (tulle gras) and padded dressing, leaving the fingers mobile.

Aftercare

1. Reduce the dressing as soon as is practical and commence early mobilization.
2. Remove the sutures at 7–10 days.

PYOGENIC INFECTIONS OF THE HAND (Fig. 30.3)

Appraise

1. Pyogenic infections of the hand are common and present with cellulitis alone. Most resolve with antibiotics, elevation and rest.

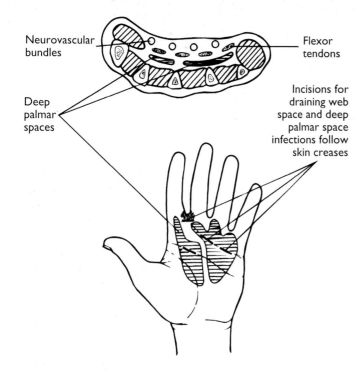

Fig. 30.4 Incisions for the drainage of web and deep palmar space infections.

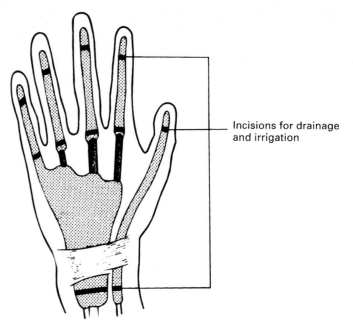

Fig. 30.5 Drainage of tendon sheath infections.

necessary. Local anaesthetic can also be instilled for postoperative pain relief.

Palmar space infections
1. When the infection is superficial, make a cruciate incision over the most tender point and cut away the corners of the skin to saucerize the lesion. Take a swab for bacteriological analysis.

> **Key point**
>
> ● Deep palmar space infections can be drained through a dorsal approach between the first and second metacarpals. Make a small stab incision and simply bluntly dissect with a clip or curved scissors to open the deep palmar space.

2. Leave a soft latex drain in situ until the drainage ceases.

Aftercare
1. Place the corner of a gauze dressing in the wound to keep it open.
2. Apply Tubigrip® to the fingers or a fluffed-up pressure dressing to the palm as appropriate and immobilize the hand with a plaster of Paris back slab with the fingers in semiflexion.
3. Elevate the hand and re-dress daily so long as the wound is draining and then leave the dressings until epithelialization is complete.

OPERATIONS ON THE NAILS

Partial avulsion of a nail

Appraise
It may be necessary to remove a portion of the nail in cases of infection or trauma. However as much of the nail should be preserved as possible, to splint any associated soft tissue or bony injury.

Action
1. Remove only that part of the nail that is separated from the nail bed, using fine scissors.
2. Apply a non-adherent dressing and Tubigrip®.

Evacuation of a subungual haematoma

Appraise
The diagnosis is usually obvious and is generally the result of a crushing injury to the finger tip. It is frequently associated with a fracture of the distal phalanx, which in theory renders this an open fracture and so you should prescribe antibiotics. Check that the nail is not dislocated from the nail bed – if it is it should be reduced.

Prepare
No specific preparation is necessary.

Action
Although there are more sophisticated devices available it is a simple matter to trephine the nail with a red-hot needle or paper clip. The blood under pressure will spurt out. Cover the hole with a sterile dressing.

Orthopaedics and trauma: lower limb

N. Goddard

Contents

TIBIAL COMPARTMENT FASCIOTOMY

Appraise

Decompression of the fascial compartments of the leg may be indicated in the following circumstances:

1. after extensive closed soft tissue injuries of the lower leg
2. after proximal vascular reconstruction following arterial injury
3. for chronic exertional compartment syndrome.

Key point

- Measure the individual compartment pressures prior to operation. This is relatively straightforward and the equipment necessary should be immediately available in almost any anaesthetic department.

You need a slit catheter (14G i.v. cannula), a length of plastic manometer tubing connected to a pressure transducer (a sphygmomanometer will do in extremis). Prepare and sterilize the skin. Instil 2 ml of 1% lignocaine into the skin and insert the catheter into the anterior compartment. When it is satisfactorily positioned withdraw the trocar. Inject a small quantity of saline into the catheter to fill the dead space. Prefill the manometer tubing with saline and connect this via a three-way tap to the slit catheter and the pressure monitor, ensuring that there are no air bubbles in the system. The three-way tap is then connected to the pressure recorder and the compartment pressure can be measured. Impending ischaemia may be considered when the compartment pressure reaches between 10–30 mmHg below the diastolic pressure. Higher pressures indicate an urgent need for fasciotomy. Impending or established compartment syndrome is a surgical emergency.

Prepare

Prepare for the anterior approach.

Access

1. The anterior and lateral compartments can be decompressed through a full-length longitudinal anterolateral skin incision lateral to the crest of the mid-tibia extending from the level of the tibial tuberosity to just proximal to the ankle.

2. Incise the fascia covering the tibialis anterior muscle and extend the incision in the fascia subcutaneously both proximally and distally so completely decompressing the anterior muscle group. By undermining the skin slightly it is possible to also decompress the lateral compartment avoiding damaging the superficial peroneal nerve. In cases of exertional compartment syndrome only, it may be possible to perform a limited decompression through a short skin incision and then extending the fascial incision with a Smillie meniscectomy knife.

3. The superficial and deep posterior compartments can be decompressed in a similar fashion using a single longitudinal posteromedial incision made just medial to the posteromedial border of the tibia.

4. Incise the deep fascia and extend the incision proximally to the level of the tibial tuberosity and distally to a point 5 cm proximal to the medial malleolus, using the same technique.

Key point

- In an emergency situation excise the middle half of the fibula, which will result in decompression of all compartments.

Closure

It is only possible to close the skin in cases of chronic exertional compartment syndrome. In acute compartment syndrome the wounds should be left open with a plan to suture the skin 3–5 days later when the swelling has subsided, using split skin grafts if necessary. It may be necessary to inspect the wound in the interim period.

Aftercare

1. Apply a compression dressing.
2. Elevate the leg.
3. Mobilization will depend on the underlying reason for the fasciotomy.

RADICAL RESECTION OF THE NAIL BED (ZADEK'S OPERATION; Fig. 31.1)

Appraise

1. This operation is suitable for chronic ingrowing toenails.
2. Do not undertake the operation in the presence of sepsis but merely remove the nail and wait for about 2 months until the sepsis has subsided.
3. Do not perform the operation in the presence of peripheral vascular disease.

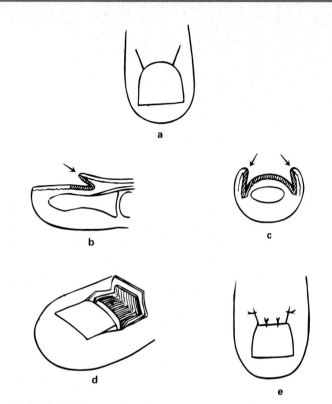

Fig. 31.1 Radical resection of the nail bed.

3. Lift the skin and subcutaneous tissue as a flap and dissect this proximally.

4. Carry the dissection under the edges of the skin incisions on either side of the terminal phalanx to the midlateral line to complete the clearance of the germinal matrix of the nail.

5. Cut across the nail bed transversely at the site of the lunula and join this transverse incision to the dissections under the nail folds.

6. Remove the block of nail bed from the surface of the proximal phalanx as far back as the insertion of the extensor tendon.

7. Check that no fragments of germinal matrix are left behind.

Closure

1. Draw the skin flap distally and suture the end to the nail bed with one or two stitches, which must be inserted carefully as they easily cut out.

2. Close the incisions on either side.

Aftercare

1. Dress the wound with a non-adherent dressing.
   2. Apply pressure with Tubigrip® bandage.
   3. Release the tourniquet.
   4. Elevate the foot for 24 hours.
   5. Allow weight bearing with or without crutches as pain permits.
   6. Remove the dressings and the stitches after 12–14 days.

FURTHER READING

Antrum RN 1984 Radical excision of the nail fold for ingrowing toenails. Journal of Bone and Joint Surgery 6B: 63–65

Henry AK 1957 Extensile exposure applied to limb surgery, 2nd edn. E & S Livingstone, Edinburgh

Rorabeck CH, Bourne RB, Fowler PJ 1983 The surgical treatment of exertional compartment syndrome in athletes. Journal of Bone and Joint Surgery 65A: 1245–1251

Zadik FR 1950 Obliteration of the nail bed of the great toe without shortening the terminal phalanx. Journal of Bone and Joint Surgery 32B: 66–67

Prepare

1. The operation may be performed under local ring-block anaesthesia with a rubber band as a digital tourniquet.

2. Clean and drape the lower leg and foot as described above, placing a shut-off towel around the instep.

Action

1. Remove the nail, if present, by separating it from the underlying nail bed with a MacDonald's elevator.

2. Make two incisions, 1 cm long, extending proximally from each corner of the nail to the transverse skin crease just distal to the interphalangeal joint.

Plastic surgery

M. D. Brough

Contents

GENERAL PRINCIPLES

Plastic surgery (Greek *plassein* = to mould) is concerned with the restoration of form and function of the human body. It is used in the repair and reconstruction of defects following damage or loss of tissue from injury or disease or from their treatment. It is used in the correction of congenital deformities. It also includes aesthetic or cosmetic surgery, which involves the treatment of developmental or naturally acquired changes in the body.

There have been many advances in plastic surgery in recent years, which have given rise to a multitude of new methods of reconstruction. These include improved techniques in microsurgery, tissue expansion, liposuction and craniofacial surgery. The most important development has been the recognition and application of axial pattern flaps. Several hundred cutaneous, myocutaneous and other flaps have now been identified but only those used most commonly will be described in this chapter.

Prepare

> **Key point**
>
> ● Plan for repair and reconstruction of tissue defects well in advance of surgery where possible. Carry out the simplest procedure to get the wound healed. Reconstruction of a defect may be primary or secondary after repair, sometimes in several stages. Make plans for each stage before embarking on the whole, so that one stage does not jeopardize a subsequent one.

1. Identify the lines of tension within the skin (Langer's lines) in the region of the proposed operation. Try to make all incisions parallel to these lines. When this is not possible, consider using a Z-plasty or local flap in closing the wound to help prevent the formation of scar contracture postoperatively.

2. Mark out a plan of the flap on the patient with a skin marker the day before operation, when using a large flap or a sophisticated reconstruction. For smaller flaps and simple incisions, mark out the area of incision on the patient after preparing the area before incising the skin. Use a fine pen and ink to mark out the lines of incision on the face. Use a broad proprietary marking pen in other areas. Try and follow these lines, as they are a useful guide once the skin has been incised and tension in the surrounding skin has changed. Be prepared, however, to make adjustments on occasions according to the circumstances.

3. While general anaesthesia is now very safe, do not forget that many operations can be carried out under regional anaesthesia or local anaesthesia. Many operations on the hand, for example, can be performed under regional anaesthesia, including cases of replantation. Large areas of split skin graft can be taken from the lateral aspect of the thigh by infiltrating the lateral cutaneous nerve of the thigh in the region of the inguinal ligament with local anaesthetic. Many other procedures can be carried out under regional anaesthesia, with the assistance of a sedative, if necessary. Many simple skin lesions can be excised under local anaesthesia. Use 1% lignocaine for this purpose. For excision of small lesions in the head and neck region, where the skin is highly vascular, use 2% lignocaine with 1:80 000 adrenaline. Wait 5 minutes after injecting the mixture, as this provides a relatively avascular field as well as anaesthesia. For extensive excisions of the face or scalp when the patient is under general anaesthesia use a more dilute solution of 0.5% lignocaine with 1:200 000 adrenaline.

Technique

Sutures
1. On the face, approximate the deep dermis of the skin edges with interrupted 5/0 polyglactin 910 sutures. Accurately appose the skin edges with 6/0 interrupted nylon sutures. Remove them on the third or fourth postoperative day. If they remain longer, suture marks form and these may prove impossible to remove without producing a more ugly scar.

2. Elsewhere on the body, approximate the deep dermis of the wound edges with 3/0 polyglactin 910 sutures and use subcuticular polypropylene sutures whenever possible, tying a knot at either end to prevent slipping. Leave these sutures in for 10 days or longer if there is a tendency for the scar to stretch because of its site.

Instruments

1. Respect tissues and their viability by handling them with care and using the appropriate instruments. For surgery of the skin, learn to support the skin with skin hooks or fine-toothed forceps. Do not crush it by holding it with non-toothed forceps.

2. For accurate suturing, use a fine needle-holder with a clasp that you find comfortable. Needle-holders with their own cutting edges require much practice before they can be used effectively. They are useful when many interrupted sutures are required and the accuracy of these is not crucial to the overall result.

3. Microvascular surgery requires specialized instruments.

Drains

When moving large flaps use large suction drains at the donor site, which has a large potential cavity.

Diathermy

1. Beware of unipolar diathermy when coagulating vessels near the skin. The burnt tissue may be visible and painful.

2. Always use a bipolar coagulator for fine work and flaps. The current from a unipolar machine could destroy the vessels in the base of a flap as it is being raised.

Skin cover

1. Close skin wounds primarily to provide ideal skin cover following incisions of the skin, excisions of skin lesions and simple lacerations.

2. Use split skin grafts to repair wounds with significant skin loss, to avoid skin closure with tension, or following trauma with an appreciable degree of crush injury to the local tissues. Skin graft survival depends on adequate vascularity of the base of the wound.

3. Use skin flaps, which carry their own blood supply with them and are temporarily self-sufficient, in primary or secondary repair or reconstruction. Use them as primary cover for vital structures such as exposed neurovascular bundles or for structures that have an inadequate blood supply to support a graft, such as bare bone, bare cartilage, bare tendons and exposed joints.

Skin closure

Appraise

Employ primary skin closure following simple skin incisions, surgical excision of small skin lesions and to repair simple lacerations. It should not be carried out if the tension in closing the wound causes blanching of the skin.

Action

1. Whenever possible, make incisions in the direction of the tension lines, particularly on the face.

2. For excisions, mark the skin in ink, planning to excise the minimal necessary amount of tissue. Draw an ellipse with pointed ends around this mark, parallel to the tension lines (Fig. 32.1a).

3. On the face, inject the surrounding tissue with 2% lignocaine and 1:80 000 adrenaline and wait 5 minutes for both components to take effect.

> ### 🔑 Key points
>
> - If the skin edges have been crushed, do not further insult them with sutures but carefully trim away dead skin and apply a simple dressing. Close the skin after a delay of 24–48 hours.
>
> - Beware of skin that has been degloved or torn from its fascial base. Resect it primarily or, if possibly viable, replace and re-examine at 48 hours, resecting it then if there is absence of bleeding when it is cut.

4. Make a vertical cut through the skin along the lines of the ellipse and take adequate clearance of the lesion in depth.

5. Undermine the skin edges beneath the layer of subcutaneous fat to facilitate approximation of the edges without tension (Fig. 32.1b).

6. Place a skin hook in each end of the wound and ask your assistant to draw them apart. This manoeuvre approximates the edges (Fig. 32.1c).

7. Close the wound in layers.

8. Apply a small dressing, or use no dressing at all if practical.

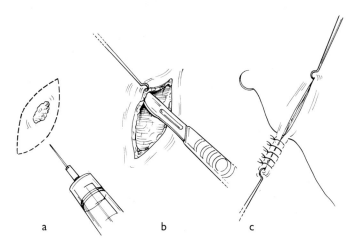

Fig. 32.1 Simple excision of skin lesion: (a) the skin is marked and surrounding skin infiltrated with local anaesthetic; (b) undermining the lateral skin margin; (c) the wound ends are distracted with skin hooks to help approximate the edges of the wound.

SKIN GRAFTS

Appraise

1. A skin graft is a piece of skin detached from its donor site and transferred to a recipient site. It may contain part of the thickness of the skin (a split skin graft or Thiersch graft) or the full thickness of the skin (a Wolfe graft).

2. A skin graft depends for its survival on receiving adequate nutrition from the recipient bed. Thus, thin split skin grafts survive more readily than thick split skin grafts or full-thickness grafts.

3. If there is a poor vascular bed or infection, no graft will survive. In these cases prepare the graft bed appropriately with dressings (see below), or consider using a flap.

4. Choose an appropriate donor site for each individual patient.

Small split skin graft

Appraise

1. A split skin graft is a sheet of tissue containing epidermis and some dermis taken from a donor site. It is obtained by shaving the skin with an appropriate knife or blade. A layer of deep dermis is preserved at the donor site and, when dressed appropriately, this is re-epithelialized from residual skin adnexae.

2. Use a small split skin graft to repair traumatic loss of small areas of skin from the hand or fingers, and occasionally in other parts of the body. Avoid using them on the tips of the thumb and index fingers since they tend to become hyperaesthetic.

3. Choose the donor site carefully. On the upper limb take skin from the medial aspect of the arm where the donor site will be inconspicuous and not from the forearm where an ugly resultant scar may be visible.

Action

1. Mark out on the medial aspect of the arm an area of skin that is more than sufficient to cover the recipient site.

2. Inject 2% lignocaine and 1:80 000 adrenaline intradermally into and beyond the marked area and wait for 5 minutes.

3. Lubricate the marked area with liquid paraffin.

4. Grip the arm on the lateral aspect with your left hand so that the skin that is marked out becomes tense, with a convex surface.

5. Cut the graft from the marked area using the Da Silva knife (Fig. 32.2).

6. Dress the donor site with a calcium alginate dressing, one layer of paraffin gauze, several layers of dressing gauze and a crepe bandage.

7. Apply the split skin graft directly on to the recipient site, spread it and anchor it using a minimal number of sutures.

8. Apply paraffin gauze, dressing gauze and a crepe bandage.

9. Re-dress the graft at 5 days.

10. Re-dress the graft donor site at 10 days.

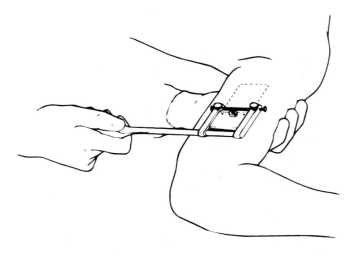

Fig. 32.2 Taking a small split skin graft with a Da Silva knife.

Large split skin graft

Appraise

1. Use these grafts following extensive skin loss from burns, trauma or radical excisional surgery.

2. The recipient site must be adequately prepared to ensure a good take of the graft. Grafts take best on exposed muscle or well-prepared granulation tissue. They do not take reliably on exposed fat where there is a poor vascular supply.

3. The take of a graft can be improved in certain circumstances by meshing it (see below), quilting it (see below), or by delaying its application and then exposing it (see below).

4. Use an electric dermatome, if available, to harvest the graft using the same principles outlined below.

Prepare

1. Following 'cold' surgical excisions, obtain haemostasis with pressure. Try to avoid using diathermy, as skin grafts do not take over diathermy burns.

2. Where subcutaneous fat is exposed, suture the overlying skin down to the muscle or deep fascia to cover it.

3. For infected wounds, take swabs for bacterial culture and prepare the recipient site with dressing of Eusol and paraffin. Change them 3–4 times a day. The recipient site is ready to receive a graft when healthy, compact, red granulation tissue is evident with minimal exudate.

> **Key point**
>
> - Do not apply grafts in the presence of β-haemolytic streptococci group A. If this organism is present, eradicate it with regular dressing changes and appropriate systemic antibiotics before grafting.

4. Choose the donor site most readily available to provide a large area of skin graft; this is usually the thigh. In young people, use the inner aspect of the thigh, where the donor site will be hidden. In elderly people, use the outer aspect of the thigh, where the skin is slightly thicker, so that if healing is delayed the wound can be easily managed.

Action

1. Prepare both recipient and donor sites by applying skin antiseptic.

2. Get your assistant to spread a large swab on the side of the thigh opposite to the proposed donor site. With his hand on the swab he supports the thigh and tenses the skin at the donor site by gripping the skin firmly with the swab.

3. Set the blade on the Watson knife to take the appropriate thickness of skin graft. Use a medium setting at first and then adjust accordingly.

4. Apply liquid paraffin on a swab to the donor site and along the knife blade.

5. Ask your assistant to hold the edge of a graft board at the starting point with his other hand (Fig. 32.3).

6. Cut a skin graft with the Watson knife, holding a board in the non-cutting hand and advancing this a few centimetres in front of the knife. Start with the knife at 45° to the skin and once the blade has

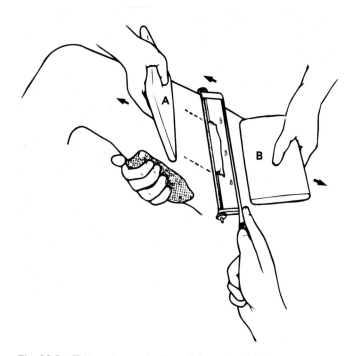

Fig. 32.3 Taking a large split skin graft from the thigh, the surgeon advances board A in front of the knife as it progresses along the thigh. The assistant tenses the skin of the thigh in his right hand, using a large swab to prevent his hand from slipping, and tenses the skin behind the knife using board B.

entered the dermis rotate it axially so that it runs just parallel with the skin surface. Use a 'sawing' action with the knife, advancing the blade only a few millimetres at a time. When an adequate length of skin has been harvested, turn the blade upwards and cut the graft off with one firm movement. If the graft is not detached with this movement, cut along its base with a pair of scissors.

7. Place the skin graft, outer surface downwards, on a damp saline swab and make sure that sufficient skin has been harvested. If in doubt, take another strip of split skin.

8. Dress the donor site with calcium alginate dressing, one layer of paraffin gauze, dressing gauze, cotton wool and a crepe bandage.

9. Apply the skin graft to the donor defect. Make sure that the graft is placed with its cut surface applied to the wound. The outer surface is opaque, the inner surface is shiny. Spread it, using two pairs of non-toothed forceps.

10. Cut off the surplus skin at the wound edge, leaving a margin of 3 mm around the periphery.

11. If the skin has been applied where a satisfactory compression dressing can be employed, do not use sutures.

12. Dress with several layers of paraffin gauze, dressing gauze, wool and crepe bandage, immobilizing the joints above and below the graft with a bulky dressing.

13. In areas where it is difficult to apply a compression dressing, immobilize the graft with interrupted sutures at the edge or insert a circumferential continuous suture around the graft.

14. Dress with paraffin gauze, dressing gauze, wool and strips of adhesive dressing.

15. Keep the graft site elevated postoperatively.

16. For grafts on the lower limb below the knee, do not allow the grafted area to be dependent for 7 days unless the graft is meshed. Then arrange progressive mobilization with compression support to the leg and foot including the graft.

Meshed grafts

Appraise

1. Meshed grafts are useful for providing skin cover to large areas, particularly when there is a limited area of donor skin, as often occurs in extensive burns.

2. Their take is more reliable as any underlying seroma, that collects escapes through the interstices of the graft, leaving the graft elements intact.

3. They are effective in covering irregular surfaces as they can be moulded to these.

4. Their main disadvantage is that the resultant appearance is less satisfactory than a sheet graft.

Action

1. Prepare the donor site in the usual way.

2. Harvest long, thin strips of split skin graft, as described above.

3. Dress the donor site.

4. Pass the skin graft through the skin mesher. It may need to be placed on a carrier for this, depending on the type of instrument (Fig. 32.4).

5. Apply the mesh graft directly on to the recipient site using two pairs of non-toothed forceps.

6. Spread the skin out appropriately to cover all suitable recipient areas.

7. Suture the graft with continuous sutures at the periphery only if the area is difficult to dress.

8. Dress the area with a calcium alginate dressing, one layer of paraffin gauze, dressing gauze, cotton wool and crepe bandage.

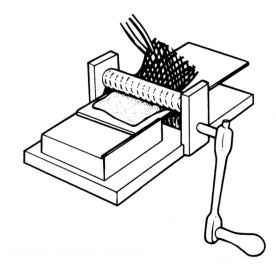

Fig. 32.4 Meshing a split skin graft. The skin graft has been placed on a plastic carrier and is being passed through the skin mesher. The cut skin, elevated at one corner by a pair of forceps, can be stretched to three times its original size or more, depending on the carrier used.

9. Re-dress at 4 or 5 days.

10. Continue to re-dress at approximately 3-day intervals until the interstices have epithelialized.

Full-thickness grafts

Appraise

1. Full thickness grafts give better cosmetic results than split thickness grafts as they contract less. The quality of the skin is better but they need a very good vascular bed to survive.

2. Their most common application is on the face following excision of small lesions, and the best results are achieved in the eyelid region and around the medial canthus.

3. They can occasionally be used on the hand, but are not generally used elsewhere, as large grafts leave a large primary defect.

4. The best donor sites are those with surplus skin so that the skin can be closed primarily with an insignificant scar. The most common donor areas are postauricular, pre-auricular, upper eyelid, nasolabial and supraclavicular skin.

Action

1. Mark the area of skin to be removed and measure it.

2. Mark out a similar area in the donor site, allowing an extra 2.5 mm or more at each margin for the contour difference that will be present at the recipient site.

3. Plan an ellipse at the donor site around the proposed graft to allow primary closure.

4. Inject local anaesthetic at the excision and donor sites.

5. Create the defect at the recipient site.

6. With a size 15 blade, cut around the margins of the planned donor skin.

7. Raise the full ellipse of skin and subcutaneous tissue.

8. Undermine the skin edges at the donor defect and close this primarily.

9. Place the skin graft on to a wet saline swab, skin surface down.

10. Using small, curved scissors, cut the subcutaneous fat off the skin graft and excise the redundant skin.

11. Place the skin graft into the defect and suture the edges at the periphery. Leave the suture ends long.

12. Use tie-over sutures to fix the dressing of paraffin gauze and proflavine wool.

13. Apply a pressure dressing for 24 hours, if possible.

14. Dress the donor site.

15. Plan to re-dress the recipient site at one week.

RANDOM PATTERN SKIN FLAPS

Introduction

1. Skin flaps are used to repair or reconstruct defects where there is an inadequate blood supply to support a skin graft. They survive on their own blood supply which they bring with them and this may be beneficial to the recipient site. It may help by introducing a new blood supply to an avascular area following irradiation, or to a fracture site where there is delayed union.

2. The quality of the skin in a skin flap is almost normal and its texture and cosmetic appearance is much better than a graft. A skin flap may, however, lose its nerve supply and have its vascular supply and lymphatic drainage partly compromised in its transfer.

3. Until relatively recently, all skin flaps were based on a random vascular pattern. It was recognized that flaps with a length greater than their base would survive in certain areas. It is now realized that the reason for this survival is that these flaps had, unknowingly, been based on an axial pattern basis.

4. Special terms are traditionally used in relation to flaps. Delay indicates partial division of a flap at its base and resuturing. This procedure encourages an improved blood supply to the flap from the opposite attachment. Complete division at the base carried out a few days later is then safer. After a flap has been transferred safely, the bridging portion may be divided. The two ends are trimmed and one is sutured into the new recipient area while the other is replaced in the donor site. This is referred to as in-setting.

5. When planning a flap, it is useful to employ a sheet of sterile paper or other similar material to act as a template. This can be cut to shape and used as a trial flap.

Z-plasty

Appraise

1. Z-plasties are used for releasing linear contractions. These usually develop along linear scars that traverse Langer's lines.

2. These linear contractions are often most evident when crossing the concavity of the flexor aspect of a joint, but they can occur on extensor surfaces and in other areas unrelated to joints.

Action

1. Draw a line along the full extent of the contracture (Fig. 32.5).

2. From one end, draw a line at 60° to the first line and of the same length.

3. From the opposite end, draw a line at 60° on the opposite side of the line for the same length.

4. Incise along the central line and excise any scar tissue.

5. Incise along the two lateral lines through the full thickness of skin and subcutaneous tissue.

6. Raise the flaps so formed, lifting the skin and subcutaneous tissue as one, holding the tip of each flap with a skin hook.

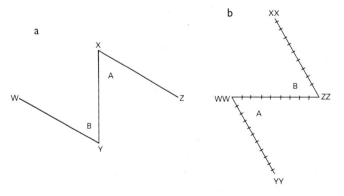

Fig. 32.5 Z-plasty. Contracture along X–Y is released to XX–YY by raising and interchanging flaps A and B. The distance W–Z is shortened to WW–ZZ.

7. Interchange the two skin flaps.

8. If the flaps do not meet comfortably, undermine the skin and subcutaneous tissue around the periphery of the wound to allow them to lie correctly.

9. Suture the tips of the two flaps into place first.

10. Suture the remaining edges of the flaps.

11. Dress the wound.

Technical points

1. The angle of the Z-plasty can be varied according to circumstances.

2. If the scar contracture is particularly long, use two or more Z-plasties, either in series or at intervals along the length of the contracture.

3. For scar contractures across a web space, use a W-plasty (Fig. 32.6). This consists of two Z-plasties, placed in reverse direction to each other, meeting at the base of the web space.

Transposition flap

Appraise

1. Small transposition flaps on the face have long been used. It is well recognized that in this region, because of the vascularity of the skin, flaps with a large length-to-breadth ratio can be used safely.

2. Transposition flaps allow skin from an area of abundance to be moved to a defect where primary closure is inappropriate.

3. On the face, there is an abundance of skin appropriate for transposition flaps in the nasolabial area, the glabellar area and the upper eyelid.

4. In other parts of the body, many axial pattern flaps are used as transposition flaps.

Action

1. Mark out the defect in ink.

2. Plan the transposition flap in an adjacent area with superfluous skin and mark this out (Fig. 32.7).

3. Check that the margin of the flap most distal from the defect is long enough from the fulcrum at its base to reach the most distal part of the defect. This is the limiting factor of the flap.

4. Excise the lesion to create the defect.

5. Raise the flap, including skin and subcutaneous tissue, and support the tip of the flap on a skin hook.

6. Transpose the flap into the defect and check that it fits.

7. Undermine the edges of the donor site defect and also the edges of the excision area to allow the flap to sit more comfortably in the defect.

8. Close the donor defect in layers.

9. Suture the flap in place.

10. Leave the flap exposed if possible, to monitor it.

Rhomboid flap

Appraise

1. A rhomboid flap is, as its name suggests, a flap with the shape of an equilateral parallelogram.

2. The rhomboid flap is most useful when the appropriate ellipse for excision of a defect is at right angles to Langer's lines. It has a similar effect to a transposition flap carried through 90°.

Action

1. Mark out the area of the defect.

2. Around this, draw the smallest possible rhomboid with equal sides.

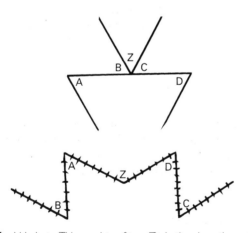

Fig. 32.6 W-plasty. This consists of two Z-plasties along the same contracture placed in reverse direction and meeting at the central point. Flaps A and B are interposed and flaps C and D are interposed. Flap Z stays in the same place but is raised during surgery to permit undermining at its base to allow it to stretch.

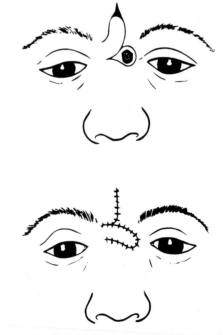

Fig. 32.7 Transposition flap. A lesion in the region of the medial canthus is excised and a transposition flap from the glabellar region is used to reconstruct the defect. A small triangle of skin at the apex of the flap is discarded and the donor site is closed primarily.

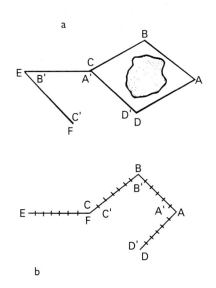

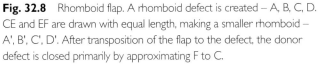

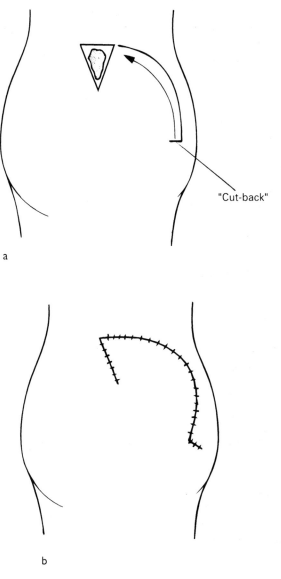

a

"Cut-back"

b

Fig. 32.8 Rhomboid flap. A rhomboid defect is created – A, B, C, D. CE and EF are drawn with equal length, making a smaller rhomboid – A', B', C', D'. After transposition of the flap to the defect, the donor defect is closed primarily by approximating F to C.

3. Draw two further lines of equal length as shown in Fig. 32.8.
4. Excise the lesion.
5. Transpose the flap, as shown in the diagram.
6. Undermine the edges.
7. Close the donor defect.
8. Suture the flap in place.

Rotation flap

Appraise
1. These are large flaps used to close relatively small defects.
2. They use excess skin at a distance from the defect and borrow small amounts of skin from a large area.
3. Their principal use is for borrowing skin from the neck to take up to the face. They can be used on the scalp and in treating sacral pressure sores.

Action
1. Mark out the skin defect.
2. Draw an isosceles triangle around the defect, with the apex of the triangle at or pointing towards the centre of the arc of rotation of the flap (Fig. 32.9).
3. Draw the arc of the rotation flap.
4. Raise the skin and subcutaneous tissue of the flap.
5. Undermine the skin at the edge of the defect and along the skin margin opposite the flap.
6. Rotate the flap into the defect.
7. Suture the flap.
8. If necessary, excise a wedge of tissue along the skin edge opposite the flap to assist rotation. A 'cut-back' into the flap at the opposite end of the arc of the flap from the defect may also help.

Fig. 32.9 Rotation flap. A sacral ulcer is created into a triangular defect and a flap from the buttock is rotated into this. A small cut-back allows greater mobility in rotation.

Advancement flap

Appraise
Advancement flaps are most commonly used on the face to preserve feature lines or structures of the face. They can be used on the forehead or for defects of the eyebrow. Frequently, in these situations, bilateral advancement flaps are used simultaneously to reconstruct one defect.

Action
1. Mark out the defect.
2. Mark out the smallest possible square or rectangle enclosing this defect, with lines parallel and at right angles to Langer's lines.
3. Extend the marks of the sides running parallel to Langer's lines in each direction from the defect, thus delineating two flaps (Fig. 32.10).

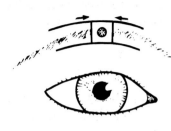

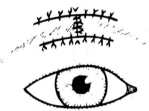

Fig. 32.10 Advancement flap. A defect in the eyebrow is excised and two advancement flaps, one from each side, are raised and advanced to meet each other over the defect. The natural lines of the eyebrow are preserved.

4. Create the defect.
5. Elevate the flaps and advance them towards each other.
6. Suture them together.
7. Suture their sides.

AXIAL PATTERN SKIN FLAPS

1. If a flap is designed around a recognized artery and vein, with these vessels passing down its central axis, it may be safely transferred with a very large length to breadth ratio. Indeed, the breadth need only be the artery and vein alone, providing they remain patent.

2. Many of the superficial muscles of the body have one principal vascular hilum, and these muscles can be rotated about the hilum on a single pedicle. It has further been realized that the skin overlying these superficial muscles receives its vascular supply from them. Consequently the muscle with its overlying skin can be transposed as a single unit, forming a myocutaneous flap. A large number of these flaps have been described, but only two commonly used ones will be described.

Latissimus dorsi flap (Fig. 32.11)

Appraise
1. The most useful application of this flap is as a myocutaneous flap in breast reconstruction and reconstruction of chest wall defects. It can be used in pharyngeal reconstruction and for defects of the back up to and just above the nape of the neck.

2. It can be used as a muscle flap alone to cover a large defect, or the muscle can be used to transfer a small island of skin (as in breast reconstruction) or a large island of skin. If a large island is transferred, primary closure of the donor site is not possible.

3. The flap has wide application in free tissue transfer (see below).

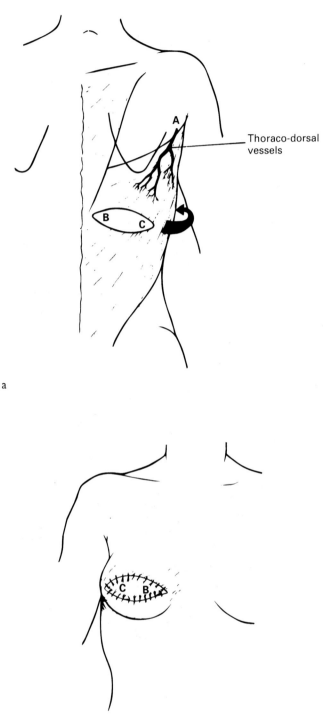

Fig. 32.11 Latissimus dorsi flap. The skin overlying the right latissimus dorsi flap is elevated from the muscle, leaving a central elliptiform island of skin attached to the muscle. The muscle is freed from its peripheral and underlying attachments and passed subcutaneously to the defect on the anterior chest wall, pivoted on its insertion A where the thoracodorsal vessels enter the muscle (a). In breast reconstruction, the muscle is sutured into the region of the reconstructed breast and the island of skin inserted into the mastectomy scar. A prosthesis is inserted beneath the flap (b).

4. The flap is based on the thoracodorsal vessels, and these enter the muscle just below its insertion into the humerus.

TRAM flap (Fig. 32.12)

Appraise

1. The transverse rectus abdominis muscle (TRAM) provides an alternative flap for breast reconstruction to a latissimus dorsi muscle. It has the advantage that it can normally transfer sufficient autologous tissue to avoid the necessity of using an implant.

2. The flap can also be used for reconstructing chest wall defects and defects of the perineum. In either of these circumstances the skin paddle may be taken in the vertical plane (a vertical rectus abdominis muscle or VRAM flap) with the skin paddle lying completely over the muscle.

3. The flap may be used as a pedicled flap based either on the superior deep epigastric vessels for breast reconstruction or chest wall defects or on the inferior deep epigastric vessels for perineal defects.

TISSUE EXPANSION

Appraise

1. The principle of tissue expansion is exemplified by the stretched abdominal wall resulting from pregnancy.

2. A tissue expander (Fig. 32.13) is inserted beneath the deep fascia or superficial muscle and expanded serially by injections of saline into an attached reservoir to stretch the overlying skin.

3. Following expansion the expander is removed and the surplus skin is used to cover the adjacent defect.

4. Expanders are most effective when placed on a bone base. They are particularly effective when placed on the calvaria to expand scalp and on the chest wall to expand skin for breast reconstruction. They have limited value in limbs.

> 🔑 **Key point**
>
> • Do not use tissue expanders under badly scarred or irradiated skin.

5. There are some more sophisticated tissue expanders available specifically designed for breast reconstruction. Some of these have a double lumen, one of which is filled with silicone. Others have a reservoir that can be detached from a valve linking it to the expander, allowing the expander to be left in situ.

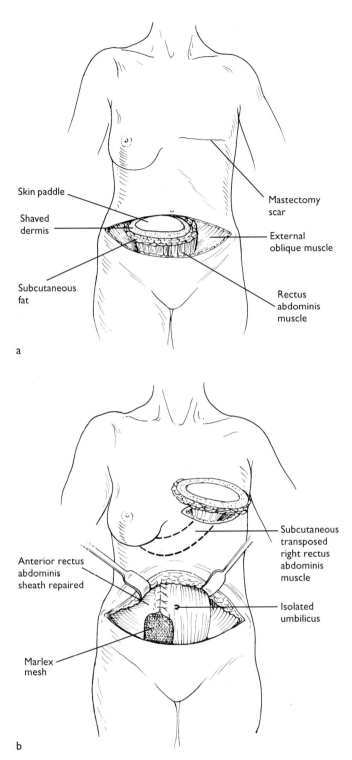

Skin paddle
Shaved dermis
Subcutaneous fat
Mastectomy scar
External oblique muscle
Rectus abdominis muscle

a

Anterior rectus abdominis sheath repaired
Marlex mesh
Subcutaneous transposed right rectus abdominis muscle
Isolated umbilicus

b

Fig. 32.12 TRAM flap. Being used for a left breast reconstruction, the flap is isolated in the abdomen with a skin paddle, a surrounding area of shaved dermis and subcutaneous fat lying over and adjacent to the right rectus abdominis muscle. The remaining skin and subcutaneous fat from the larger ellipse is excised (a). After division of the lower part of the right rectus abdominis muscle, the flap is transferred on the upper part of the muscle and passed subcutaneously into the opened mastectomy wound. The anterior rectus sheath of the upper part of the muscle is closed and the defect of the anterior sheath below this is repaired with Marlex mesh (b).

Tissue expander
Round reservoir with flat metallic base

Fig. 32.13 Tissue expander and reservoir.

MICROVASCULAR SURGERY

1. Microvascular surgery involves the anastomosis and repair of small vessels.

2. It has clinical application in cases of replantation and free tissue transfer.

3. The surgery is highly specialized. Operations may take many hours and require special instruments in addition to an appropriate microscope.

4. This surgery should be carried out in specialized units.

Replantation

Appraise

Replantation may be considered following accidental amputation or devascularization of any of the following parts:

1. limbs proximal to the ankle or wrist joints: this is called macro-replantation
2. parts of limbs distal to the ankle or wrist joint: this is called microreplantation
3. the ear
4. the scalp
5. the penis
6. composite pieces of facial tissue.

BURNS

Appraise

> **Key point**
>
> ● Patients with burns involving 15% of the body surface area (10% in children) or severe burns of the face or hands should be treated in a specialized burns unit. Patients with any significant inhalation burn should also be admitted to a specialized unit.

1. The treatment of patients with extensive burns is complex and ideally these patients should be treated initially in an intensive care unit.

2. Carefully assess to discover the type of burn, extent, depth, state of patient including co-morbidity.

3. Initiate appropriate local and general management.

Superficial burns

Action

1. Clean the burn wound and remove the roof of all blisters.

2. Expose superficial burns of the face but apply sterile liquid paraffin to reduce crusting.

3. For burns of the perineum, clean these and expose but apply silver sulphadiazine cream. Nurse the patient without dressings on a sterile sheet on a low air loss or water bed but keep him warm.

4. Cover superficial burns of other areas with two layers of paraffin gauze and a bulky absorptive dressing. Leave this dressing for 1 week unless it becomes soaked, when you should change it. Change the dressing at 1 week and subsequently twice a week until the wound is healed.

Deep dermal burns

1. Tangentially shave with a graft knife between the second and fifth day.

2. Continue to shave until punctate bleeding is evident from the surface.

3. Achieve haemostasis with pressure and apply a split skin graft.

4. Re-dress at 4 days.

5. When fully healed, measure and apply a pressure garment. This is an elasticated garment specifically measured for the individual to cover the area of the burn wound. Advise the patient to wear this for 6 months or longer if necessary to minimize hypertrophy and contracture of the resulting scars.

6. If you do not have facilities or expertise for the above surgery, treat the burn conservatively and re-dress twice each week.

7. Treat areas that are not healed at 3 weeks as full-thickness burns.

Extensive full-thickness burns

Escharotomy

1. Note the areas of full-thickness burns that are circumferential around digit, limb or trunk. If the viability of the distal part is jeopardized, or if respiration is hindered as with partial circumferential burns of the chest wall, carry out an escharotomy.

2. Give an appropriate intravenous dose of diazepam.

3. Take a scalpel and incise along the full length of the full thickness burn, allowing subcutaneous fat to bulge out of the escharotomy wound.

4. Repeat the longitudinal escharotomy at different sites of the circumference until satisfactory perfusion of the distal part is restored.

5. Dress the wounds with paraffin gauze or silver sulphadiazine cream.

Action

1. Identify a suitable area, not exceeding 20% of the body area, to treat primarily.

2. Identify a suitable donor site for the skin graft.

3. Excise the chosen area of full thickness burn with a scalpel and be sure that the resultant bed consists of viable tissue. It is often safer to excise all subcutaneous fat to leave a graft bed of deep fascia. Achieve haemostasis.

4. Harvest a split skin graft and mesh this (see above).

5. Apply the mesh graft to the burn wound site and dress with several layers of paraffin gauze and an absorbent dressing.

6. Re-dress after 4 days.

7. Do not excise burn tissue between the fifth and the 12th day post-burn, as the patient may be in an unsuitable catabolic state.

8. Do not excise further burn until the donor site has healed and is ready for reharvesting, or another donor site is available.

Small areas

1. Operate between the second and fifth day.

2. Excise all burn tissue and apply a split skin graft.

3. If the viability of subcutaneous fat is in doubt, excise this down to the deep fascia.

4. If the viability of the tissue is still in doubt, dress the wound and bring the patient back to the theatre 48 hours later. Re-assess viability at this second operation. Excise further if necessary and graft.

5. Re-dress after 4 days.

OTHER WOUNDS

Infected wounds that should not be closed primarily arise in a multitude of different situations. Two common causes presenting to plastic surgeons include pressure sores and necrotizing fasciitis. Their management is described below.

Wounds from pressure injuries

Appraise

1. Pressure injuries are common and difficult to detect in the early stages of development. The tissues between the skeleton and an external surface are compressed, causing a variable degree of ischaemia, which may be sufficient to cause necrosis. Necrosis may involve the superficial skin, the full thickness of skin or all the tissues overlying the skeleton.

2. Pressure injuries can occur in many sites but are most frequently found in well-recognized 'pressure areas' over the backs of the heels and around the pelvis, over the ischial tuberosity, the sacrum and the greater trochanter.

3. They result from the patient lying on or against a hard surface for a prolonged time. They may occur when the patient is comatose or under general anaesthesia or when the area is insensate, as in diabetic neuropathy or paraplegia. They are more likely to occur in these circumstances if the patient is thin, poorly nourished, cachectic and relatively immobile. Some surgical patients are therefore at particular risk.

4. There may be no significant evidence of the injury for some time after the event. Usually the first sign is erythema in the damaged area. Blistering usually indicates a superficial injury only. If the damage is deep the skin colour changes to blue and then to black as a thick eschar develops over a period of many days. This remains dry for several weeks before the necrotic tissue starts to separate.

5. Spontaneous separation of the underlying necrotic tissue may take many weeks or even months. When the necrotic tissue has separated, the wound will heal by secondary intention. A residual sinus will persist if necrotic tissue remains buried or if the underlying bone becomes infected.

6. As many patients with these injuries are debilitated, the above process may take many months and treatment is aimed at accelerating the healing process without insulting the patient further with unnecessary surgery.

Action

1. Avoid these injuries by identifying those patients particularly at risk.

2. Attend to their general health, specifically their nutrition and other medical disorders.

3. Take appropriate precautions when they are on the operating table and when in bed on the ward. Use one of the many specialized mattresses or beds to distribute the weight of the patient where possible. If these are not available the nursing staff may need to assist a change of position of the patient at least every 2 hours.

4. Cover superficial wounds with non-adherent dressings such as paraffin gauze and change on alternate days until healed.

5. Cover hard eschar with simple protective dressings only, or leave exposed if appropriate.

6. When the eschar starts to separate use a debriding agent such as Eusol and paraffin dressings changed daily.

7. Assist separation of the eschar by using a forceps and scissors during a dressing change. Repeat this with every change of dressing and avoid formal debridement in theatre and an unnecessary general anaesthetic.

8. Take wound swabs at regular intervals to monitor the organisms present but use antibiotics sparingly, for example if there is evidence of surrounding cellulitis.

9. Advise the patient to have a regular bath or shower, if appropriate, to help clean the wound and improve the patient's morale.

10. When a cavity is established use a vacuum dressing. After irrigating and cleaning the wound with saline, insert the foam dressing, introduce the drain and cover with an occlusive dressing. Apply negative pressure to the drain via the pump and leave for 2–3 days before repeating.

11. If a vacuum pump is not available, change the dressings to calcium alginate when the necrotic tissue has separated and a surface layer of red granulation tissue is evident. Change this daily.

12. If a large cavity persists consider introducing a large cutaneous or myocutaneous flap (see above, Rotation flap).

13. Also consider continuing with dressings until healed, avoiding surgery and allowing uninterrupted mobilization.

Necrotizing fasciitis

Appraise

1. This is a rare condition but one that must be recognized early if the patient is to survive.

2. There is a focal point where the infection commences, and this often arises from a surgical intervention.

3. The condition results usually from the symbiotic effect of the coincidental occurrence of an aerobic staphylococcus and an anaerobic streptococcus.

4. The bacteria appear to spread initially and preferentially along fascial planes. The overlying subcutaneous fat and skin are subsequently rendered ischaemic and necrotic.

Action

1. Look out for:

a. unexpected local cellulitis
b. rapidly expanding cellulitis
c. deteriorating general condition.

2. Take wound swabs and blood specimens for culture of organism and sensitivities

3. Commence on appropriate antibiotics.

4. Mark the edge of the area of erythema on the skin.

5. If the area of erythema is seen to progress beyond the marked line within a few hours, take the patient to theatre immediately.

6. Use a cutting diathermy to remove all skin showing erythema as well as underlying subcutaneous fat and deep fascia.

7. Remove any tissue suspicious of being involved in the infective process.

8. Dress the wound with gauze soaked in saline and further absorbent dressings, leaving the skin adjacent to the wound available for inspection.

9. Take the patient back to theatre after 24 hours or earlier if there are signs of progression of the disease.

10. Carry out further debridement of infected tissue.

11. Repeat this after a further 24 hours, remaining vigilant until all signs of infection have been eradicated.

12. When the patient is stable, consider covering the residual defect with split skin grafts or skin flaps or a combination of these.

SCARS

Hypertrophic scars

1. These present as red, raised, broad, hard, itchy scars that are unsightly and uncomfortable. They develop a few months after the wound has healed.

2. Beware of excising or revising them unless there was failure of primary healing or unless a marked contraction has developed. Simple excision of the scar alone will probably cause a larger one to develop.

3. Inject the scar tissue only with triamcinolone.

4. Repeat the injections at monthly intervals for 3–6 months or longer if necessary until the scar is soft.

5. Avoid excessive injections and avoid injecting the triamcinolone into the surrounding skin. This may cause skin atrophy.

6. If the scars are extensive, fit and apply a pressure garment as early as possible. Advise the patient to wear this garment for 6–12 months.

7. A pressure garment is a synthetic elastic garment that is specifically measured to fit part of an individual.

8. In applying pressure to a scar, it modifies the maturation and limits hypertrophic scar formation, provided it is applied early.

9. Pressure garments are most useful in reducing hypertrophic scar formation and preventing the development of contractures, particularly from burn wounds.

10. They are also used in controlling progressive lymphoedema.

Keloids

1. Keloids have a different histological appearance from hypertrophic scars.

2. They are most commonly found in patients of African origin but can be found in all races.

3. Excision of keloids, like excision of hypertrophic scars, only temporarily cures the problem. A larger lesion will develop in its place and this treatment is to be condemned.

4. Treatment with triamcinolone, as used for hypertrophic scars (see above), reduces the size of most keloids but does not eliminate them. This may, however, be the best treatment.

5. Excision of the whole keloid followed by radiotherapy to the resultant scar can be very effective. This requires expertise in radiotherapy but may not be suitable for young patients.

LASER SURGERY

Lasers are being used to treat an increasing number of skin lesions. These fall into four principal groups.

1. Vascular lesions
2. Pigmented lesions
3. Tattoos
4. Skin resurfacing.

PROSTHETIC IMPLANT MATERIALS

Appraise

1. All implants must be inserted under strict aseptic techniques.

2. Implants require good-quality soft tissue cover to prevent ulceration of the overlying skin.

3. If subsequently exposed, most implants will become infected and require removal. Later replacement when the infection has been eradicated may be possible.

4. All implants develop a surrounding fibrous capsule. This may be useful but is a disadvantage with a breast prosthesis as the fibrous capsule may contract and distort the prosthesis.

5. Several inert metals are used in reconstruction:

a. Titanium plates are used in cranioplasty.
b. Gold weights are inserted into the upper eyelid in facial palsy to improve function by assisting closure.
c. Stainless steel, vitallium and tantalum are occasionally used.

6. Hard plastics used in reconstruction include: methyl methacrylate, used in cranioplasty; polyethylene, used as a mesh in abdominal wall repair; and polypropylene. Proplast®, a combination of two polymers, polytetrafluoroethylene and pyrolytic graphite, is used to augment the cheek and the chin.

7. Silicone is a general term for a class of polymers with long chains of dimethyl siloxane units $[-CH_3-Si-O-CH_3]$. These are manufactured in many forms, including liquids, gels, resins, foams, sponges and rubbers.

8. Silicone implants are used in facial bone augmentation, small joint replacement in the hand and as a stent to reconstruct tendon sheaths prior to tendon grafting.

9. Silicone implants are commonly used in breast augmentation or reconstruction. Some breast implants consist of a silicone gel contained within a silicone elastomer shell. Others are made using a cohesive gel that maintains their shape. A textured surface modifies the fibrous reaction of the body and capsule contracture is reduced. There is no scientific evidence to show that any silicone breast implant has a significant carcinogenic risk and although these implants may leak there is no evidence that the silicone that does leak causes any serious complication.

FURTHER READING

McGregor IA, McGregor AD 1995 Fundamental techniques of plastic surgery and their surgical applications, 9th edn. Churchill Livingstone, Edinburgh. An excellent manual of basic techniques in plastic surgery, ideal for young trainees in the specialty and general surgeons.

Paediatric surgery

L. Spitz and I. D. Sugarman

Contents

GENERAL CONSIDERATIONS IN NEONATAL SURGERY

Introduction

To obtain optimal results, neonatal surgery is best practised by fully trained paediatric surgeons working in large specialist centres. The concentration of clinical material in such centres offers experience in the management of a wide variety of congenital abnormalities and facilitates the organization of training and research programmes. Support is provided from experts in nursing, anaesthesia, radiology, pathology and paediatric medicine, all essential for a satisfactory outcome.

1. The neonatal circulation is unstable and any noxious stimulus may result in renal or intestinal ischaemia or intracranial haemorrhage.

2. The ratio of surface area to weight in the neonate is twice that of the adult and this exposes the infant to genuine risks of dehydration from excessive insensible fluid loss accompanied by hypothermia, the latter enhanced by radiated losses, especially from the head.

3. The neonatal kidney is immature and can only function within a limited homeostatic range. The diuretic response is weak and circulatory overload can easily occur following excessive intravenous fluid administration, which may also cause reopening of the ductus arteriosus, resulting in hypoxia and severe heart failure.

4. Liver functions, particularly detoxifying enzyme systems, are restricted and hyperbilirubinaemia easily develops.

5. Low immunoglobulin levels and reduced leucocyte activity result in poor resistance to infection, bacteraemia rapidly progressing to meningitis.

6. Infection compounds any cardiac, renal or hepatic failure. Progressive multiorgan failure rapidly develops, the correction of which is difficult.

Preoperative preparation

1. Cross-match one unit of fresh packed cells.

2. Administer vitamin K, phytomenadione 1 mg intramuscularly, if this was omitted in the immediate postnatal period.

3. Check the blood glucose using Dextrostix®. Correct hypoglycaemia by giving 50% glucose intravenously.

4. Correct any acid/base and fluid imbalance.

5. In all emergencies, keep the stomach empty through a large (8F) nasogastric tube.

6. Ensure good intravenous access through a cannula conveniently sited for the anaesthetist.

7. Use ECG, pulse, blood pressure and oxygen saturation monitors. Monitors for measuring partial pressures of oxygen and carbon dioxide in inspired and expired gases are also available.

8. For very sick infants, continuously record blood pressure through a transduced intra-arterial cannula, which also facilitates intermittent blood gas analysis and assessments of serum electrolyte and haemoglobin concentrations.

9. Use a central venous cannula when blood loss is expected to be massive or when peripheral venous access is limited, but measurements of central venous pressure are of limited value in this age group.

10. Keep the infant normothermic. Radiant heat losses, especially from the head, must be limited by wrapping the head and limbs in aluminium foil and losses from convection must be limited by restricting the movement of personnel in the theatre and by swaddling the patient in warm gamgee. A thermostatically controlled warm air blanket should be placed below the patient. The ambient temperature of the theatre should be kept at 26°C with doors closed to prevent draughts.

THE ABDOMINAL OPERATION

> 🔑 **Key points**
>
> - Because of the relatively wide, truncated abdomen, greater access is afforded by transverse than longitudinal incisions.
>
> - A recommended 'general purpose' incision is a transverse, muscle-cutting, supra-umbilical incision extending across right and left rectus abdominis muscles.

Access

1. Place the prepared infant supine on the operating table.

2. Make a long, transverse skin incision, 1–2 cm above the umbilicus, with a scalpel.

3. Divide the subcutaneous fat and fascia with cutting diathermy to limit blood loss.

4. Similarly, divide the anterior sheath of left and right rectus abdominis muscles.

5. Coagulate the superior epigastric vessels on the deeper surface of each rectus abdominis muscle.

6. Divide the posterior sheath and fascia down to the peritoneum.

7. Open the peritoneum on either side of the midline.

8. Identify, clamp and divide the relatively large umbilical vein. Ligate both ends of the vein with 0000 polyglycolic acid.

9. After assessment, the incision may be readily extended, using cutting diathermy, into the oblique muscles of the abdominal wall at either, or both, ends of the incision.

Closure

1. It is unnecessary to close the peritoneum.

2. Close the muscles and fascia en masse with either continuous or interrupted sutures of 000 or 0000 polyglactin 910, polyglycolic acid or polydioxanone.

3. Close the skin with a continuous subcuticular suture of 00000 polyglycolic acid, polydioxanone or polyglactin 910.

4. When wound infection is expected, omit the subcuticular suture and close with adhesive tapes.

5. Do not use tension sutures or through-and-through skin sutures because the cosmetic results are unacceptable.

INGUINAL HERNIA

Appraise

1. In the paediatric age range inguinal hernia is generally due to failure of closure of the processus vaginalis. The hernia may be complete (to the scrotum) or incomplete (confined to the inguinal region). Operation is indicated in all cases.

2. Inguinal hernias become irreducible in up to 30% of infants, the peak incidence being between the ages of 6 and 12 weeks. Strangulation is rare in the neonatal period but, when it does occur, there is appreciable postoperative morbidity and a high mortality rate.

3. If the hernia becomes irreducible, pressure upon the spermatic cord causes testicular ischaemia, and infarction may occur after as little as 4 hours. Up to 25% of neonates with an irreducible hernia develop severe testicular ischaemia.

4. Premature babies are particularly prone to develop complications. Herniotomy should be carried out at a stage when the infant has gained sufficient weight to warrant discharge from hospital or as soon as complications occur. These small infants often have hydrocephalus following intraventricular haemorrhage and have bronchopulmonary dysplasia associated with the need for prolonged mechanical ventilation. The help of an experienced paediatric anaesthetist is invaluable and sometimes operation can be performed only by using spinal or epidural anaesthesia. These patients are prone to all of the complications associated with 'persistent fetal circulation' and postoperative deaths do occur, even with elective operation in a regional centre.

5. In infants under the age of 6 months, the tissues are thin and friable so operative difficulties are common. Treatment is best left to paediatric surgeons.

6. Before embarking upon operation for an inguinal hernia, ensure that the ipsilateral testis is in the scrotum, otherwise orchidopexy is indicated at the same time as herniotomy.

7. Performing an orchidopexy on an infant under the age of 6

months with an irreducible hernia is a particularly difficult operation that must not be attempted by a surgeon without special training unless there are exceptional circumstances.

8. Except in children with neuromuscular disorders, herniotomy rather than herniorrhaphy is the treatment of choice.

Herniotomy through the inguinal canal

1. Make an incision 2 cm long in a skin crease midway between the deep ring and pubic tubercle.

2. Divide the subcutaneous fat and Camper's fascia using scissors.

3. Incise Scarpa's superficial fascia with scissors and retract it.

4. Clear a small patch of external oblique aponeurosis over an area of 2 cm^2, at least 1 cm above the inguinal ligament.

5. Incise the external oblique aponeurosis with scissors or a scalpel and retract the edges. Do not open the external inguinal ring.

6. Dissect into the inguinal canal, keeping close to the posterior surface of the external oblique aponeurosis.

7. Soon the ilioinguinal nerve will come into view, and this provides a useful landmark.

8. Using a mosquito artery forceps, split the fibres of the cremaster muscle overlying the spermatic cord just inferior to the ilioinguinal nerve.

9. Gently grasp the internal spermatic fascia with a mosquito forceps and use this to deliver the spermatic cord from its bed while pushing away the adherent fibres of the cremaster muscle with a delicate non-toothed dissecting forceps.

10. Pass the index finger of the non-dominant hand behind the cord and use it and the thumb to rotate the cord so that its posterior aspect comes into view.

11. Using a non-toothed dissecting forceps, split the internal spermatic fascia overlying the vas and vessels in a longitudinal direction.

12. Gently sweep the vas and vessels away from the sac. Do not hold the vas or vessels with the forceps because a crush injury may occur.

13. Place an artery forceps across the sac, and divide the sac distal to the forceps. Allow the distal part of the sac to fall back into the wound.

14. Dissect the vas and vessels from the proximal part of the sac until the inferior epigastric vessels are seen.

15. Rotate the artery forceps to twist the neck of the sac, so ensuring that there is no bowel or omentum within it.

16. Ligate the sac flush with the deep ring using a 0000 polyglycolic acid suture, and then transfix the sac just distal to this tie. Ligation prior to transfixation and ligation prevents the needle from causing a split in the sac, which may spread across the deep ring and on to the peritoneum of the anterior abdominal wall, and so prevents the embarrassing escape of intestines or omentum at a difficult site to repair.

17. Allow the vas and vessels to drop back into the inguinal canal.

18. Close the inguinal canal with two or three sutures.

19. Approximate the Scarpa's fascia with one central suture.

20. Close the skin with a subcuticular stitch. If 0000 polyglycolic acid is used, the whole operation may be accomplished using but one suture. Alternatively, close the skin with adhesive skin tapes.

21. Gently pull the testis to the bottom of the scrotum to ensure that it does not become caught in the superficial inguinal pouch, necessitating an orchidopexy.

physiological saline and potassium (10 mmol KCl/500 ml 0.9% saline)

5. Check that serum potassium levels are above 3.5 mmol/l before arranging operation.

Anaesthesia
Although local anaesthesia has been used for pyloromyotomy with great success, general endotracheal anaesthesia by an experienced paediatric anaesthetist is superior.

Access
1. The infant lies supine on the operating table, protected from cold.
2. Site the transverse incision, 3–4 cm long, in the right hypochondrium midway between the costal margin and the palpable inferior margin of the liver. The medial end of the incision ends 1–2 cm from the midline.
3. Having incised the skin with the scalpel, divide the subcutaneous tissue and muscles using cutting diathermy to limit blood loss.
4. Open the peritoneum.
5. Retract the inferior margin of the liver superiorly by means of a broad malleable retractor protected by a moist gauze swab.
6. Identify the greater curvature of the stomach directly or after applying gentle traction on the transverse mesocolon.
7. *Do not attempt to withdraw the pyloric tumour by applying direct traction on the mass*; this results in serosal tears and haemorrhage.
8. Deliver the greater curvature of the body of the stomach into the wound.
9. Apply gentle traction on the greater curvature until the firm, white, glistening pyloric tumour is brought into view. Ease it out of the peritoneal cavity and into the wound.
10. Identify the pyloric vein of Mayo. This marks the distal end of the pyloric canal.

Action (Fig. 33.1)
1. Make an incision 1–2 mm deep with a scalpel on the anterior surface of the pyloric tumour in the relatively avascular plane midway between the superior and inferior borders. Extend the incision from the pyloric vein of Mayo through the pyloric canal and on to the hypertrophied body of the stomach.
2. Using firm but gentle pressure on the incised pylorus with a MacDonald dissector, the blunt handle of a scalpel or a blunt artery forceps, split the hypertrophied muscle down to the submucosa.
3. Split the pyloric mass from end to end using a pyloric spreader (Denis Browne) or blunt artery forceps. Ensure that all the fibres of the pyloric tumour are split.
4. Bubbles of air or bile at the duodenal end of the incision signify a perforation of the mucosa, most common in the duodenal fornix.
5. Close a perforation with a few interrupted 0000 or 00000 chromic catgut sutures and cover with omentum.

Aftercare
1. Except in small premature babies, the procedure is carried out on a day-case basis and there are no special postoperative precautions.
2. A slight fever on the first postoperative night is a normal response to surgery.

ORCHIDOPEXY

Appraise
1. Incidence of an undescended testis is approximately 3% at birth, falling to 1% at 1 year of age.
2. If either bilateral or unilateral associated with a hypospadias, perform chromosomes to rule out intersex.
3. If a testis is impalpable, laparoscopy is the investigation of choice to assess the presence or absence of the testis, and its site.
4. If there are bilateral impalpable testes, which are confirmed at laparoscopy to be intra-abdominal, bring one testis down at a time. This can either be by a Fowler–Stephens procedure (ligating the testicular vessels and relying on the spermatic fascia for vascularity of the testis) or microvascular transfer.
5. In the 'ascending testis' a testis that was normally sited in the scrotum 'ascends' with age. The incidence of this unknown, but the condition is probably commoner than suspected.
6. The operation for the undescended testis should be performed between the age of 1 and 2 years.

PYLORIC STENOSIS

Appraise
1. This occurs predominantly in male infants (M:F = 4:1) around the second to fourth week of life.
2. The cardinal features are projectile non-bilious vomiting, failure to thrive and constipation.
3. The diagnosis is established by palpating the pyloric 'tumour' in the right hypochondrium.
4. Confirmation by ultrasound examination is performed when doubt about the diagnosis remains after examination.

Prepare
1. Measure serum urea, electrolytes and acid/base status.
2. Correct hypochloraemia and hypokalaemia with intravenous infusion of half-physiological saline adding potassium (10–15 mmol KCl/500 ml 0.45% saline).
3. It is unnecessary to correct the alkalosis, which resolves spontaneously with the saline infusion.
4. Prohibit all milk feeds and leave a nasogastric tube on free drainage, replacing nasogastric losses millilitre for millilitre with

6. Haemorrhage from the incised pylorus is mainly due to venous congestion. Bleeding usually ceases once the pylorus is returned to the abdominal cavity. If bleeding persists, use diathermy coagulation.

Closure

1. Close the wound en masse using interrupted 0000 polyglycolic acid sutures.

2. Approximate the skin with a continuous subcuticular 00000 polyglycolic acid or chromic catgut suture.

Aftercare

1. Many surgeons commence feeds within 4–6 hours of operation. There is evidence that gastric peristalsis is ineffective at this stage and vomiting is common.

2. Continue intravenous fluids for 12–24 hours.

3. Starting with 15–20 ml of dextrose saline, reintroduce feeds cautiously 12 hours after operation. Gradually increase the volume until normal milk feeds are being offered at 24–48 hours.

4. The infant is ready for discharge from hospital on the second to fourth postoperative day.

5. If a perforation of the mucosa occurred, withhold feeds for 24 hours while continuing nasogastric decompression and intravenous fluids.

FURTHER READING

Hutson JM, Beasley SW (eds) 1988 The surgical examination of children. Heinemann Medical Books, Oxford.

Lister J, Irving IM (eds) 1990 Neonatal surgery, 3rd edn. Butterworths, London.

Spitz L, Nixon HH (eds) 1988 Paediatric surgery. In: Dudley H, Carter D, Russel RCG (eds) Rob and Smith's Operative surgery, 4th edn. Butterworths, London.

Welch KJ, Randolph JG, Ravitch MM et al (eds) 1986 Paediatric surgery, 4th edn. Year Book Medical Publishers, Chicago.

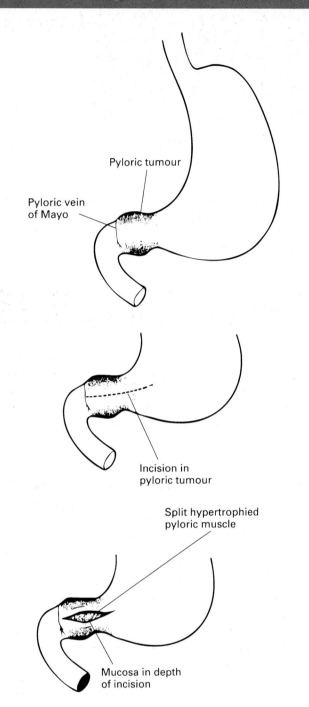

Pyloric tumour

Pyloric vein of Mayo

Incision in pyloric tumour

Split hypertrophied pyloric muscle

Mucosa in depth of incision

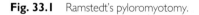

Fig. 33.1 Ramstedt's pyloromyotomy.

Upper urinary tract

C. G. Fowler and I. Junaid

Contents

INTRODUCTION

1. Urology has developed as a separate discipline in part by the sophistication of the endoscopic procedures, demanding specialist skills. In the UK, general surgeons no longer perform occasional urological procedures and urologists infrequently undertake general surgical emergencies.

2. In an emergency, or in the absence of specialist colleagues, general surgeons may need to operate to save life or correct severe morbidity. Moreover, routine inguinoscrotal and genital procedures such as circumcision, hydrocele repair, orchidopexy and excision of epididymal cysts are performed both by urologists and general surgeons.

3. You should be capable of treating acute retention.

ACUTE PYONEPHROSIS (OBSTRUCTED INFECTED KIDNEY)

Appraise

1. An acutely ill patient is liable to die from septicaemia and its consequences. Underlying obstruction may be due to a stone, a congenital hold-up at the pelviureteric junction or, much less commonly, a tumour within or outside the urinary tract. Confirm the diagnosis with plain abdominal X-ray and ultrasound examination. The urine contains organisms that can also be cultured from the blood.

2. *Ultrasound guided percutaneous nephrostomy* is usually the best way to drain an obstructed infected kidney. Aspiration helps to establish that the tube is in the correct position and also provides a specimen of pus for culture. Initially, the rate of drainage may be disappointing. Output often increases as renal function recovers.

3. Open surgery is indicated only if the appropriate expertise is unavailable, if it is impossible to introduce a satisfactory percutaneous drain, or when the pus in the kidney is too thick to be aspirated through the small-calibre tube used for percutaneous nephrostomy. Drain the

kidney by open surgery if the cause of the obstruction is a calculus in the ureter or renal pelvis; it is sensible to operate to remove the obstruction. If not, open placement of the nephrostomy tube may be necessary. This is not a simple procedure, so do not undertake it lightly.

OPEN NEPHROSTOMY FOR ACUTELY OBSTRUCTED KIDNEY

Prepare

1. Promptly rehydrate the patient and administer a broad-spectrum antibiotic intravenously. Manage a severely ill patient in an intensive care unit for monitoring, and respiratory and circulatory support if necessary.

2. Place the patient on the side with the affected kidney uppermost, allowing you to make an incision below the 12th rib and expose the convex border of the kidney.

Action

1. Occasionally the pus-filled calyces 'point' on the surface of the kidney like ripe abscesses. Make an incision through the parenchyma at this point, which will release a satisfying gush of pus.

2. More commonly, the calyces are impalpable because the overlying renal tissue is stiff and oedematous. Try using a large-bore needle on a syringe to locate the pus-filled collecting system. A more certain method is to enter the collecting system through the renal pelvis. Find the renal sinus and gently clear away the fat by blunt dissection to reveal the posterior surface of the renal pelvis. Follow the capsule over the convex posterior border of the kidney, keeping towards the lower pole. Make a small transverse pyelotomy.

3. Introduce a malleable silver probe, with a hole at the end, through the pyelotomy and manoeuvre it to puncture the cortex from within a lower pole calyx. Tie the tip of a size 18F tube drain or Foley catheter to the probe with a suture and pull it back into the renal pelvis.

4. Close the pyelotomy and anchor the catheter to the capsule using 3/0 or 4/0 absorbable sutures. Bring out the nephrostomy tube through the abdominal wall with as straight a course as possible, to facilitate changing the tube if necessary.

OBSTRUCTED KIDNEY CAUSED BY AN IMPACTED STONE

Appraise

1. Obstruction of a kidney for a few days does not usually cause serious harm. However, if there is infection or there is no function in the contralateral kidney, there is an urgent need to drain the kidney.

2. The obstruction may be due to an impacted stone at the pelvi-ureteric junction or in the lower ureter. The diagnosis is usually made with the plain abdominal X-ray and ultrasound scan or an intravenous urogram.

3. A patient presenting with an acutely obstructed kidney is best relieved using a percutaneous nephrostomy. If radiological expertise is not available, then perform an open nephrostomy.

URETEROLITHOTOMY FOR A LOWER URETERIC CALCULUS

Action
1. Select the appropriate incision for the location of the stone as shown on the X-ray. Make an oblique muscle-splitting or muscle-cutting incision on the lateral side of the anterior abdominal wall down to the peritoneum. You can extend the incision upwards or downwards as necessary.

2. Sweep the peritoneum medially to expose the retroperitoneal structures. Identify the ureter and impacted stone within it. Try not to dislodge the stone while palpating it. Place wet nylon tapes proximally and distally to prevent it slipping up to the kidney or downwards.

3. Make a vertical ureterotomy over the stone a few millimetres longer than the calculus and remove it using a Watson–Cheyne dissector. Close the ureterotomy by loosely approximating the adventitia with a few interrupted, absorbable sutures. Leave a soft tube drain in the vicinity.

RUPTURE OF THE KIDNEY

Appraise
1. The majority of injuries are from blunt trauma due to falls, road traffic accidents and sports. Penetrating injuries are associated with gunshot and stab wounds; these are often multiple, associated with trauma to bowel, pancreas and spleen. Most blunt injuries are managed conservatively. Penetrating injuries usually require surgery.

2. Resuscitate the patient. If there is haematuria in a patient with a history of trauma, order an intravenous urogram (IVU), followed by computerized tomography (CT) scan if there is poor visualization or disruption.

Action
1. Employ a midline transabdominal incision to give access to the abdominal organs and kidneys. Explore the abdomen and palpate the retroperitoneal structures. If you encounter a large pulsatile expanding haematoma, first gain control of the renal pedicle. Eviscerate the small intestine and incise the peritoneum over the aorta, exposing the vena cava and aorta. Identify the renal artery(ies) and vein(s) and place vessel loops around them to gain control.

2. Now open the perirenal fascia of Gerota to expose the kidney. Sometimes the kidney can be repaired, with closure of the collecting system defects and excision of devitalized tissue. If the kidney cannot be preserved, perform nephrectomy. Provided that the contralateral kidney has been confirmed intact and functioning, prefer nephrectomy to attempting a difficult repair, with attendant risks.

REPAIR OF DAMAGED URETER

Assess
If inadvertent surgical ureteric injury is recognized at the operation, repair it immediately. For this reason always check to exclude any possible damage.

Action
1. Mobilize both ends of the divided ureter to make sure that these are accessible for anastomosis.

2. Place a double pigtail stent with one end in the renal pelvis and the other in the urinary bladder. If a double pigtail stent is not available, splint the anastomosis with a small-calibre (6F or 8F) paediatric feeding tube.

3. Open out the ends like a broad, flat-bladed spatula, i.e. spatulate, and hold the ends between stay sutures (Fig. 34.1). Anastomose them using small interrupted sutures of 4/0 or 5/0 chromic catgut.

4. Leave a size 18F tube drain in the vicinity of the ureteric anastomosis.

5. Remove the stent or tube splint after about 10 days.

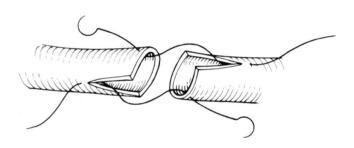

Fig. 34.1 Spatulated ureteroureterostomy.

DRAINAGE OF A PERINEPHRIC ABSCESS

Appraise
1. This usually develops in diabetic, debilitated or immunocompromised patients, and is often associated with renal cortical abscess or pyonephrosis.

2. The safest procedure is preliminary drainage followed by nephrectomy.

Action
1. Position the patient as for nephrectomy

2. Make a small incision below the 12th rib or where the abscess is pointing on the skin.

3. Deepen the incision to the perinephric space. Pus usually starts to pour out as you reach the space.

4. Sweep your forefinger around in the perinephric space to break all the septa.

5. Leave a wide-bore soft plastic tube drain in this cavity and secure it to the skin.

6. Close the wound lightly with interrupted monofilament nylon sutures.

Lower urinary tract

C. G. Fowler and I. Junaid

Contents

SUPRAPUBIC CYSTOTOMY DRAINAGE

Appraise

1. A suprapubic tube is used to drain the bladder if it is impossible or inappropriate to pass a urethral catheter.

2. A suprapubic cystostomy is often a routine alternative to urethral catheterization but is particularly indicated when the urethral route is closed by trauma (urethral disruption) or stricture. Use local anaesthesia unless the patient is already under general anaesthetic or deeply unconscious.

> **Key point**
>
> - A 'stab' suprapubic cystostomy can be performed safely only if the bladder is full. If it is not palpable, order an ultrasound scan to check that the bladder contains urine. If the bladder is empty, wait until it fills.

Action

1. Prepare and drape the patient, who lies supine. Select a point 2–3 cm above the pubic symphysis. Infiltrate local anaesthetic through the skin, subcutaneous tissues and linea alba. There is a 'give' as the needle enters the bladder and clean urine can be drawn back into the syringe. This indicates the depth and direction of your suprapubic access to the bladder.

2. A variety of disposable suprapubic catheters come packaged with instructions for use. Some are threaded over a sharp obturator rather like a knitting needle. Advance the assembly of needle and catheter carefully until you feel a 'give' that indicates that the tip is in the lumen of the bladder. Confirm this by noting when urine flows back between the catheter and its introducer. Now advance the tube into the bladder before removing the needle.

Another type has a disposable plastic trocar, which is used to establish a track into the bladder through which a catheter can be passed. With the patient lying flat, aim downwards and slightly caudally.

3. When you reach the bladder, take care to thread a sufficient length of catheter into the bladder so that it stays in when the bladder collapses.

> **Key point**
>
> - Be wary of the sudden loss of resistance that indicates that the end of the introducer is in the bladder. If you are using too much force, you may find yourself impaling the posterior wall of the bladder and even the rectum!

4. Secure the catheter. Many are equipped with a balloon or a preformed 'pigtail' end that curls up in the bladder.

5. With a very scarred suprapubic area, particularly when the bladder is not palpable, it may be preferable to formally expose the bladder and sew in the suprapubic catheter.

a. Make a 3–4 cm transverse or vertical incision 3 cm above the symphysis pubis. Expose the anterior rectus sheath and incise the linea alba muscles in the midline. Hold the rectus muscles apart with retractors and use the index finger to develop the space between the posterior surface of the pubic bone and the anterior bladder wall.

b. Pick up the bladder with two tissue forceps. If there is retropubic scarring it may be difficult to identify the bladder. However, it is safe to continue in a downward and backward direction provided the bladder is distended.

c. Divide the bladder wall between the forceps and enter the bladder. Pass in a selected catheter such as a large Foley, and inflate the balloon. Close the bladder wall around the catheter with one or two all-coats 2/0 chromic catgut sutures.

d. Appose the rectus muscles with absorbable sutures. It is permissible to bring the catheter out of the skin incision.

e. Fix the catheter to the skin with a suture.

CYSTOSCOPY

Appraise

1. There are really very few indications for you, as a general surgeon, to cystoscope a patient.

2. However, you may be forced to pass an instrument, usually a rigid one, in order to relieve clot retention. It is therefore necessary to understand the technique of passing a rigid cystoscope. It is very similar to that of passing a metal urethral dilator.

Action

1. Place the patient in the lithotomy position.

2. Use general anaesthesia when possible.

3. Clean and appropriately drape the patient.

4. Check the cystoscope for lighting and irrigation.

5. If you are inexperienced, it is safer to insert the cystoscope under direct vision, using a 0° or 30° rod-lens telescope, with the irrigation running. The whole of the urethra can be visualized as the instrument is inserted and you are less likely to cause damage. This is particularly important following post-prostatectomy secondary haemorrhage, which requires evacuation of the clots. In this situation, 'blind' passage of the cystoscope can be difficult and its tip may well undermine the trigone.

6. If it is necessary to pass a large 27F resectoscope sheath in order to clear the clot, try to use a visual obturator so that you can insert it under vision. If this is not available and you have to insert the sheath 'blind', obtain a preliminary view of the urethral anatomy using the cystoscope to help you know where you are going.

MANAGEMENT OF SUPERFICIAL URINARY EXTRAVASATION

Appraise

This may follow injury during urethral dilatation or develop behind an anterior urethral stricture. It is uncommon but produces extensive necrosis of subcutaneous tissue and skin. Colles' fascia limits posterior migration of fluid, and its attachment to the inguinal ligament stops spread down the thighs. Urine fills the subcutaneous tissues of the scrotum and penile shaft, ascending up the abdominal wall. If the urine is not already infected it will certainly become so.

Action

1. Divert the urinary stream by suprapubic cystostomy drainage. Make as many incisions as are necessary in the skin of the perineum, scrotum, penile shaft and abdominal wall to let out infected urine and necrotic tissue. Use a specific antibiotic if the sensitivity is known, or administer a broad spectrum one.

2. If Fournier's gangrene is developing, you must excise all necrotic tissue and start an intensive course of antibiotics (see p.65). Even in expert hands the outlook is poor.

EMERGENCY TREATMENT OF RUPTURED URETHRA

Appraise

1. Such injuries are often seen in victims of multiple trauma. They may result from direct perineal injury that damages the bulbous or penile urethra, or be associated with pelvic ring fractures. If possible, gently perform an ascending urethrogram using aqueous contrast solution.

Ruptured bulbous urethral damage from 'falling astride' injuries and posterior urethral injuries resulting from pelvic trauma require specialist skills, so limit your intervention to performing suprapubic cystostomy drainage if necessary.

TRAUMATIC RUPTURE OF THE BLADDER

Extraperitoneal rupture can follow lower abdominal blunt trauma when the bladder is full; diagnosis is by cystogram, using aqueous contrast medium. Treat it conservatively by inserting a urethral catheter and administering broad-spectrum antibiotics. Intraperitoneal rupture does not usually occur in isolation.

FURTHER READING

Blandy J 1986 Operative urology, 2nd edn. Blackwell Scientific, Oxford

Blandy J, Fowler C (eds) 1996 Urology, 2nd edn. Blackwell Scientific, Oxford

Renvall S, Nurmi M, Aho A 1989 Rupture of the urinary bladder: a potentially serious condition. Scandinavian Journal of Urology and Nephrology 23: 185

Webster GD, Mathes GL, Selli C 1983 Prostatomembranous urethral injuries: a review of literature and a rational approach to their management. Journal of Urology 130: 898

Male genitalia

C. G. Fowler and I. Junaid

Contents

CIRCUMCISION

Appraise

Circumcision is most commonly performed for cultural reasons. The strictly medical indications are few and include phimosis, paraphimosis, recurrent balanoposthitis and carcinoma of the penis.

Prepare

1. Circumcision in infants is traditionally performed without anaesthesia but the justification for this must be open to question.

2. A penile ring block can be used, injecting a mixture of lignocaine and bupivacaine adjusted to the patient's body weight. Do not use adrenaline.

3. Alternatively, circumcision can be performed under general or spinal anaesthesia.

Action

1. Grasp the tip of the dorsal surface of the foreskin in the midline with a small artery forceps and gently pull it downwards until it is held on the stretch.

2. If phimosis is particularly severe, use a second pair of artery forceps as a dilator to enlarge the opening.

3. Using a silver probe in the infant, or artery forceps in the adult, gently free the foreskin from the glans so that it can be completely retracted, leaving no adhesions or inspissated smegma behind. Wash it with non-spirituous solution.

4. Pull the foreskin down over the glans and apply two straight artery forceps side by side in the midline on the dorsal surface of the foreskin. Divide it between these two (Fig. 36.1a).

5. Continue the incision in the same direction with straight scissors about 3–6 mm short of the corona, according to the size (Fig. 36.1b).

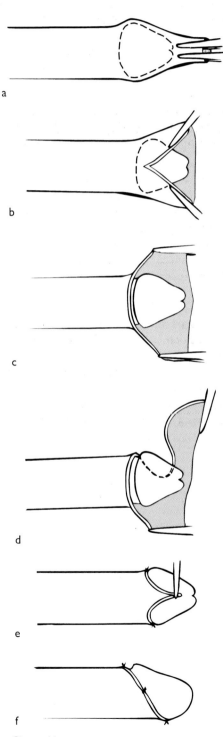

a

b

c

d

e

f

Fig. 36.1 Circumcision.

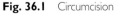

6. From the apex of this incision, cut laterally until the incision reaches the lateral border of the glans (Fig. 36.1c).

7. Now carry the incision towards the frenulum, making sure that both surfaces of the foreskin are cut together. This ensures that the undersurface of the glans is not denuded of skin (Fig. 36.1d).

Alternative method

1. A more elegant alternative method is particularly useful for adults.

2. Grasp the tip of the foreskin between two haemostats and gently stretch it over the glans.

3. Make a circumferential incision in the penile skin at the level of the corona using a blade, taking care not to sever the veins that lie just below the skin. Divide the veins between haemostats and ligate them.

4. Make an incision through the dorsum of the foreskin to expose the glans penis followed by a second circumferential incision in the skin of the inside surface of the prepuce about the 0.5 cm from the corona. Free the foreskin by cutting the connective tissue that remains, until it is attached only by the frenulum.

5. Place a small artery forceps across the frenulum, so catching the inverted-V extension of skin and frenulum together, and excise the foreskin (Fig. 36.1e).

6. Transfix the frenulum and apex of the shaft skin with a fine chromic catgut stitch and tie it firmly, releasing the artery forceps. Leave one end of the suture long to act as a stay suture.

7. Search for, pick up and ligate with fine catgut all the bleeding vessels. There is usually an artery on each side of the shaft of the penis that tends to retract.

8. Bring the two layers of the foreskin together with absorbable sutures. Leave a long end to the suture placed at the dorsal position so it can also act as a stay stitch. Appose by gentle traction on the two stay sutures, the cut edges of the foreskin, ready for suturing. Avoid using too many sutures (Fig. 36.1f).

? Difficulty?

1. Do not pull downwards on the foreskin once the initial two artery forceps have been applied, or you will remove too much skin.

2. Never use diathermy.

3. An adherent foreskin may be very difficult to separate from the glans. It may even require sharp dissection, particularly with long-standing phimosis in adults following repeated infections, or in balanitis xerotica obliterans.

4. Always make sure all bleeding is stopped. Infants cannot tolerate blood loss.

Aftercare

1. Dressings usually fall off and are unnecessary. A loose dressing is all that is needed.

2. In particular, avoid sewing dressings in place. Baby boys have been known to lose the glans penis through ischaemia caused by tight dressings or by constricting threads from a dressing.

3. Permit gentle bathing from the second postoperative day.

4. Warn the patient (or parents) that it will take several weeks for the penis to heal and achieve the final cosmetic result.

PARAPHIMOSIS

Appraise

1. In paraphimosis, the retracted foreskin causes a constriction that interferes with venous and lymphatic return from the glans penis. The resulting oedema makes it even more difficult to reduce the paraphimosis.

2. It is often possible to reduce paraphimosis by gentle but prolonged squeezing of the swollen glans penis and manipulation of the foreskin.

3. If this fails, operation is indicated.

Prepare

It is usual to use general anaesthesia but the penile ring block described on page 249 works well.

Action

1. Hold the penis on the fingers of one hand, placing the thumb uppermost on the glans.

2. Depress the glans downwards to expose the constricting band. In long-standing paraphimosis the resulting oedema makes it exceedingly difficult to identify this ring clearly.

3. Transect the ring longitudinally with a small knife. This incision should be of sufficient length and depth to release the constriction and so enable the paraphimosis to be reduced.

4. Leave the incision wide open, covered with loose dressings.

Proceed to formal circumcision when all inflammation and oedema has settled.

ADULT HYDROCELE

Excision of hydrocele

This procedure is suitable for very large or thick-walled hydroceles.

Action

1. Grasp the scrotum firmly with one hand and stretch the skin over the hydrocele.

2. Choose an appropriate area between the vessels in the skin to make a transverse incision. The vessels usually run transversely. Carry the incision through all layers of the scrotum. Make the incision long enough to allow the entire scrotal contents to be delivered. The scrotal skin stretches easily, so this incision need not be of great length. Secure all bleeding points.

3. Use dissecting scissors and clean all the coverings off the hydrocele sac until it is completely free.

4. Incise the sac and allow the fluid to escape. Continue the incision until the testicle can be freely delivered.

5. Excise the sac only, keeping close to the testicle.

6. Run a fine continuous haemostatic catgut suture along the cut edge of the sac.

7. Secure all small bleeding points with fine catgut suture.

8. Return the testicle to the scrotum.

9. Grasp the dartos muscle at each end of the incision with tissue forceps. Elevate them to bring the muscle into view.

10. Approximate the dartos muscle with a continuous catgut suture. This gathers the muscle together and with it the skin, obviating the need for skin sutures.

11. Apply a firm scrotal support, or use a 10cm crepe bandage to wind around the scrotum to minimize any subsequent swelling.

12. With a very adherent sac, which needs scissors dissection to free it from the scrotum, it may be difficult to stop all oozing. Do not hesitate to use a drain in these circumstances.

13. An alternative technique is Jaboulay's operation. Instead of running a haemostatic suture along the cut edge of the sac, suture the edges together behind the epididymis.

Lord's procedure

Appraise

Lord's procedure is particularly good when the sac is relatively thin-walled. It has the advantage of requiring only a small incision in the scrotal skin and in the hydrocele sac itself, minimizing bleeding.

Action

1. Incise the scrotum down to and including the hydrocele sac, securing all bleeding points in the incision.

2. Widen the incision only until it is big enough to deliver the testis.

3. Deliver the testis, everting the hydrocele sac behind it.

4. Using interrupted sutures, pick up the edge of the sac and gather up the sac wall with a series of bites according to the sac size, finally taking a bite of the tunica.

5. When all these sutures are in place, tie them, so bunching up and obliterating the hydrocele around the testis.

6. Finally close the scrotal incision.

7. Apply a scrotal support.

TORSION OF THE TESTICLE

Appraise

> **Key points**
>
> - A swollen painful testis in a boy is a torsion until proved otherwise.
> - Never delay operation: every minute counts. Never be tempted to leave the good side for another time; the child may leave the district and never return to hospital.

Prepare

1. Carefully counsel the boy and his parents. Seek consent for exploration, orchidectomy if the testis is necrotic and fixation of the contralateral side.

2. Counselling includes the information that the insertion of a testicular prosthesis can be considered in the future if the testis has to be removed.

Action

1. Incise the scrotum transversely as described for hydrocele operations. Continue the incision in depth until the testicle and cord can be delivered.

2. Untwist the torsion and wrap the testicle in a warm pack.

3. Make a similar incision in the other side of the scrotum and deliver the non-twisted testicle, noting any abnormal anatomy that may be present.

4. With a fine nylon stitch, take a firm bite of the tunica of the testicle and anchor it to the side-wall of the scrotum. Do this at both upper and lower poles taking care to avoid the vas, the epididymis and the blood supply to the testis.

5. Close the scrotal incision on the non-twisted side.

6. Remove the pack from the twisted testicle and examine it carefully for viability. If it is obviously dead and remains black, it must be removed. Place a strong artery forceps across the cord and then remove the testicle and tie the cord with strong catgut.

7. If there is any hope of viability, return the testicle to the scrotum, fixing it with fine nylon sutures as described for the other side.

ORCHIDECTOMY

Appraise

1. Indications for simple orchidectomy are severe recurrent attacks of epididymitis, chronic epididymitis, unsalvageable testicular trauma, testicular infarction, and in the management of prostatic carcinoma. Discuss the possibility of inserting a testicular prosthesis.

2. Plan to include involved, attached, inflamed skin. Enter the scrotal sac through healthy skin. Deliver the testis. Apply gentle traction, clean the cord to free 4–6 cm and doubly clamp it at the upper level. Doubly tie above the upper clamp. Transect the cord below the upper clamp and gently dissect out the testis. Leave the wound open to drain freely if there is infection, otherwise insert sutures to close the skin.

TESTICULAR TRAUMA

Unless there is increasing pain and swelling, support, rest and painkillers may suffice. Explore if there is increasing size and pain to evacuate a haematoma, repair a torn tunica albuginea or simply excise a shattered testicle.

EXCISION OF EPIDIDYMAL CYSTS

Excise epididymal cysts only when they become uncomfortably large. Removal of epididymal cysts is relatively contraindicated in the young or unmarried, as it often renders that side sterile. The condition is multiple, so warn patients that recurrent cysts are likely.

Action

1. Incise the scrotum as described for excision of a hydrocele sac.

2. Deliver the testicle along with its appendages, including the cysts. Remember that cysts are often multiple and commonly occur in the upper pole of the epididymis.

3. With blunt and scissors dissection, holding the testicle with one hand, or using an assistant to hold it, clean off all the adventitial tissue surrounding the cyst.

4. Using the same scissors dissection, completely excise the cyst or else marsupialize it by cutting off the whole protruding surface.

5. If there are very many cysts it is best to excise that part of the epididymis bearing them. Oversew the raw area left after this manoeuvre with fine chromic catgut.

6. Return the testicle to the scrotum and continue as described for hydroceles.

A Lord's type of procedure, as described for hydrocele, is often practical for large simple epididymal cysts. Be sure, however, that further cysts are not present.

VASECTOMY FOR STERILIZATION

Appraise

1. This is an operation which causes more irritating, usually trivial, postoperative complaints leading to litigation in the courts than any other urological procedure. For this reason alone it is important to explain exactly to the patient and his wife what is entailed.

2. Warn the patient that any operation on the scrotum is liable to pain, swelling and infection. Very exceptionally this may be so severe as to necessitate re-exploration.

3. Warn the patient that pain can be experienced well after the operation, due to a small amount of sperm leaking and setting up an irritating area in the scrotum, which can lead to little painful lumps. Exceptionally, these may need to be excised.

4. Sterilization is not immediate and the store of sperm must be exhausted first. This usually takes 2–3 months. To be absolutely certain, it is generally accepted that a seminal count should be performed at 3 months and 4 months; only when two consecutive completely negative counts are obtained with a month in between is it safe to pronounce the patient sterile. If the counts are equivocal, it is safer to re-explore.

5. Warn the patient that recanalization can occur. It is rare, occurring in between 1 and 2 per 1000 vasectomies. It can occur years after vasectomy and is not due to surgical error or omission. If the partner shows signs of pregnancy, she must seek appropriate advice. Early recanalization can be deduced from the equivocal postoperative sperm counts.

Key point

- Make sure the detailed consent form covers all these points, that it is understood and signed.

---

6. Warn the patient that, if a local anaesthetic proves unsatisfactory, then the procedure must be abandoned and will be performed under a general anaesthetic at a later date.

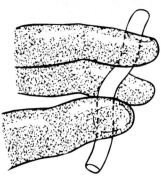

Fig. 36.2 Vasectomy: identifying the vas.

Action

1. Grasp the upper part of the scrotum between the first two fingers and the thumb so as to be able to roll the scrotal skin between them.

2. Feel the hard round structure of the vas and roll it away from the other structures of the cord (Fig. 36.2).

3. Grip the vas between the middle finger, which invaginates the scrotum, and the thumb on the outside. Move the index finger nearer to the thumb. Now spread the index finger and thumb apart, so holding the vas firmly across the invaginated middle finger. This presents the vas in relief.

4. Make a 1 cm cut into the scrotal skin in the direction of the vas. The cut should go down to the vas, cutting through the adventitia that covers it.

5. Still firmly holding the vas, grasp it with tissue holding forceps (Alliss) or better still with ring forceps specially designed to encircle the vas. It is helpful to make a longitudinal cut deliberately down through the immediate cover-ings of the vas so that its glistening white muscular coat is in view before applying forceps around it.

6. Release the finger and thumb. The vas now protrudes from the incision, held by the forceps.

7. Force an artery forceps under the vas to separate a length of it from its coverings and to be doubly sure that it cannot escape back into the scrotum.

8. Apply artery forceps about 3 cm apart on the vas and excise the segment between them. Tie each end with no. 1 catgut, burying the lower end deep in the scrotum. Incorporate the tied upper end into the subcutaneous tissues when closing each wound. This separates the two ends as widely as possible.

9. Repeat the procedure on the other side.

10. Send the excised segments for histological confirmation.

Difficulty?

1. Do not attempt this operation under local anaesthesia unless the patient, and the scrotum, are relaxed.

2. If you lose the vas in the scrotum, try again. Never be tempted to grope blindly for structures in the scrotum.

3. If it is difficult, do not be satisfied with simple division; stop and start again at another time, carefully explaining the reason to the patient.

Neurosurgery

R. S. Maurice-Williams

Contents

GENERAL PRINCIPLES

🔑 Key point

- Before operating on the brain or spinal cord, remember that central nervous tissue is easily damaged and, once damaged, cannot regenerate.

Access to the brain

Burr holes

1. These can be carried out rapidly but are mainly of diagnostic value. Use them to establish whether there is any haematoma on the brain surface in that part of the head or whether the brain is under tension. Realize that a burr hole exposes only a tiny part of the surface of the intracranial contents and that nearby or deep pathology may be present without anything abnormal being found. Burr holes seldom give sufficient access to allow definitive treatment of important lesions. For this reason, always place your scalp incisions and burr holes so that they can be converted either into an osteoplastic flap or into a craniectomy, if more room is needed.

2. Apart from the use of multiple exploratory burr holes after a head injury, a single burr hole may be used to biopsy a cerebral tumour, drain a cerebral abscess or tap the lateral ventricles in acute hydrocephalus.

Craniotomy

An osteoplastic flap is turned and is replaced at the end of the operation. A craniotomy is the best way of exposing a wide area of the intracranial contents above the tentorium.

Craniectomy

A burr hole is extended by removing bone around it, leaving a defect that remains at the end of the operation. Avoid a craniectomy on the skull vault as the bone defect will require plastic repair later. There are two situations where a craniectomy can be fashioned without the need for later surgery:

1. A craniectomy is the usual mode of exposing the posterior fossa contents. The bone defect is covered over by the thick suboccipital muscles.
2. The outer wall of the middle fossa may be removed by a 'subtemporal craniectomy' to provide access to an arterial extradural haematoma or a swollen temporal lobe. At the end of the operation the defect is concealed by suturing the temporalis muscle over it.

SCALP LACERATIONS

Appraise

1. An unsutured small scalp laceration can pump out a great deal of blood over a short period of time, so arrest any bleeding from the scalp as soon as is practicable after injury with a temporary single layer of through-and-through sutures.

2. If the patient has been struck on the head with a heavy object, X-ray the skull to ensure that the laceration does not cover a depressed skull fracture.

Action

1. Shave adequately and closely round the laceration before exploring it.

2. The scalp is very vascular and heals well, seldom getting infected, so do not excise the contused edges of the laceration in such an enthusiastic manner that you produce a scalp defect or cannot get the edges together without tension.

3. If the galea has been breached, always close the scalp laceration in two layers of interrupted 3/0 silk sutures.

a. The wound edges are held together by galeal sutures, 1 cm apart, inverted so that the knots face inwards. Cut the loose ends very short so that they cannot work their way out through the skin.

b. Insert skin sutures 1.0–1.5 cm apart, passed through all the layers of the scalp and tied fairly tightly to arrest bleeding from the scalp layers. These sutures may be removed on the fifth postoperative day. Do not insert small sutures closer together than 1 cm or you may produce necrosis of the wound edges.

4. Transfer a patient with severe scalp loss to a special unit where plastic and neurosurgical facilities are available.

DEPRESSED SKULL FRACTURE

Appraise

1. The purpose of elevating a depressed skull fracture is to reduce the risk of infection, so only compound depressed skull fractures require elevation. Depressed fractures with overlying skin intact should be left alone. In occasional cases the dislocation of the skull contour may be so great that elevation is required for cosmetic reasons.

2. Excise the overlying scalp laceration if it is badly contused. Extend the incision to give access to the whole depressed area. Scrape the scalp off the underlying bone and hold the incision wide open with self-retaining retractors. Clear the pericranium away with a periosteal elevator to reveal the whole depressed area.

3. Make a burr hole just outside the edge of the visibly depressed region in order to expose dura not involved in the depression.

4. Insert a periosteal elevator into the burr hole, slide it gently between the bone and the dura and ease out the depressed fragment. Remove dirt, debris, and any small flakes of bone from the wound, and send them for bacteriological culture. If the dura is intact, leave it. If it is lacerated, extend the laceration in order to inspect the brain beneath. Gently remove any indriven bone or debris, and clear away pulped or clearly necrotic brain tissue by a combination of irrigation and gentle suction. Arrest bleeding points with gently applied diathermy.

5. Finally, irrigate the whole wound with hydrogen peroxide solution and 20 ml of physiological saline containing 20,000 units of penicillin and 50 mg of streptomycin.

6. Close the dura with 3/0 silk sutures. Cover any gaps in the closure with two layers of Surgicel©.

MISSILE WOUNDS OF THE BRAIN

Appraise

1. The energy of a missile is transmitted to the object it strikes. The small size of an entry hole may conceal massive disruption of the intracranial structures.

2. Decide whether active treatment is likely to lead to a worthwhile outcome. The prognosis is poor following through and through wounds, if the patient has been deeply unconscious with fixed dilated pupils from the time of injury, or has persistent hypotension which cannot be explained by blood loss.

3. Do not operate until the patient has been resuscitated and you have obtained good quality X-rays to show the position of the fragments of missile, bone and debris. Cross match blood and start a broad spectrum antibiotic.

4. The underlying principle is to minimize the risks of infection and cerebral swelling by removing all indriven debris and devitalized brain tissue. Access is through a generous craniectomy that encompasses the entry wound. Open the dura widely. Using saline irrigation and gentle suction pick out indriven bone, debris, pieces of missile and pulped brain. Coagulate bleeding vessels. Irrigate the debrided track with hydrogen peroxide solution and with 20,000 units of penicillin dissolved in physiological saline.

5. Close the dura with 3/0 silk sutures. Excise any contaminated wound edges of scalp then close it with two layers of 3/0 silk sutures.

FURTHER READING

Collins REC, Cashin PA 1999 General surgeons and the management of head injuries. Annals of the Royal College of Surgeons of England 81: 151–153

Gynaecological surgery

M. E. Setchell

Contents

GENERAL CONSIDERATIONS

Preoperative care

> #### 🔑 Key points
>
> - Nowhere is informed consent more important than in gynaecological surgery. Give a full explanation of the probable operative procedure and its consequences, particularly if future fertility is likely to be affected; if the woman wishes, keep the partner informed as well.
>
> - Keep shaving of pubic and vulval hair to a minimum; it is particularly uncomfortable when it is regrowing.
>
> - Patients should stop taking the oral contraceptive pill 6 weeks before elective major gynaecological surgery. Menstruation is not a contraindication to gynaecological surgery, nor indeed to thorough examination
>
> - Remember that pregnancy predisposes to thromboembolism, and use prophylactic heparin readily.

Prepare

1. *Positioning of patient.* Vaginal operations are carried out in the lithotomy position. Laparoscopy is best carried out with the patient in Lloyd–Davies stirrups, with steep head-down tilt. Abdominal operations are carried out with the patient supine and 5–10° of head-down tilt.

2. *Catheterization.* Empty the bladder by catheterization before all abdominal procedures, laparoscopy included. Separate the labia and swab the urethral meatus with antiseptic solution. Without allowing the labia to close again, pass a silver or plastic catheter well into the bladder. Now let the labia approximate and press firmly and continuously suprapubically. When the urine flow ceases, gradually withdraw the catheter, taking care not to allow air to be sucked into the bladder.

SURGERY OF ECTOPIC PREGNANCY

Appraise

1. A classic ruptured ectopic pregnancy is easily diagnosed by the findings of severe abdominal pain, guarding and rebound, and hypovolaemic shock. A tubal abortion or slowly leaking ectopic pregnancy is less easy to diagnose, and ultrasound scanning (using a transvaginal probe), together with a rapid β-hCG assay, often helps to make the diagnosis.

2. Laparoscopy is not often required to confirm the diagnosis of ruptured ectopic pregnancy but will always be required in the less acute forms of tubal abortion or slow leakage. In non-ruptured cases, laparoscopic salpingotomy and aspiration of the pregnancy is the treatment of choice if future pregnancy is desired (Fig. 38.1).

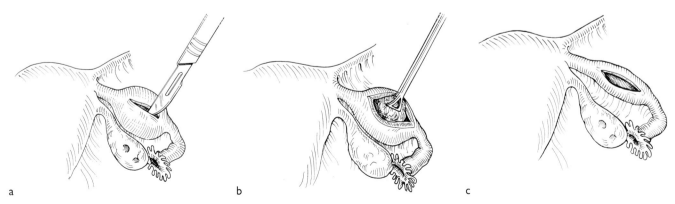

a   b   c

Fig. 38.1 Conservative management of an ectopic pregnancy; a similar technique applies to both a laparoscopic and an open approach: (a) incision over antimesenteric border of tube with needle diathermy; (b) removal of the trophoblast tissue with grasping forceps and suction/irrigation cannula; (c) salpingotomy left to heal without suturing after ensuring haemostasis.

3. Once the diagnosis of ruptured ectopic has been made, take the patient to the operating theatre as soon as possible. Do not wait for blood to be cross-matched or hope that the patient's condition will improve. She will improve only when the fallopian tube is clamped.

Prepare

1. Order a full blood count, group and save serum (if not cross-matching), and secure intravenous access as soon as ectopic pregnancy is suspected.

2. If the patient is shocked, take her to theatre for immediate laparotomy; in less acute forms arrange for laparoscopy with a view to conservative laparoscopic surgery.

Salpingectomy or salpingotomy by laparotomy

Appraise

This is the standard treatment for a ruptured ectopic pregnancy and is the method of choice unless you have acquired training and skill in laparoscopic surgery. If the patient has appreciable signs of surgical shock, proceed to laparotomy forthwith.

Access

Make a generous incision, either midline or Pfannenstiel (if you are used to this incision).

Action

1. As soon as the peritoneal cavity is open, aspirate blood with the sucker.

2. Pass a hand into the pelvis and bring the uterus with its appendages up into the wound. Identify the ruptured tube. Place one or more clamps across the mesosalpinx and another clamp across the cornual end of the tube, then excise the damaged tube. In most cases it is neither necessary nor desirable to remove the ovary. Doubly ligate the pedicles beneath the clamps, using chromic catgut or polyglactin 910.

3. If the tube has not ruptured, and future pregnancy is desired, make a 1 cm linear incision over the swollen portion of the tube and aspirate the trophoblast as described for laparoscopic salpingotomy. You do not need to close the tube.

4. Inspect the contralateral tube and ovary. The other tube may have a hydrosalpinx or haematosalpinx but do not be tempted to tamper with it. Bilateral tubal pregnancy is excessively rare. Carefully record the state of the pelvis.

5. Before closing the abdomen, aspirate and swab out as much blood as possible, and estimate the volume of blood loss. Washing the peritoneal cavity with Hartmann's solution may help to reduce adhesion formation.

Postoperative

1. Obtain as accurate an estimate as possible of the amount of blood aspirated from the peritoneal cavity, and replace it with blood transfusion if the loss exceeds 1 litre.

2. Use central venous pressure monitoring to gauge blood and fluid replacement if there has been severe shock.

3. Administer prophylactic antibiotics such as cephradine and metronidazole or co-amoxiclav for three doses if tubal rupture and substantial haemoperitoneum has occurred.

PREGNANCY AND EMERGENCY SURGERY

The presence of a pregnancy may cause considerable confusion in the diagnosis of an acute abdomen and may make access more difficult at laparotomy. It should not, however, deter you from performing emergency abdominal operations when necessary.

Appendicitis

The appendix is pushed upwards and outwards during pregnancy, so that the physical signs of appendicitis may be considerably altered. Because the large pregnant uterus may prevent the normal walling-off of acute appendicitis, generalized peritonitis occurs more readily. Make a gridiron incision above and lateral to the normal site, or consider a right paramedian incision if there is doubt about diagnosis.

Cholecystitis

Acute cholecystitis and biliary colic are not uncommon in pregnancy, but the symptoms may be atypical, simulating hyperemesis or indigestion of pregnancy. If you make the diagnosis of gallbladder disease in pregnancy, prefer to wait until after delivery before carrying out cholecystectomy. If there is a need to perform the operation during pregnancy, prefer to carry it out in the middle trimester.

Red degeneration of a fibroid

Pregnancy and fibroids often coexist, and a fibroid growing rapidly during pregnancy may undergo red degeneration. This is an extremely painful condition; sometimes the pain is so severe that exploratory laparotomy is carried out. Once the diagnosis of fibroids is confirmed, *do not attempt to remove the fibroids*, as myomectomy in pregnancy is attended with catastrophic haemorrhage and loss of the fetus. The only exception to this rule is if a pedunculated fibroid has undergone torsion and is gangrenous.

Placental abruption

The condition of abruptio placentae (premature detachment of the placenta) results in severe abdominal pain and uterine tenderness, which may or may not be accompanied by vaginal bleeding. A major degree of abruption causes profound shock and usually results in fetal death. Lesser degrees may cause diagnostic difficulty. Tenderness is localized over the uterus, and in the severe form the uterus acquires a characteristic woody-hard feel to it. Unless labour occurs spontaneously, induce it with prostaglandins and amniotomy (puncture of the fetal membranes)

Rectus sheath haematoma

Occasionally, a spontaneous haematoma occurs in the rectus sheath as a result of spontaneous haemorrhage from the inferior epigastric vessels in pregnancy. A tender mass appears in the abdominal wall. Treat the condition conservatively.

Ear, nose and throat

M. P. Stearns

Contents

FOREIGN BODIES IN THE THROAT

Appraise

Fish bones lodge at any level, often in the tonsil or vallecula. More substantial fragments (chicken, rabbit and chop bones) usually stick in the postcricoid region or upper oesophagus. Rarely, occluding foreign bodies (sweets, meat bolus) can cause airway obstruction, leading to sudden death. Dentures (often broken) impact in the mid-oesophagus. A stricture, benign or malignant, may obstruct even a small bolus, such as a pea or piece of potato.

Action

1. Inspect the throat carefully, using a headlight and tongue depressor. Look for the tip of a buried fish bone in the tonsil or base of the tongue. Use a fine pair of angled forceps to grasp and remove the bone. It may be helpful to anaesthetize the throat using lignocaine spray as a topical local anaesthetic.

2. If you cannot see the foreign body directly, use a laryngeal mirror (as in indirect laryngoscopy) to examine the back of the tongue and laryngopharynx. A bone in these sites can often be retrieved *under visual control* with angled forceps. Have the patient hold his own tongue as far out as possible (grasping it with a gauze swab). Use your left hand for the mirror and right hand for the forceps (if you are right handed). You *must* be able see the forceps closing on the foreign body accurately.

3. If mirror examination shows a foreign body deep in the pyriform fossa or postcricoid space, or if a radiograph shows it in the hypopharynx or upper oesophagus, then carry out direct endoscopy under general anaesthesia. Use a laryngoscope or short oesophago-scope and suitable forceps to bring the foreign body into the lumen of the endoscope. Take care not to push a sharp object through the visceral wall. Try to rotate it so that its most traumatic aspect is disimpacted and will either trail harmlessly, or be inside the endoscope, during withdrawal.

? Difficulty?

Do not attempt to remove from the oesophagus a denture bearing sharp hooks. This requires special expertise. It may be necessary to cut the denture into two pieces.

RELIEF OF UPPER AIRWAY OBSTRUCTION

Appraise

1. Immediately relieve respiratory obstruction from major facial or laryngeal trauma, laryngopharyngeal tumours and impacted foreign bodies.

2. Ensure that there is a clear airway if the patient is comatose. If necessary, assist respiration with mouth-to-mouth breathing, or using an Ambi bag, a laryngeal mask or endotracheal intubation. If necessary, ventilate the patient.

3. An obstructed airway can frequently be expanded using positive pressure by mouth-to-mouth respiration, or through a face mask or oral tube, thus providing an adequate passage for air or oxygen.

⚷ Key points

- Identify the cause of obstruction

- Eliminate the cause if possible, or

- Pass an endotracheal tube through or past it, or

- Perform laryngotomy or tracheostomy to get below the obstruction. A totally obstructed patient can be partially relieved by inserting one or more large-bore hypodermic needles through the cricothyroid membrane

Laryngotomy (cricothyrotomy)

1. Lie the patient supine with extended neck.

2. Make a horizontal stab incision between the cricoid and thyroid cartilages. Press the blade backwards until you feel the point enter the airway and air begins to hiss in and out through the wound with respiration (Fig. 39.1).

3. With no loss of time, remove the knife and insert a small tube, curved downwards, inside the tracheal lumen. A correctly designed laryngotomy tube is flattened somewhat, so as to lie neatly between the cartilages, but if none is available use *any* type of tube, metal, rubber or plastic – even unsterile, if it maintains the airway.

4. An improvised tube is difficult to keep in a correct position so control it manually until a stable airway can been established.

5. Unless the cause of acute asphyxia is quickly curable (e.g. removal of impacted foreign body, or angioneurotic oedema), perform an elective tracheostomy within 48 hours and close the laryngotomy incision.

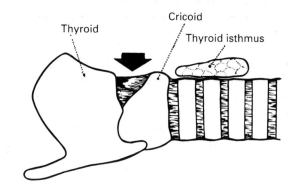

Fig. 39.1 Emergency laryngotomy. Incision through cricothyroid membrane.

Emergency tracheostomy

Appraise (2, 3, 4)

Always prefer laryngotomy to tracheostomy because it is quicker and there is less haemorrhage. *Very rarely* (e.g. if a subglottic lesion precludes laryngotomy and defies intubation even with a rigid bronchoscope) you must perform emergency tracheostomy.

Prepare

1. Lie the patient supine with extended neck by placing a sand bag or a 1 litre bag of fluid for intravenous infusion beneath the shoulders. Ensure the head is in a central position.

2. Deliver oxygen by face mask to give a few more minutes operating time.

3. If there is time, inject local anaesthetic such as 1% lignocaine with 1:100 000 adrenaline.

Action

1. Cut vertically from the lower border of the thyroid cartilage in the midline to the suprasternal notch. Deepen the incision and extend it between the strap muscles. Feel the first tracheal ring with the left index finger.

2. Then divide the thyroid isthmus to expose the anterior tracheal wall. Profuse bleeding can be controlled by pressure from an assistant. Decide quickly whether there is time to clamp major bleeding points before incising the trachea vertically through the second, third and fourth rings.

3. Insert a tracheal dilator to secure an airway. Introduce a tracheostomy tube. A cuffed tube prevents further aspiration of blood and allows ventilation, but it is slightly more difficult to insert.

4. Now control the worst of the bleeding. Use a tracheal suction catheter through the tube to clear blood which has already been aspirated into the trachea.

Postoperative

Subsequent decisions and procedures depend upon the cause of the obstruction and the patient's general condition. Monitor respiration and pulse during, and for several hours after, such a crisis. Institute assisted ventilation and/or cardiac resuscitation immediately post-operatively if necessary.

Elective tracheostomy (3, 4)

1. This procedure is considerably easier to perform, in controlled conditions, on an appropriately prepared and anaesthetized patient. Either local or general anaesthesia may be used.

2. Ensure that you have available a correct-sized tracheostomy tube. If it has a cuff, test it for leaks. If you intend to ventilate the patient, use a plastic, cuffed tube, not a metal tube. Check also that the connections from tube to anaesthetic equipment are correct.

Action

1. Inject the surgical area with a solution of 1/200 000 adrenaline to help achieve haemostasis. Make a horizontal skin-crease incision halfway between the cricoid cartilage and the suprasternal notch.

2. Separate the pretracheal muscles vertically and divide the thyroid isthmus between artery clips. Pretracheal vessels just below the cricoid may need to be diathermized. Ligate the inferior thyroid veins, since diathermy is unreliable. Ligate or oversew the edges of the thyroid isthmus and expose the anterior tracheal wall.

3. Having established haemostasis make a 1–2 cm vertical incision, centred on the third or fourth tracheal ring (Fig. 39.2).

Do not excise segments or cut flaps because there is a risk of subsequent stenosis. In addition, a tracheal flap may obstruct the passage of a tube.

🔑 Key point

- Insert a strong stitch through the cut tracheal edge on each side and leave the ends long, protruding through the skin wound. These can be used to draw the trachea forwards and open the incision in it to facilitate the reintroduction of a tube. This is particularly useful in paediatric tracheostomies. If a patient is accidentally extubated and the tube cannot be rapidly replaced, fatal respiratory obstruction can occur.

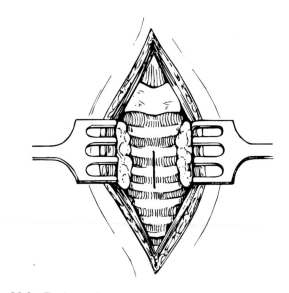

Fig. 39.2 Elective tracheostomy.

4. Hold the tracheal incision open with a tracheal dilator. Ask the anaesthetist to withdraw the endotracheal tube to the subglottic level. Now insert, for example, a cuffed plastic tracheostomy tube. Inflate the cuff just sufficiently to prevent leakage around it when the anaesthetist inflates the patient's lungs. Over-inflation of the cuff can lead to subsequent tracheal stenosis. The anaesthetist can now connect the tubing to the tracheostomy tube and withdraw the endotracheal tube. Have the endotracheal tube left until now, so that if there is any difficulty in inserting the tracheostomy tube, or if the cuff bursts, the anaesthetist can continue to ventilate the patient through the endotracheal tube.

5. Close the skin *loosely* around the tube. Loose suturing allows drainage of any blood and also helps prevent air emphysema developing around the incision

Complications

1. Haemorrhage can occur from the thyroid isthmus and the inferior thyroid veins. Ensure that the surgical field is dry before closing up.

2. In young infants the brachiocephalic vein may rise above the suprasternal notch, so take care to avoid injuring it.

Oral and dental

I. M. Laws

Contents
General principles of oral surgery

GENERAL PRINCIPLES OF ORAL SURGERY

Prepare
1. Make sure you have good illumination.
2. Arrange for adequate suction apparatus.
3. Make sure your assistant is efficient and can anticipate.

Anaesthesia
1. Most minor procedures such as tooth extraction, biopsy, removal of salivary calculi and suturing of lacerations can be carried out using local analgesia. Local anaesthetics are available in 2 ml glass cartridges, the most common of which contain 2% lignocaine with adrenaline. Use 3% prilocaine with felypressin for patients sensitive to adrenaline. These cartridges fit into a syringe with a disposable needle.
2. In the upper jaw, deposit 1.5 ml of solution over the apex of the offending tooth on the buccal side and about 0.5 ml on the palatal side. In the lower jaw, a similar technique may suffice for the anterior teeth. For the posterior teeth, an inferior alveolar and lingual nerve block is required at the lingula of the mandible, along with a long buccal nerve block at the anterior edge of the ramus of the mandible. Regional nerve block can also be used in the maxilla. Refer to appropriate literature before attempting these blocks.
3. The depth of analgesia may not be sufficient in the presence of inflammation but can be increased by depositing a few drops of anaesthetic solution into the periodontal membrane of the tooth.
4. General anaesthesia is often preferable in the treatment of children, patients who have fluctuant abscesses and where there is a history of allergy to local anaesthetic. Intravenous sedation may be required for nervous adults.

General anaesthesia should be administered by a person other than the surgeon. The anaesthetic should be maintained through a nasal endotracheal tube. Insert a moist pack into the oropharynx to prevent the inhalation of blood and debris during the treatment. Remember to remove the pack at the end of the operation.

The jaws should be held apart with a prop or gag and the head stabilized in a rubber ring or horseshoe. Care should be taken not to dislocate the jaw. The lips are easily scuffed when operating because of the drying effects of the anticholinergic drugs used in general anaesthesia. Keep them moist or lightly coated with petroleum jelly.

Haemostasis
Post-extraction haemorrhage is often due to torn or unsupported mucosa.
1. Remove excess clot.
2. Suture tightly across the socket. Repair any lacerations.
3. Apply pressure with a gauze pad for 10 minutes.
4. If bleeding continues, press a resorbable haemostatic material (e.g. oxidized cellulose) into the socket.
5. Sit the patient up at least 45°. Consider sedation.
6. Control secondary haemorrhage with pressure and treat the infection with antibiotics (systemic and/or local) and 6% hydrogen peroxide mouthwashes.
7. Medical reasons for prolonged bleeding must be treated according to their cause, e.g. haemophilia, thrombocytopenia or hepatic cirrhosis.
8. Patients taking the anticoagulant warfarin should be given 5% tranexamic acid as a mouthwash. Flush the socket with the liquid then insert some oxidized cellulose and suture the socket. The mouthwash is used to bathe the mouth four times per day for 5 days. If the prothrombin time is within the normal therapeutic range the warfarin need not be stopped if only a few teeth are to be removed.

Suturing
1. Use a half-circle 22–24 mm needle with a reverse cutting edge.
2. Use 000 sutures. Silk is easy to use but must be removed. Catgut is suitable for mucoperiosteum but rapidly becomes unticd on mobile mucosa such as tongue, lip and cheek. Polyglactin 910 remains intact in the mouth for 3–4 weeks and produces minimal reaction but has irritating knots and ends. Nylon must be removed and is uncomfortable.
3. Use a needle-holder with a ratchet to avoid dropping the needle into the pharynx.
4. Insert the needle into the mucosa 3–5 mm from the edge, taking greater care on the more friable lingual edge.
5. The mucosal edges can rarely be approximated over a socket without excessive removal of bone. If you wish to apply even tension, insert mattress sutures.
6. Tie knots with the needle-holder rather than fingers. This is easier if the tail of the suture material is kept short.
7. Remove non-resorbable sutures after 5–7 days.

Aftercare
1. During the healing period, there may be constant discomfort and anxiety as the mouth continues to be used for eating, swallowing, salivation and speaking. Moderate analgesics usually suffice to control the pain. Aspirin mixture, used as a gargle, relieves a sore throat caused by an endotracheal tube and packing to make

swallowing more comfortable. Ice packs applied to the skin for the first 4–6 hours reduce the swelling and subsequent discomfort.

2. A soft diet may be required for the first few days because the patient may have difficulty in opening the mouth wide and have reduced power when chewing.

3. Patients who have had their fractured jaws fixed together require special care in the early postoperative hours to avoid inhalation of vomit. Blood is often swallowed after oral surgery, causing vomiting. Ensure that the stomach is empty preoperatively and administer an antiemetic such as prochlorperazine or metoclopramide. Keep a suction machine and wire-cutters by the bedside and show the nurses which wires to cut in an emergency.

4. Prophylactic antibiotics are given routinely when bone surgery is carried out.

FURTHER READING

Archer WH 1975 Oral surgery. WB Saunders, Philadelphia

Howe GL 1990 The extraction of teeth, 2nd edn. John Wright, Bristol

Hutchison I, Lawlor M 1990 Major maxillofacial injuries. In: ABC of trauma. British Medical Journal 301: 595–599

McGowan DA 1999 An atlas of minor oral surgery: principles and practice. Martin Dunitz, London

Moore JR 1991 Principles of oral surgery, 4th edn. Manchester University Press, Manchester

Rowe NL, Williams JL 1994 Maxillofacial injuries, 2nd edn. Churchill Livingstone, Edinburgh

Ward-Booth P, Hausaman J, Schendel S 1999 Maxillofacial surgery. Churchill Livingstone, Edinburgh

Ophthalmology

J. D. Jagger and D. Abrams

Contents

FOREIGN BODIES

Appraise

Intraocular foreign bodies

> 🔑 **Key point**
>
> • These require specialist intervention if it is available; the important thing for you to recognize is the possibility of the condition.

A foreign body is particularly likely to be missed where the entry wound is small and the initial disturbance minimal. Here the history of something going into the eye, especially while hammering and chiselling, and the absence of a foreign body on superficial inspection should prompt an X-ray of the orbit. Most small intraocular foreign bodies are sterile, and once the condition is recognized no harm will accrue from delay until dealt with in more favourable conditions. If large, a foreign body may cause a penetrating injury that needs to be dealt with in itself.

Subtarsal foreign bodies

1. Remove these by everting the upper eyelid after instilling proxymetacaine, amethocaine, oxybuprocaine or cocaine. Have a cotton-wool swab to hand *before starting*. Ask the patient to look down and to keep doing so. Grasp the upper lid lashes with the thumb and forefinger of one hand and pull the lid down and forwards. With an orange stick, press the upper edge of the tarsal plate downwards (some 4 mm from the lid margin) and then lift the lashes so as to rotate the lid over the orange stick, which pushes the tarsal plate down and under the lid margin at the same time.

2. Once the eyelid is everted, keep hold of the lashes and press them against the eyebrow, instructing the patient the while to keep looking down. Remove the orange stick and use the hand released to remove the foreign body with the cotton-wool swab. Return the lid to its normal position by withdrawing both hands and asking the patient to look up.

Corneal foreign bodies

1. If you suspect the foreign body to be deep in the cornea, do not tackle it yourself, as manipulation may push it into the anterior chamber. To remove superficial corneal foreign bodies, first anaesthetize the eye. A good light, focused on the cornea, and magnification are essential.

2. Very superficial foreign bodies may be brushed off by a cotton-wool swab. Embedded foreign bodies require to be needled out. Insert a 19G disposable needle tangentially to the cornea to get behind the foreign body – in other words do not go directly for it, enter the cornea a little to the side. Lever the foreign body out. Sometimes rust is left behind; attempt to pick it out, but do not try too hard. If the rust is slight and milk-chocolate in colour, leave it; it will disappear itself. If it is darker, however, get as much out as comes easily. More may need to be removed after a period of a few days' softening up.

3. Pad the eye after putting in an antibiotic ointment. Put in a mydriatic according to the degree of manipulation – i.e. very easy removal, no mydriatic; moderately easy, homatropine 2% drops; very difficult, atropine 1% drops. See the patient daily till healed and fluorescein-stain-free.

BURNS

1. *Chemical burns*. The immediate treatment is removal of any matter mechanically and, particularly, copious irrigation using any harmless fluid to hand. Do not hunt for specific antidotes. Antibiotic/steroid ointments are applied as well as atropine if the cornea is involved, and the conjunctival fornices should be kept patent to prevent symblepharon by twice-daily rodding with a glass rod. Always admit patients with lime burns for observation as the effects may be delayed and half-hourly drops including vitamin C may be required.

2. *Thermal burns*. Those affecting the lids are treated as skin burns elsewhere, but problems of ocular protection may arise.

INFECTIONS AROUND THE EYE

Pyogenic infections

1. Avoid incision wherever possible but, in conditions where extreme tense swelling due to pus is causing severe pain, obey the surgical maxim of 'where there's pus, let it out'.

2. This situation arises in the lids (styes and more particularly infected meibomian cysts), in the lacrimal apparatus (acute dacryocystitis) and, very rarely, for a pointing orbital cellulitis. Whenever

possible, incise lid abscesses from the inner aspect. Anaesthetize the lid by infiltrating 1% lignocaine with adrenaline into the lid substance, both subcutaneously and subconjunctivally. Evert it (Fig. 41.1) and incise at right angles to the lid margin through the tarsal plate. Do not curette any meibomian granulations such as would be done for a non-infected cyst.

3. For acute dacryocystitis a local anaesthetic may not be necessary if it is obviously pointing. Incise from below the inner palpebral ligament down and out for 15 mm parallel to the orbital margin. A drain is not necessary.

4. Infections of the eyeball itself may be localized, as for example a pyogenic corneal ulcer, or widely disseminated, as when a metastatic infection lodges in the choroid, spreading thence to the vitreous and all parts of the eye.

5. A corneal ulcer may perforate and require a conjunctival flap to cover it and help it to heal. It may also be accompanied by pus in the anterior chamber (hypopyon), which, if unresponsive to intense local and systemic chemotherapy, may require sampling by paracentesis for microscopy and culture. The use of superglue may act as an emergency treatment of corneal perforation. Anaesthetize the eye first with amethocaine. Apply 2–3 drops of superglue to the perforation after drying it with a sterile swab and cover with a bandage contact lens.

6. Severe destructive infection or endophthalmitis is treated by chemotherapy and steroids systemically and locally; failure to control it may require removal of the eye.

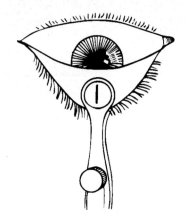

Fig. 41.1   Everting the lower lid, with a chalazion clamp.

FURTHER READING

Collin JRO 1993 A manual of systematic eyelid surgery. Churchill Livingstone, Edinburgh

Easty DL (ed) 1990 Current ophthalmic surgery. Baillière Tindall, London

Roper-Hall MJ (ed) 1989 Stallard's eye surgery, 7th edn. John Wright, Bristol

Willshaw H 1993 Practical ophthalmic surgery. Churchill Livingstone Edinburgh

Index

Venous (system)/veins 193–6
  varicose 193–6
Ventilation, artificial 12–13
Veress needle 49–50
Viral infection in high-risk patients 5
Virilizing syndromes 179

W-plasty 234
Warren distal splenorectal shunt 158
Wedge excision of the lip 207
Wounds (accidental/injurious) *see also* Blunt injuries; Penetrating
    injuries; Trauma
  open 214–16
  sucking 202

Wounds (surgical)
  closure *see* Closure
  contamination and infection *see* Contamination and infection
  from pressure injuries 239
  see also Skin
Wrist, ganglion of dorsum 223–4

Z-plasty 233–4
Zadek's operation 227–8
Zenker's diverticula 76
Zollinger–Ellison syndrome 154

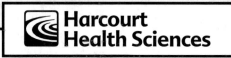